William,
324 Pop
Milford, CT   06460

1997
YEAR BOOK OF
DRUG THERAPY®

Statement of Purpose

The YEAR BOOK Service

The YEAR BOOK series was devised in 1901 by practicing health professionals who observed that the literature of medicine and related disciplines had become so voluminous that no one individual could read and place in perspective every potential advance in a major specialty. In the final decade of the 20th century, this recognition is more acutely true than it was in 1901.

More than merely a series of books, YEAR BOOK volumes are the tangible results of a unique service designed to accomplish the following:

- to *survey* a wide range of journals of proven value
- to *select* from those journals papers representing significant advances and statements of important clinical principles
- to provide *abstracts* of those articles that are readable, convenient summaries of their key points
- to provide *commentary* about those articles to place them in perspective

These publications grow out of a unique process that calls on the talents of outstanding authorities in clinical and fundamental disciplines, trained literature specialists, and professional writers, all supported by the resources of Mosby, the world's preeminent publisher for the health professions.

The Literature Base

Mosby and its Editors survey more than 1,000 journals published worldwide, covering the full range of the health professions. On an annual basis, the publisher examines usage patterns and polls its expert authorities to add new journals to the literature base and to delete journals that are no longer useful as potential YEAR BOOK sources.

The Literature Survey

The publisher's team of literature specialists, all of whom are trained and experienced health professionals, examines every original, peer-reviewed article in each journal issue. More than 250,000 articles per year are scanned systematically, including title, text, illustrations, tables, and references. Each scan is compared, article by article, to the search strategies that the publisher has developed in consultation with the 270 outside experts who form the pool of YEAR BOOK editors. A given article may be reviewed by any number of editors, from one to a dozen or more, regardless of the discipline for which the paper was originally published. In turn, each editor who receives the article reviews it to determine whether or not the article should be included in the YEAR BOOK. This decision is based on the article's inherent quality, its probable usefulness to readers of that YEAR BOOK, and the editor's goal to represent a balanced picture of a given field in each volume of the YEAR BOOK. In addition, the editor indicates when to include figures and tables from the article to help the YEAR BOOK reader better understand the information.

Of the quarter million articles scanned each year, only 5% are selected for detailed analysis within the YEAR BOOK series, thereby assuring readers of the high value of every selection.

The Abstract

The publisher's abstracting staff is headed by a seasoned medical professional and includes individuals with training in the life sciences, medicine, and other areas, plus extensive experience in writing for the health professions and related industries. Each selected article is assigned to a specific writer on this abstracting staff. The abstracter, guided in many cases by notations supplied by the expert editor, writes a structured, condensed summary designed so that the reader can rapidly acquire the essential information contained in the article.

The Commentary

The YEAR BOOK editorial boards, sometimes assisted by guest commentators, write comments that place each article in perspective for the reader. This provides the reader with the equivalent of a personal consultation with a leading international authority—an opportunity to better understand the value of the article and to benefit from the authority's thought processes in assessing the article.

Additional Editorial Features

The editorial boards of each YEAR BOOK organize the abstracts and comments to provide a logical and satisfying sequence of information. To enhance the organization, editors also provide introductions to sections or individual chapters, comments linking a number of abstracts, citations to additional literature, and other features.

The published YEAR BOOK contains enhanced bibliographic citations for each selected article, including extended listings of multiple authors and identification of author affiliations. Each YEAR BOOK contains a Table of Contents specific to that year's volume. From year to year, the Table of Contents for a given YEAR BOOK will vary depending on developments within the field.

Every YEAR BOOK contains a list of the journals from which papers have been selected. This list represents a subset of the more than 1,000 journals surveyed by the publisher and occasionally reflects a particularly pertinent article from a journal that is not surveyed on a routine basis.

Finally, each volume contains a comprehensive subject index and an index to authors of each selected paper.

The 1997 Year Book Series

Year Book of Allergy, Asthma, and Clinical Immunology: Drs. Rosenwasser, Borish, Gelfand, Leung, Nelson, and Szefler

Year Book of Anesthesiology and Pain Management®: Drs. Tinker, Abram, Chestnut, Roizen, Rothenberg, and Wood

Year Book of Cardiology®: Drs. Schlant, Collins, Gersh, Graham, Kaplan, and Waldo

Year Book of Chiropractic®: Dr. Lawrence

Year Book of Critical Care Medicine®: Drs. Parrillo, Balk, Calvin, Franklin, and Shapiro

Year Book of Dentistry®: Drs. Meskin, Berry, Kennedy, Leinfelder, Roser, Summitt, and Zakariasen

Year Book of Dermatologic Surgery®: Drs. Greenway, Papadopoulos, and Whitaker

Year Book of Dermatology®: Drs. Sober and Fitzpatrick

Year Book of Diagnostic Radiology®: Drs. Federle, Gross, Dalinka, Maynard, Rebner, Smirniotopolous, and Young

Year Book of Digestive Diseases®: Drs. Greenberger and Moody

Year Book of Drug Therapy®: Drs. Lasagna and Weintraub

Year Book of Emergency Medicine®: Drs. Wagner, Dronen, Davidson, King, Niemann, and Roberts

Year Book of Endocrinology®: Drs. Bagdade, Braverman, Horton, Kannan, Landsberg, Molitch, Morley, Nathan, Odell, Poehlman, Rogol, and Ryan

Year Book of Family Practice®: Drs. Berg, Bowman, Davidson, Dexter, and Scherger

Year Book of Geriatrics and Gerontology®: Drs. Beck, Burton, Ostwald, Rabins, Reuben, Roth, Shapiro, and Whitehouse

Year Book of Hand Surgery®: Drs. Amadio and Hentz

Year Book of Hematology®: Drs. Spivak, Bell, Ness, Quesenberry, Wiernik, and Blume

Year Book of Infectious Diseases®: Drs. Keusch, Barza, Bennish, Poutsiaka, Skolnik, and Snydman

Year Book of Medicine®: Drs. Klahr, Cline, Petty, Frishman, Greenberger, Malawiste, Mandell, and O'Rourke

Year Book of Neonatal and Perinatal Medicine®: Drs. Fanaroff, Maisels, Stevenson

Year Book of Nephrology, Hypertension, and Mineral Metabolism: Drs. Schwab, Bennett, Emmett, Hostetter, Kumar, and Toto

Year Book of Neurology and Neurosurgery®: Drs. Bradley and Wilkins

Year Book of Nuclear Medicine®: Drs. Gottschalk, Blaufox, Neumann, Strauss, and Zubal

Year Book of Obstetrics, Gynecology, and Women's Health: Drs. Mishell, Herbst, and Kirschbaum

Year Book of Occupational and Environmental Medicine®: Drs. Emmett, Frank, Gochfeld, and Hessl

Year Book of Oncology®: Drs. Ozols, Cohen, Glatstein, Loehrer, Tallman, and Wiersma

Year Book of Ophthalmology®: Drs. Wilson, Augsburger, Cohen, Eagle, Flanagan, Grossman, Laibson, Maguire, Nelson, Penne, Rapuano, Sergott, Spaeth, Tipperman, and Ms. Salmon

Year Book of Orthopedics®: Drs. Sledge, Poss, Cofield, Dobyns, Griffin, Springfield, Swiontkowski, Wiesel, and Wilson

Year Book of Otolaryngology–Head and Neck Surgery®: Drs. Paparella and Holt

Year Book of Pathology and Laboratory Medicine: Drs. Mills, Bruns, Gaffey, and Stoler

Year Book of Pediatrics®: Dr. Stockman

Year Book of Plastic, Reconstructive, and Aesthetic Surgery®: Drs. Miller, Cohen, McKinney, Robson, Ruberg, Smith, and Whitaker

Year Book of Podiatric Medicine and Surgery®: Dr. Kominsky

Year Book of Psychiatry and Applied Mental Health®: Drs. Talbott, Ballenger, Breier, Frances, Meltzer, Schowalter, and Tasman

Year Book of Pulmonary Disease®: Dr. Petty

Year Book of Rheumatology®: Drs. Sergent, LeRoy, Meenan, Panush, and Reichlin

Year Book of Sports Medicine®: Drs. Shephard, Alexander, Drinkwater, Eichner, George, and Torg

Year Book of Surgery®: Drs. Copeland, Bland, Deitch, Eberlein, Howard, Luce, Seeger, Souba, and Sugarbaker

Year Book of Thoracic and Cardiovascular Surgery®: Drs. Ginsberg, Wechsler, and Williams

Year Book of Urology®: Drs. Andriole and Coplin

Year Book of Vascular Surgery®: Dr. Porter

1997

The Year Book of
DRUG THERAPY®

Editors

Louis Lasagna, M.D.

Dean of the Sackler School of Graduate Biomedical Sciences, and Academic Dean, School of Medicine, Tufts University, Boston

Michael Weintraub, M.D.

Director, Office of Drug Evaluation, Food and Drug Administration*

* The opinions and assertions contained herein are the private views of the author and are not to be construed as official or as reflecting the views of the Food and Drug Administration or the Federal Government of the United States.

Mosby

St. Louis Baltimore Boston Carlsbad Chicago Naples New York Philadelphia Portland

London Madrid Mexico City Singapore Sydney Tokyo Toronto Wiesbaden

Mosby

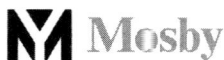

Dedicated to Publishing Excellence

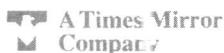

A Times Mirror
Company

Vice President and Publisher, Continuity Publishing: Kenneth H. Killion
Director, Editorial Development: Gretchen C. Murphy
Developmental Editor: Bernadette Buchholz
Acquisitions Editor: Li Wen Huang
Project Specialist, Editing: Denise M. Dungey
Assistant Project Supervisor, Production: Sandra Rogers
Freelance Staff Supervisor: Barbara M. Kelly
Illustrations and Permissions Coordinator: Steven Ramay
Director, Editorial Services: Edith M. Podrazik, B.S.N., R.N.
Information Specialist: Terri Santo, R.N.
Circulation Manager: Lynn D. Stevenson

1997 EDITION
Copyright © May 1997 by Mosby–Year Book, Inc.

Printed in the United States of America
Composition by Reed Technology and Information Services, Inc.
Printing/binding by Maple-Vail

Mosby–Year Book, Inc.
11830 Westline Industrial Drive
St. Louis, MO 63146
Customer Service: customer.support@mosby.com
www.mosby.com/Mosby/CustomerSupport/index.html

Editorial Office:
Mosby–Year Book, Inc.
161 North Clark Street
Chicago, IL 60601
series.editorial@mosby.com

International Standard Serial Number: 0084–3733
International Standard Book Number: 0–8151–5295–7

Table of Contents

Journals Represented

Mosby and its Editors survey more than 1,000 journals for its abstract and commentary publications. From these journals, the Editors select the articles to be abstracted. Journals represented in this YEAR BOOK are listed below.

Acta Dermato-Venereologica
Acta Obstetricia et Gynecologica Scandinavica
Acta Paediatrica
Allergy
American Family Physician
American Heart Journal
American Journal of Cardiology
American Journal of Emergency Medicine
American Journal of Epidemiology
American Journal of Gastroenterology
American Journal of Hematology
American Journal of Hypertension
American Journal of Kidney Diseases
American Journal of Medical Quality
American Journal of Medicine
American Journal of Obstetrics and Gynecology
American Journal of Psychiatry
American Journal of Public Health
American Journal of the Medical Sciences
American Surgeon
Anaesthesia and Intensive Care
Anesthesia and Analgesia
Anesthesiology
Annals of Allergy, Asthma, & Immunology
Annals of Emergency Medicine
Annals of Internal Medicine
Annals of Pharmacotherapy
Annals of Rheumatic Diseases
Annals of Thoracic Surgery
Archives of Dermatology
Archives of Disease in Childhood
Archives of Neurology
Archives of Pediatrics and Adolescent Medicine
Archives of Surgery
Arthritis and Rheumatism
Australian and New Zealand Journal of Medicine
Blood
Bone Marrow Transplantation
British Heart Journal
British Journal of General Practice
British Journal of Psychiatry
British Journal of Surgery
British Medical Journal
Canadian Journal of Anaesthesia
Canadian Journal of Psychiatry
Canadian Medical Association Journal
Cancer

Cephalalgia
Chest
Circulation
Clinical Endocrinology (Oxford)
Clinical Infectious Diseases
Clinical Nephology
Clinical Pharmacology and Therapeutics
Contraception
Critical Care Medicine
Diabetes Care
Diabetologia
Digestive Diseases and Sciences
Drug and Alcohol Dependence
Endocrine Journal
European Heart Journal
European Journal of Clinical Pharmacology
European Journal of Haematology
European Respiratory Journal
European Urology
Family Medicine
Fertility and Sterility
Gastroenterology
Genitourinary Medicine
Gut
Headache
Hepatology
Infection Control and Hospital Epidemiology
International Journal of Artificial Organs
International Journal of Cancer
International Journal of Geriatric Psychiatry
International Journal of Obesity
Journal of Allergy and Clinical Immunology
Journal of Bone and Joint Surgery (American Volume)
Journal of Bone and Mineral Research
Journal of Clinical Endocrinology and Metabolism
Journal of Clinical Epidemiology
Journal of Clinical Microbiology
Journal of Clinical Oncology
Journal of Clinical Pharmacology
Journal of Clinical Psychopharmacology
Journal of Emergency Medicine
Journal of General Internal Medicine
Journal of Gerontology
Journal of Heart and Lung Transplantation
Journal of Human Hypertension
Journal of Neurology
Journal of Neurology, Neurosurgery and Psychiatry
Journal of Neurosurgery
Journal of Pain and Symptom Management
Journal of Pediatric Hematology/Oncology
Journal of Pediatrics
Journal of Pharmacology and Experimental Therapeutics

Journal of Rheumatology
Journal of Urology
Journal of the American Academy of Dermatology
Journal of the American Board of Family Practice
Journal of the American College of Cardiology
Journal of the American Geriatrics Society
Journal of the American Medical Association
Journal of the National Cancer Institute
Kidney International
Lancet
Mayo Clinic Proceedings
Medical Care
Medical Journal of Australia
Nephrology, Dialysis, Transplantation
Nephron
Neurology
New England Journal of Medicine
New Zealand Medical Journal
Obstetrics and Gynecology
Ophthalmology
Oral Surgery, Oral Medicine, Oral Pathology, Oral Radiology Endodontics
Pain
Pediatric Infectious Disease Journal
Pediatric Research
Pharmacotherapy
Postgraduate Medical Journal
Psychosomatic Medicine
Scandinavian Journal of Rheumatology
Scandinavian Journal of Urology and Nephrology
Southern Medical Journal
Sports Medicine
Surgical Neurology
Therapeutic Drug Monitoring
Thorax
Thyroid
Transplantation
Urology
Western Journal of Medicine

STANDARD ABBREVIATIONS

The following terms are abbreviated in this edition: acquired immunodeficiency syndrome (AIDS), cardiopulmonary resuscitation (CPR), central nervous system (CNS), cerebrospinal fluid (CSF), computed tomography (CT), deoxyribonucleic acid (DNA), electrocardiography (ECG), health maintenance organization (HMO), human immunodeficiency virus (HIV), intensive care unit (ICU), intramuscular (IM), intravenous (IV), magnetic resonance (MR) imaging (MRI), and ribonucleic acid (RNA).

NOTE

The YEAR BOOK OF DRUG THERAPY® is a literature survey service providing abstracts of articles published in the professional literature. Every effort is made to assure the accuracy of the information presented in these pages. Neither the editors nor the publisher of the YEAR BOOK OF DRUG THERAPY® can be responsible for errors in the original materials. The editors' comments are their own opinions. Mention of specific products within this publication does not constitute endorsement.

To facilitate the use of the YEAR BOOK OF DRUG THERAPY® as a reference tool, all illustrations and tables included in this publication are now identified as they appear in the original article. This change is meant to help the reader recognize that any illustration or table appearing in the YEAR BOOK OF DRUG THERAPY® may be only one of many in the original article. For this reason, figure and table numbers will often appear to be out of sequence within the YEAR BOOK OF DRUG THERAPY®.

Introduction

Sir Austin Bradford Hill was one of the fathers of the modern controlled clinical trial, having been involved in the famous United Kingdom study of the value of parenteral streptomycin in treating pulmonary tuberculosis. In November 1965 Hill gave the Heberden Oration, which was published in March 1966 in the *Annals of the Rheumatic Diseases*, vol 25, pp 107–113. It deserves to be read in its entirety by anyone interested in the assessment of drug effects, because it remains valid today.

Here are some quotes from that admirable Oration:

> Given the right attitude of mind, there is more than one way in which we can study therapeutic efficacy. Any belief that the controlled trial is the only way would mean not that the pendulum had swung too far but that it had come right off its hook.
>
> [T]he controlled trial does not tell the doctor what he wants to know. It may . . . show without any doubt that treatment A is *on the average* better than treatment B . . . that result does not answer the practicing doctor's question what is the most likely outcome when this drug is given to a particular patient?
>
> Can we identify the individual patient for whom one or the other of the treatments is the right answer? Clearly that is what we want to do and present-day investigators ought to give far more attention to the problem. There are very few signs that they are doing so.
>
> Certainly we are never going to learn how to treat depressions, or any other illness, just from double-blind sampling in a statistician's office. The statistician's office merely provides an experimental design upon which to hang the skilled clinical observations that must characterize *any* form of inquiry into therapeutic efficacy . . . There is no question of replacing valuable clinical observation by a series of mathematical symbols. Those who think so have the myopia of Don Quixote; they mistake the scaffold for the house.
>
> . . . the object of [the statistician's] life must be professional suicide. Once the clinician has grasped the simple techniques that have been brought to his aid, the statistician has no further part to play. Along with the old soldier he can fade away, contentedly, if sometimes wistfully.

Read the whole article, gentle reader. It's remarkable.

Louis Lasagna, M.D.

1 General Information

Are Single-dose Toxicology Studies in Animals Adequate to Support Single Doses of a New Drug in Humans?
Monro A, Mehta D (Pfizer Central Research, Groton, Conn)
Clin Pharmacol Ther 59:258–264, 1996   1–1

Objective.—Because the majority of new chemical entities do not progress beyond phase I or phase II clinical studies, many potentially useful drugs are never brought to market. Even though phase I studies have excellent safety records, much time and money is spent doing required preclinical toxicology studies in 2 animal species. Reducing the scope of these animal studies could significantly accelerate drug development, primarily by reducing the amount of bulk chemical that has to be synthesized.

Toxicology Guidelines: History and Current Situation.—The guidelines, issued by the FDA more than 25 years ago, have only recently been receiving systematic review. Europe and Japan have no official guidelines for preclinical toxicology studies in animals.

Proposed Strategy.—Single-dose human studies would give more reliable information than repeated dose studies in animals by providing information about bioavailability, pharmacokinetics, and pharmacodynamic and toxic end points. Such studies would require only small amounts of compound. Based on the information obtained, multidose clinical studies or additional toxicologic studies could be conducted.

Nature of Safety Concerns in Single-Dose Human Studies.—Acute toxic events such as cardiovascular, respiratory, and CNS effects cause the greatest concern. The most common events observed, however, are skin or hypersensitivity reactions.

Preclinical Studies That Best Address Clinicians' Concerns.—Adverse events that affect the function of the individual are of prime concern to clinicians. Exhaustive animal tissue analysis provides little useful clinical information. The carcinogenic threat or reproductive hazard of a single dose is extremely small. Highly toxic entities would be eliminated in initial animal testing.

Function in Nonclinical Surrogates.—There is poor correlation between adverse effects seen in animals and humans. Adverse effects seen with repeated dosing may not be observed in single-dose studies or may obscure adverse reactions that occur with a single dose. Because animals generally clear drugs from their systems faster than humans, pharmacokinetic results in animals are not reliable indicators for dosing regimens in humans. Single-dose studies would also reduce metabolic complications that sometimes arise with multidose studies. Study designs should emphasize safety, reduce the need for histopathologic examination to a few key organs, and restrict animal studies to male animals because single-dose human studies are restricted to males.

Conclusion.—There is a good scientific rationale for using time- and money-saving single-dose human clinical studies.

▶ A lot of drug candidates never get beyond phase I (the earliest exposure of humans—often healthy volunteers—to the agent). As these authors point out: "...the first dose in humans is often the make-or-break point in the life of a potential new drug."

This paper argues that we now do too much unnecessary animal study before proceeding to the first dose, and that less preclinical work would save money and time without compromising quality.

L. Lasagna, M.D.

Success Rates for New Drugs Entering Clinical Testing in the United States
DiMasi JA (Tufts Univ, Boston)
Clin Pharmacol Ther 58:1–14, 1995   1–2

Introduction.—Developing drugs is a risky and time-consuming matter. In a considerable majority of cases, research on new chemical entities (NCEs) is abandoned after clinical testing without obtaining marketing approval. The clinical success rates achieved for new drugs are a key indicator of how effectively pharmaceutical companies are proceeding from the point where new drugs are available for clinical testing to approval of these drugs for marketing.

Methods —Information on NCEs was obtained from a Center for the Study of Drug Development database derived from a survey of 36 pharmaceutical firms in the United States for the years 1963 to 1989. These firms filed a total of 1,943 investigational new drug applications. Most NCEs were self-originated, whereas 389 were identified as licensed.

Findings.—For most of the period surveyed, the predicted final success rates were intermediate between current rates and the maximum possible rates. Predicted success rates for the years 1964 to 1969 were within 1.2% of the maximum rate. Success rates for filings in the early 1980s were modestly less than rates for the late 1970s, but very close to the success rates achieved in the early 1970s. There was little change over time in the proportion of new drug applications that will be approved. Most CNS agents filed in the late 1970s failed. In contrast, above-average success rates were achieved for antineoplastic and anti-infectious agents. Current success rates are highest for medium-sized pharmaceutical firms and lowest for small firms, but predicted final success rates are very similar.

Final Word.—It will be important to ascertain what underlying factors are responsible for observed changes in clinical success rates of new drugs.

▶ This is an important and helpful paper. The main reason it is helpful is that it will serve as a basis of a pre–Prescription Drug User Fee Act analysis of drugs and their success rate. Actually, all bets are off as the FDA is decreasing new drug application approval times. As this paper shows, the new drug application time is very important, because 82.2% of drugs reaching this stage eventually achieve approval. The reasons for longer times for small firms, the so-called boutique or niche firms, may be that they are trying to get more innovative drugs approved.

I believe that the specific medication candidates for approval will have to be examined to see whether they were more innovative than blockbuster drugs. One key point made by DiMasi is that better screening in basic pharmacologic work may be leading to shorter development times, with the possibility of simultaneously looking for really important medications. There always will be medications with minor improvements ("me-too drugs"), but very important medications as well will be in development, particularly in the hot areas such as AIDS and neurologic disease, and even in the biotechnical area.

M. Weintraub, M.D.

A Survey of Physician Knowledge of Drug Costs
Hoffman J, Barefield FA, Ramamurthy S (Univ of Texas Health Sciences Ctr, San Antonio)
J Pain Symptom Manage 10:432–435, 1995   1–3

Introduction.—The cost of prescription drugs is an important factor in the growing cost of health care, and the price of drugs has been shown to affect medication compliance. Physicians do not have ready access to information on drug costs, and previous studies have suggested that they have inadequate knowledge in this area. Physicians' knowledge of the actual prices of 1 frequently used class of drugs was evaluated in a survey study.

Methods.—Information on the actual price to the patient for 12 nonsteroidal anti-inflammatory drugs was gathered by surveying a random sample of pharmacies. Then, pain clinic and orthopedic physicians in the same area were asked to estimate these costs. Response rates were 52% from pharmacies and 67% from physicians.

Results.—The pharmacies' medication prices varied widely. For all 12 drugs, the difference between the highest and lowest price quoted for a 30-day supply was more than $20, with the difference reaching as high as $72 for 1 drug. Of the 95 responding physicians, 81% said that the cost of drugs was an important consideration. However, their estimates of drug costs declined within the pharmacy price range in only 38% of cases. Just 25% of the physicians gave an in-range estimate for at least half of the medications. Most of the physicians' estimates were significantly correlated with the pharmacies' mean prices.

Conclusions.—Physicians have inadequate knowledge about the costs of the medications they prescribe. Efforts are needed to make information on pharmacy prices more readily available and to increase physicians' knowledge of these prices. The result could be lower overall costs for prescription medications, and possibly increased patient compliance.

▶ For a long time we have known that physicians do not know how much medications cost. The question is, "Should they?" I believe the answer is that they should have a general indication in their heads as to which medications are more expensive and which are less expensive. One problem with knowing a lot about medications and their costs is that, in some pharmacies, the price for drug A can be very, very high, much higher than in any other pharmacy. At the same time in that very same pharmacy, the cost for drug B can be very, very low, much lower than at any other pharmacies, even than in pharmacies having a lower cost for drug A. Of course, that is the American system, and, in fact, it is enforced by the inability to set prices. However, it is unlikely that the range of ibuprofen prices would increase from less than $10 to more than $30 or that the cost of salsalate would range from $8 to almost $30. Of course, the champion of this particular study would be tolmetin, which ranged from $24 to $96. In this investigation, the vast majority of physicians believed that the price of the drug was very important, but they did not even know the cost of the medication that they most frequently prescribed. This is another area in which we must do better.

M. Weintraub, M.D.

Lessons From International Experience in Controlling Pharmaceutical Expenditure: I. Influencing Patients
Freemantle N, Bloor K (Univ of York, England)
BMJ 312:1469–1471, 1996   1–4

Background.—In response to increasing costs in health care systems, several national governments have developed policies aimed at controlling drug costs by controlling both the supply of and demand for drugs. The impact of these policies was investigated by examining the literature dealing with policies to reduce patient demand for drugs.

Methods.—Evaluative studies of international policies to control drug costs and improve the cost effectiveness of drugs were identified with both computer and hand searches. Studies that met predetermined quality criteria were reviewed, including randomized studies and nonequivalent group designs with pre-post measures.

Results.—Policies used to depress demand for drugs include the following interventions: copayments (requiring payment of a proportion of the cost by patients), patient caps (which limit the number of prescriptions reimbursed per patient), and withdrawal of reimbursement for certain drugs. These policies have been shown to reduce the use of both nonessential drugs and essential drugs such as antihypertensive drugs and drugs for heart conditions, diabetes, and thyroid conditions. In addition, there were increases in health care costs related to reduced use of essential drugs, such as acute psychiatric services and nursing home institutionalization. There were patterns of increased use of drugs with uncertain efficacy in attempts to substitute for drugs withdrawn from reimbursement. Some of these substituted drugs may have risks of habituation and adverse effects.

Conclusion.—It is unlikely that policies to restrict prescription drug use will adequately contain costs or improve the cost-effectiveness of use of particular drugs. Patients may instead switch to use of less effective drugs and services. These policies may, therefore, have substantial deleterious effects of patient care.

▶ Organizations, whether they are political or private, seem to always want to control drug costs. They actually forget that drugs are among the most cost-effective of all treatments. It seems to me that we can even stand a little bit of overprescribing—not a lot, but some overprescribing—to make sure that patients are covered with the best drug. I do not want to be accused of condoning poor prescribing, because I don't. But I do think that studies have shown us, over and over again, that the control of medications results in a decrease in essential as well as nonessential drugs. Whenever we challenge a prescribing practice or a medical practice of any kind—such as mothers being kept in the hospital for *x* days after having given birth—we really have to have a very good basis for challenging those practices.

M. Weintraub, M.D.

Lessons From International Experience in Controlling Pharmaceutical Expenditure: III. Regulating Industry
Bloor K, Maynard A, Freemantle N (Univ of York, England; Nuffield Provincial Hosps' Trust, London)
BMJ 313:33–35, 1996   1–5

Background.—The authors have been reviewing recent policies for controlling drug spending in developed countries. Efforts to influence the behavior of physicians and patients were examined in the first 2 articles in this series. Industry regulatory policies for controlling pharmaceutical spending were examined in this article.

Policies to Regulate Industry.—Governmental control of licensing; reimbursement; prices, including reference pricing; and profits were the focus of the review. The problem with efforts to control price and profit is that they do not include incentives for promoting cost-effective drug use, instead emphasizing cost containment and the profitability of domestic industry. Price negotiations and reference pricing systems may help to encourage cost-effectiveness by permitting a premium price only for drugs with evidence of important therapeutic benefit. However, unless a carefully monitored economic evaluation is made, price controls appear to be a crude cost-containment method. Although no studies comparing the impact of various price control policies have been conducted, such studies are feasible. In Australia, price negotiations are carried out with knowledge of the cost-effectiveness of new products. In contrast, the British system seeks to control profits rather than prices or reimbursement, and, thus, carries no incentives for improving cost-effectiveness.

Discussion.—Efficient resource utilization requires measures for encouraging cost-effective drug use that take both the price and use of drugs into account. Increased efficiency and patient benefit may be possible if carefully monitored economic evaluations are performed.

▶ This is the third in a series of papers describing different approaches to controlling drug costs in developed countries. They all deserve careful reading in their original versions. Regulating drug prices does not seem to be a very effective way to control health care costs.

L. Lasagna, M.D.

The Impact of Immunosuppressive Regimens on the Cost of Liver Transplantation: Results From the U.S. FK506 Multicenter Trial
Lake JR, Gorman KJ, Esquivel CO, et al (Univ of California, San Francisco; Putnam Associates , Burlington, Mass; California Pacific Med Ctr, San Francisco; et al)
Transplantation 60:1089–1095, 1995   1–6

Purpose.—Orthotopic liver transplantation is an expensive and resource-intensive procedure. Efforts to lower the costs of liver transplantation will necessitate accurate assessment of the actual costs, identification of the main factors contributing to cost, and identification of ways to reduce cost without adversely affecting outcomes. As part of a multicenter study of the costs of liver transplantation, the costs associated with tacrolimus vs. cyclosporine (CsA)-based primary immunosuppression were investigated.

Methods.—The analysis looked at average 1-year posttransplant charges for patients in the U.S. Multi-center Prospective Randomized Trial Comparing FK-506 to Cyclosporine in Liver Transplantation. All first-year inpatient charges, including readmissions, were assessed; professional and outpatient costs were not included.

Results.—Two hundred sixteen patients completed the trial. The average length of stay was 7 days shorter for the patients receiving tacrolimus than for those receiving CsA. In addition, the average 1-year cost was about $19,000 lower in the tacrolimus group. The cost differential seemed to stem largely from differences in the rejection profiles of the 2 immunosuppressive regimens: severe rejection was less likely to develop in patients receiving tacrolimus. As the incidence and severity of rejection increased, so did the average length of stay and the costs of transplantation. No significant differences were found in patient or graft survival.

Conclusions.—For recipients of orthotopic liver transplants, immuno-suppression with tacrolimus is more cost-effective than CsA. The difference is largely related to the differing rejection profiles of the 2 immuno-suppressive agents and is not associated with any difference in clinical outcomes. Resource utilization in liver transplantation is linked to the incidence and severity of rejection: more frequent and severe rejection leads to more ICU readmissions, longer hospital stays, more laboratory tests, and more antirejection medications, and thus to higher overall transplantation costs.

▶ Studies of this sort are being increasingly carried out, because of our cost-containment environment. This one shows the benefit (medically as well as economically) of putting liver transplant recipients on an effective immunosuppressive regimen.

L. Lasagna, M.D.

Teaching Information Mastery: Evaluating Information Provided by Pharmaceutical Representatives
Shaughnessy AF, Slawson DC, Bennett JH (Harrisburg Hosp, Pa; Univ of Virginia, Charlottesville)
Fam Med 27:581–585, 1995   1–7

Background.—Pharmaceutical representatives (PRs) play a major role in the continuing education of family physicians as well as in the education of residents. There is debate over how the information provided by PRs should be incorporated into the residency curriculum. Residents must understand the sales process so that they can separate the useful information provided by PRs from that which could mislead them. A structured curriculum was designed to teach evaluation of PRs' presentations.

Methods.—The curriculum was implemented to prepare residents to evaluate the information provided by PRs and to address the faculty's conflicts in attempting to rebut claims made during a sales presentation. The Pharmaceutical Representative Evaluation Form was designed to aid in evaluating the completeness of the presented information, the general techniques of persuasion used, and the use of rational vs. nonrational appeals. In guiding discussions about PRs' presentations, the evaluation form helped residents to understand the sales process and, based on this understanding, to confirm or dispute the information presented.

Results.—Formal evaluation suggested that the residents quickly learned how to identify potential fallacies of logic and other misleading sales techniques. Responses to a pretest-posttest questionnaire showed that the residents had learned how PRs and accepting promotional items from PRs can affect their prescribing behavior. Although most PRs seemed glad that their role was perceived as educational, others found this responsibility burdensome.

Conclusions.—The curriculum evaluated helped residents to critically analyze the pharmaceutical sales process. They were thus better able to separate the "wheat from the chaff" in a valuable source of medical information. Learning to evaluate the information presented by PRs is just part of the larger process of becoming a medical information master.

▶ It's refreshing to read an article that suggests ways of profiting (intellectually) from PRs instead of cavalierly dismissing them as craven scoundrels. (Are there any uncraven scoundrels?)

L. Lasagna, M.D.

Recall Accuracy for Prescription Medications: Self-report Compared With Database Information
West SL, Savitz DA, Koch G, et al (Univ of North Carolina, Chapel Hill; Univ of Pennsylvania, Philadelphia)
Am J Epidemiol 142:1103–1112, 1995   1–8

Background.—Recall inaccuracy is a potential limitation of information collected by self-report. Self-report information was compared with database information to determine recall accuracy for prescription medications.

Methods.—Five hundred sixty patients taking a nonsteroidal anti-inflammatory drug (NSAID) or a noncontraceptive estrogen and 140 patients not taking these drugs participated. Demographic, behavioral, and drug information was obtained by telephone from 356 individuals who received an NSAID or an estrogen and 98 who did not.

Findings.—Forty-one percent of the patients with only 1 NSAID dispensation were able to recall any NSAID use, compared with 85% of those with multiple NSAID dispensations. Thirty percent were able to remember the name of the NSAID, and 15% remembered both the name and the dose. Seventy-eight percent of those taking estrogens could recall the name, but only 26% remembered the name and the dose. Age appeared to affect recall accuracy: patients aged 50 to 65 years were better able to recall the name of the NSAID than those aged 66 to 80 years. This was also true for those receiving estrogen. Sex did not influence recall accuracy. The drug name was recalled more often for agents stopped 2 to 3 years earlier than for those stopped 7 to 11 years earlier. Specificity ranged from 92% to 100%.

Conclusions.—Studies that use questionnaires to elicit past drug use will probably obtain incomplete drug histories, leading to misclassification of exposure. The quality of self-report data is affected by the respondent's age, recall interval, drug type, repetitiveness of use of the drug, and the degree of specificity required.

▶ Epidemiologists are guilty of not worrying enough about recall bias when asking people about their taking of medications. Unfortunately, pharmacy databases are also flawed sources, because the prescribing of a drug, or the filling of a prescription, tells us little about the taking of a drug. Patients often take less than they're supposed to; taking more than is prescribed is rare.

L. Lasagna, M.D.

Sample Sizes for Comparative Inhaled Corticosteroid Trials With Emphasis on Showing Therapeutic Equivalence
Zanen P, Lammers J-WJ (Univ Hosp Utrecht, The Netherlands)
Eur J Clin Pharmacol 48:179–184, 1995   1–9

Background.—Many new inhaled corticosteroids or formulations of these drugs will soon be compared with older ones to determine therapeutic equivalence. In such trials, the statistical evaluation methods will differ from the classic methods. The old approach has been replaced by the 2 one-sided tests procedure, in which a new sample size equation is derived. The important aspects of this equation are the coefficient of variation of the parameter measured, the difference between the means of the 2 groups, and the equivalence limit. This equation was used in a study estimating the number of volunteers needed in a parallel inhaled corticosteroids equivalence trial.

Methods and Findings.—Changes in the forced expiratory volume in 1 second and in the histamine concentration or dose that caused a 20% decrease in the forced expiratory volume in 1 second caused by a corticosteroid were the end points chosen. Data were extracted from published placebo-controlled trials. A range of equivalence limits and differences between the group means were defined. A large number of volunteers— between 500 and 1,000—would be needed because of the small corticosteroid effect and the high variance. For inhaled corticosteroids, the equivalence limit is not known. This needs to be defined to avoid questions on outcomes.

Conclusions.—Because of the large number of patients needed, parallel inhaled corticosteroid equivalence trials will probably need to be multi-center trials. Potential sources of bias in such studies include varying definitions of asthma, resulting in noncomparable patient groups. Such biases, in turn, will make the study findings difficult to interpret. Alternative methods for establishing therapeutic equivalence are needed.

▶ One of the best ways of showing equivalence (not by the method of poorly done studies, however) is to find an adequate number of the right kind of patients who will respond with a standardized outcome; that outcome should be easily measured. The patients would have the same level of adverse effects. Of course, such patients do not exist. Another point that is beneficial in such studies is to undertreat the patients so that they will have a reasonable "upside sensitivity." That, too, is very difficult to do because it may mean undertreating patients with severe asthma. Studying the patients more in depth may allow a better analysis of the outcome, but it increases the cost.

These authors have searched for methods of evaluating corticosteroids. They have discovered some nonpharmacodynamic parameters. In many ways, the nonpharmacodynamic methods leave much to be desired. Their only benefits are doability and cost. Unless they can be shown to be related to pharmacodynamics, their value will still be questioned. Nonetheless, this is an interesting paper, particularly because we will be faced with having to figure out some way to do these studies—if not just for new drugs, then for generic copies of old drugs.

M. Weintraub, M.D.

Crossover Trials With a Binary Response: A Powerful Method Despite the Carryover Effect

Cleophas TJM, van Lier HJJ (Merwede Hosp Dordrecht, The Netherlands; Univ Hosp Nijmegen, The Netherlands)
J Clin Pharmacol 36:198–202, 1996   1–10

Background.—The crossover design is commonly used in clinical trials. It has the advantage of avoiding between-subject variability in comparisons. However, the design assumes that treatment order does not influence treatment outcome. Therefore, only symptomatic treatments, not curative treatments, can be studied in crossover comparisons. However, some symptomatic treatments can have small curative effects. Therefore, the significance of carryover effects was examined in crossover trials with a binary response.

Methods.—A mathematical model was developed based on standard statistical tests to evaluate to what degree crossover effects can reduce the power of the reported treatment effect.

Results.—When the 2 treatments act independently, the power of detecting a treatment effect in a crossover trial involving 20–50 subjects is always greater than 94%. In situations in which the 2 treatments do not act independently, the power to detect a treatment difference is at least 74% if the first treatment is more effective. When the second treatment is more effective, the power to detect a treatment effect is enhanced.

Conclusion.—Crossover studies with a binary response do not need to be analyzed for carryover effects if the result is positive. However, testing for carryover effect may be useful if the result is negative, using the data from the first period and parallel-group analysis.

▶ This statistically oriented paper is really very important for several reasons. One thing is that it proves that the yes/no or present/absent outcome in a crossover study can really be very important for testing new drugs. When we do such a study, the outcome of interest will be understood by everybody involved. The therapeutic answer can be couched in "What are my chances for having a positive effect?" The doctor can comfortably answer, "Your chances are *x*%." Physicians should be requesting this kind of trial so that not only can the patients understand, but doctors can communicate the outcome of therapy better.

M. Weintraub, M.D.

Increasing the Number of Drugs Available Over the Counter: Arguments For and Against
Bradley CP, Bond C (Univ of Birmingham, England; Univ of Aberdeen, Scotland)
Br J Gen Pract 45:553–556, 1995   1–11

Introduction.—In recent years, many drugs that were previously available only by prescription have become available over the counter. This trend is expected to continue. The consequences of the increasing number of drugs available over the counter and guidelines for recommending their use were investigated.

Advantages and Disadvantages.—Physicians should be aware that more drugs are becoming available over the counter, and this knowledge may affect their consultations. They must ask each patient about any self-medication before deciding on treatment for the patient because interactions between over-the-counter and prescription medications are a potential problem. When the physician asks about self-medication, the patient will ask whether the physician approves. The increased use of over-the-counter medications, which are regarded as safe, suggests that patients may be taking greater responsibility for their own health. Also, because patients are buying these medicines themselves, they may be reducing costs. On the other hand, the greater availability of over-the-counter medications may prompt patients to believe that there is "a pill for every ill." In addition to the risk of drug interactions, this trend may also increase the chances of adverse drug reactions and of self-treatment in situations when medical care should be sought. A physician's recommendation to use over-the-counter drugs may also carry some legal risk.

Guidelines for Recommendation.—Several steps can be taken to avoid the pitfalls of over-the-counter drug use. First, the physician should always ask patients about their previous and current self-medication habits to help identify any potential adverse drug reactions or interactions. Second, patients need to be educated about which medications are generally safe to use, and about appropriate use of nonprescription drugs in general. Third, physicians and pharmacists need to communicate more closely regarding over-the-counter medication use. As more drugs become available on a nonprescription basis for the first time, new links must be forged between physicians, pharmacists, and patients.

Discussion.—More drugs will continue to become available on an over-the-counter basis. Important advantages and disadvantages are associated with this trend. Following the recommended guidelines will help ensure that patients, physicians, and pharmacists alike realize the benefits while minimizing the adverse consequences.

▶ More drugs are available over the counter worldwide. In the United States, the H_2 blockers for treatment of heartburn join antacids and home remedies. The availability of minoxidil, nicotine gum, naproxen sodium, and ketoprofen as well as ibuprofen for children's fever and pain, is another example of this important movement. Part of the impetus for increased over-the-counter drugs may be the medical profession's and the population's greater feelings that the average individual can, and wants to, diagnose and treat their own illnesses.

A very important point made in this paper is that not enough physicians ask their patients about the use of over-the-counter medications. The Public Health Service's *Healthy People 2000* states that 75% of physicians should ask their elderly patients about the use of over-the-counter medications. I certainly hope that more physicians and more patients communicate about over-the-counter medications. These drugs remain a valuable source of treatment for many people. However, they are real medicines and no one should forget that; neither the patient taking them nor the physician, who is watching both the general availability as well as individual medications used by a particular patient.

M. Weintraub, M.D.

The Future for Self Medication

Bradley C, Blenkinsopp A (Univ of Birmingham, England; Univ of Keele, Staffordshire, England)
BMJ 312:835–837, 1996   1–12

Objective.—The factors driving the trend toward increasing availability and use of over-the-counter (OTC) medications far outweigh the opposing factors. Current and future trends in OTC medicines are reviewed, along with their implications for health care professionals.

Trends.—The number of drugs changed from prescription-only to OTC status has greatly increased in recent years, although the formulations, dosages, and indications are not necessarily the same. Safety is the major reason for restricting the availability of drugs, but some have argued that this objection can be overcome by simply providing patients with more information. If this argument prevails, an even broader range of drugs may become available on an OTC basis in the near future. Under the "collaborative care" concept, physicians may delegate part of the continuing treatment of patients with chronic conditions to others, particularly pharmacists.

Implications.—As the trend toward self-medication gains momentum, physicians, pharmacists, and other health care professionals will have to respond actively and constructively. A more effective means of reporting adverse reactions—with increased involvement of pharmacists—will be needed. Pharmacists may see greater profits from increased sales of OTC medications, but there will also be some loss of dispensing fees. Some means of rewarding pharmacists for advising patients will be needed. Nurses are likely to play an increasing role in recommending OTC drugs.

Discussion.—As the trend toward patient self-medication grows, health care professionals must discuss their response. Improved communication among physicians, pharmacists, and nurses has the potential to create a more constructive interaction among health care professionals and patients. Alternatively, turf wars over who controls medication use could split the professions, making patients more vulnerable to the risks inherent in using medicines.

▶ There are lots of pressures pushing patients into increasing use (with or without suggestions from their physicians) of OTC medicines. Such a trend is not predictably good or bad (probably a bit of each), but we need to monitor it.

L. Lasagna, M.D.

Evaluation of Physician Intervention Letters
Rascati KL, Okano GJ, Burch C (Univ of Texas, Austin; Texas Medicaid Vendor Drug Program, Austin)
Med Care 34:760–766, 1996   1–13

Background.—Drug utilization review (DUR), devised as a method of encouraging appropriate prescribing, has been required of Medicaid agencies since passage of the Omnibus Budget Reconciliation Act of 1990. The effectiveness of mailing intervention letters to physicians whose patient profiles indicate possible inappropriate prescribing was assessed.

Methods.—Through examination of Texas Medicaid Vendor Drug claims for a 3-month period in 1993, profiles of 335 patients receiving potentially inappropriate medication were extracted. Members of the Texas DUR board agreed that for anti-ulcer therapy, no benefit was derived from the combination of 2 histamine-2 receptor antagonists (H2s) or the combination of an H2 with omeprazole; 113 patients fit this profile (H2-H2 group). A review of the literature also revealed no benefit of combining an H2 with sucralfate (222 patients, H2-S group); however, the board did not unanimously consider this use universally inappropriate, hence this patient group was analyzed separately. The intervention letters from the Texas Department of Human Services indicated the results of the literature review, recognized the need for individualized therapy, and included response forms, copies of patient profiles, and stamped envelopes. Letters were sent to the physicians of 174 randomly selected patients; 161 patients served as controls.

Results.—The response rate was 71.2%; 48.9% of the respondents agreed with the letter and 19.1% disagreed. Profiles extracted 6 months after the intervention revealed that concurrent drug therapy was still

14 / Drug Therapy

occurring for 47.7% of the patients in the intervention group and 64.4% of the patients in the control group. More physicians prescribing H2-S therapy disagreed with the letter (29.1%) than did physicians prescribing H2-H2 therapy (3.8%).

Conclusions.—The effectiveness of intervention letters for this use is supported by the high response rate, moderately high agreement with the letter, and statistically significant reduction in duplicative therapy in the experimental group.

▶ Here goes a counterintuitive argument: I am going to say that I worry a great deal about these letters. The problem with them is that physicians may comply with the letters because it is just easier to do so rather than to tell the company that sends them out (or the Medicaid group) that the doctor may have discovered a better way to treat disease X or syndrome Y. The doctor might have used expensive or forbidden medications. I really think this is a major problem because I believe in the innovativeness and inventiveness of some physicians as they try to deal with their patients. The doctors do not publish these data often enough, but I will bet they are doing a lot of very intelligent prescribing. Unfortunately, the more often people follow these letters, which really are based on deviations away from the mean on prescribing, the less we will ever know about the potential for interesting drug therapy.

M. Weintraub, M.D.

Medication Compliance After Renal Transplantation
Hilbrands LB, Hoitsma AJ, Koene RAP (Univ Hosp Nijmegen, The Netherlands)
Transplantation 60:914–920, 1995   1–14

Objective.—A major cause of late graft failure after renal transplantation is medication noncompliance. The degree of compliance with immunosuppressive and antihypertensive drugs in the first year after renal transplantation was investigated prospectively by monthly pill counts. The relationship of noncompliance to a number of demographic and clinical variables and to the occurrence of rejections was also investigated.

Methods and Findings.—One hundred twenty-seven patients involved in a randomized comparison of cyclosporine monotherapy and azathioprine-prednisone therapy were studied. Mean compliance rates were about 100%. However, there was considerable variation within and between patients. During the study year, noncompliance rates were 23% for cyclosporine, 13% for azathioprine, 23% for prednisone, 36% for atenolol, and 32% for nifedipine. The mean compliance scores for all immunosuppressive drugs were greater than those for antihypertensive agents. Compliance for prednisone was better in men than in women. No other consistent relationships between compliance and demographic factors, graft function, or quality of life were found. Compared with patients with

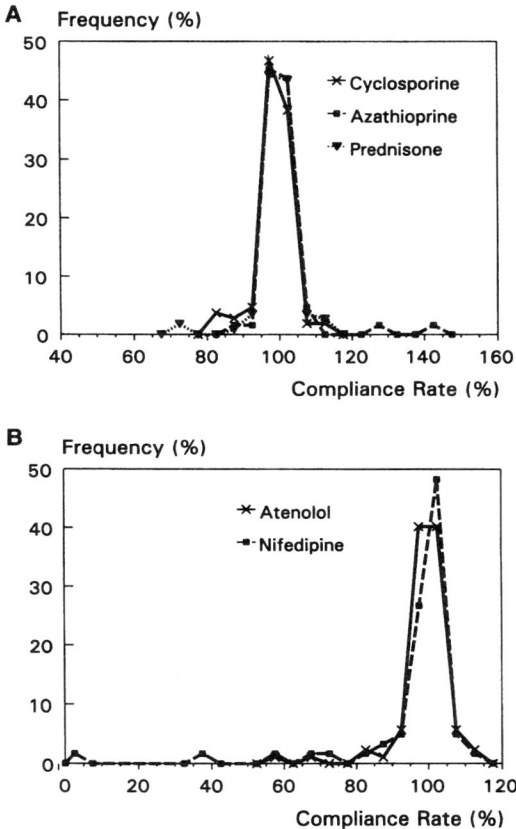

FIGURE 1.—Frequency distributions of compliance rates (number of tablets taken as a percentage of number of tablets prescribed) with (**A**) immunosuppressive and (**B**) antihypertensive drugs. The compliance rates concern the entire study period (1 year). (Courtesy of Hilbrands LB, Hoitsma AJ, Koene RAP: Medication compliance after renal transplantation. *Transplantation* 60:914–920, 1995.)

no rejection episodes, patients with 1 or more acute rejection episodes had a higher degree of undercompliance, especially for prednisone. Compliance scores improved greatly after a rejection episode (Fig 1).

Conclusions.—Compliance with medication was high in the first year after renal transplantation. Adherence to immunosuppressive treatment was better than to antihypertensive agents. Poor compliance with prednisone was correlated with a subsequent rejection episode, which then seemed to prompt compliance.

▶ The average reported rate for compliance of 100% is misleading. It is so because some patients take too little drug and others too much. In fact, there was a lot of noncompliance (13% to 36%) even by the insensitive technique of "pill counts."

L. Lasagna, M.D.

Beliefs About Steroids: User vs Non-user Comparisons
Schwerin MJ, Corcoran KJ (Naval Health Research Ctr, San Diego, Calif; Southern Illinois Univ, Carbondale)
Drug Alcohol Depend 40:221–225, 1996   1–15

Introduction.—A model of behavior describes the following progression: beliefs shape attitudes, which influence intent, which leads to behavior. Although the use of anabolic steroids (AS) is associated with several adverse effects, such use is still widespread. The differences in beliefs concerning AS between AS-using bodybuilders and non–AS-using bodybuilders were examined.

Methods.—Bodybuilders at a university were interviewed, using the Beliefs about Steroids Scale (BASS), a 40-item questionnaire. Of the 47 bodybuilders, 20 were currently or had used AS and 27 had never used AS.

Results.—There were significant differences between the users and nonusers on 35 of the 40 BASS items. The AS users had stronger beliefs about the physical effects of AS use, including strength and athleticism, and about the psychological effects of AS use, including feeling more confident, assertive, sexually aroused, and happy/optimistic. In contrast, nonusing bodybuilders had a stronger belief in the negative effects of AS use, including drug-related health problems.

Conclusions.—AS-using bodybuilders have substantially more positive attitudes regarding AS use than do bodybuilders who do not use AS. Further study is needed to determine the influence of positive expectancies on AS use.

▶ Anabolic steroids can produce all sorts of adverse effects, but users of these preparations are not deluding themselves about the benefits. They *do* build muscle mass, strength, aggressiveness, and confidence, and athletes have shown an ability to differentiate between these steroids and placebos as measured by perceptions of their own strength.[1]

L. Lasagna, M.D.

Reference

1. Crist DM, Stackpole PJ, Peake GT: Effects of androgen-anabolic steroids on neuromuscular power and body composition. *J Appl Physiol* 54:366–370, 1983.

Variation in the Practice of Dose Reduction of Chemotherapeutic Agents After Weight Loss or Amputation
O'Marcaigh AS, Betcher DL, Gilchrist GS (Mayo Clinic, Rochester, Minn)
J Pediatr Hematol Oncol 17:172–175, 1995   1–16

Background.—In patients receiving chemotherapy, the occurrence of weight loss or amputation necessitates dose reductions to avoid excessive treatment-related toxicity. Several methods are used to calculate necessary dose reductions. These include dose reduction in proportion to the decrease in body surface area or the amount of weight lost, and no dose reductions unless toxicity occurs.

Methods and Findings.—Pediatric oncologists, pediatric oncology nurses, and data managers were surveyed to determine the methods of calculating dose reductions currently used for patients who have lost weight, who have had an amputation, and who have lost further weight after amputation. Of 274 persons surveyed, 237 responded, for a rate of 80.6%. The most popular dose-reduction method was to decrease the dose in proportion to body surface area. This method was used in 88% of patients with weight loss alone, in 60% of those undergoing amputation, and in 66% of patients who had amputation and have ongoing weight loss. The chosen method of dose reduction resulted in a discrepancy of up to 37% among administered doses.

Conclusions.—Standardization is needed in chemotherapy dose-reduction methods for patients who lose weight or undergo amputations. Further research is needed to determine the best method of dose reduction in such patients.

▶ It certainly seems that this problem should have been studied at some time in the past. However, it has not been studied, and physicians and nurses are left out on a limb trying to decide the best way to adjust the dose when someone is losing weight or has an amputation. Failure to standardize the method of calculation of the dose may lead to excessive toxicity or to differences among institutions or physicians at the same institution in the amount of drug prescribed. Unfortunately, this may even affect the achievement of a good outcome.

M. Weintraub, M.D.

Effective Administration of Heparin and Antibiotic Prophylaxis
Avery CME, Jamieson N, Calne RY (Addenbrooke's Hosp, Cambridge, England)
Br J Surg 82:1136–1137, 1995   1–17

Background.—At one center, the administration of heparin and antibiotic prophylaxis was found to be inadequate, which prompted a change in departmental procedures. To determine whether this change resulted in any improvement, a follow-up audit was done.

Methods and Findings.—Heparin prophylaxis was administered to 77 patients, or 97%, undergoing elective procedures. Sixty-seven percent received the initial dose before surgery or at induction. All of 36 patients undergoing emergency procedures received heparin prophylaxis. Overall, antibiotic prophylaxis was administered to 97.1% of the patients, with 86.1% receiving the initial dose before surgery or at induction. Ninety-six percent of patients undergoing emergency procedures received prophylactic antibiotics, with 84.8% receiving the initial dose before surgery or at induction. All of these rates compare favorably with the percentages documented in the previous audit.

Conclusions.—The administration of prophylactic drugs can be improved significantly. Prophylaxis protocols should be clarified early, possibly at job orientation meetings. Good practice should be reinforced to increase awareness of the importance of heparin prophylaxis. A list of groups at risk should be provided to the nursing staff, and preoperative checklists should be carefully completed before surgery.

▶ The problem with this study is that it is confounded by duration of treatment effect. That is, not only was the same, or a similar, protocol discussed orally, but it was really repeated over the second time period. This shows that continual reminders are important and necessary to achieve success. I do not know why we need repetition, but the protocol details and goals apparently must be re-emphasized over and over again.

M. Weintraub, M.D.

Anaesthetists, Errors in Drug Administration and the Law
Merry AF, Peck DJ (Green Lane Hosp, Auckland, New Zealand)
N Z Med J 108:185–187, 1995   1–18

Objective—Anesthetists are particularly likely to be involved in legal cases arising from drug administration errors. These errors can involve the identity of an anesthetic drug or its dose or route of administration. New Zealand anesthetists were surveyed regarding the problem of anesthetic drug administration errors.

Methods—The study questionnaire was sent to a random sample of 75 New Zealand anesthetists. They were asked about the prevalence of drug administration errors, in terms of the total number of drugs that an anesthetist might administer during his or her career; preventive strategies; and the current medicolegal environment in New Zealand, where any fatal drug error could qualify as negligence and, therefore, as criminal negligence.

Results.—The response rate was 88%. Eighty-nine percent of respondents said they had made at least 1 drug administration error, and 12.5% said they had made a drug administration error resulting in patient harm. Many different preventive strategies were reported, such as labeling of syringe contents and using a syringe size code. However, none of these strategies was significantly related to the frequency of error. All of the respondents reported that they were concerned about the possibility that they could be charged with manslaughter if a patient died as a result of a medication error. Eighty-three percent believed that the current legal climate could interfere with reporting of drug errors, although 88% said that they always reported their errors.

Conclusions.—Almost all anesthetists surveyed reported making errors in drug administration, and a significant proportion of these errors resulted in patient harm. Given that such errors are bound to occur, it is not logical to treat them as criminal. Instead of looking for scapegoats, it would be better to direct efforts at finding rational ways of reducing the problem of drug administration errors.

▶ A medical school classmate of mine is very interested in and has even changed his life to the study of physician errors. He told me that airline pilots make a huge number of errors. Perhaps the pilots make mental errors. They can make physical errors or judgment errors. Fortunately, however, only very, very rarely do they result in a serious outcome. In much the same way, physicians make many errors. Thankfully, when physicians prescribe antibiotics, even if we decide on the wrong bug as having caused an infection, we probably give a drug that has a spectrum including that organism. And, when physicians make an error in judgment, fortunately the human body sometimes will heal itself in spite of or because of our therapy. The paper discusses some cases of manslaughter arising from fatal drug errors in New Zealand. After reading this, I wish my classmate would hurry up and get to the bottom of why physicians make errors and how they can be minimized.

M. Weintraub, M.D.

Screening for Clinical Laboratory Errors With Medicare Claims Data: Results for Digoxin

Winkelman JW, Mennemeyer ST (Univ of Alabama, Birmingham; Abt Associates Inc, Cambridge, Mass)
Am J Med Qual 11:25–32, 1996   1–19

Background.—Research in quality assurance has emphasized analysis of outcomes in the evaluation of the effectiveness of medical procedures. However, little has been done to evaluate the effect on outcomes of intermediate inputs in the medical process, including laboratory tests. Therefore, the performance of clinical laboratories was evaluated using downstream event monitoring, which tracks patient outcomes during a critical period after a laboratory test to examine the effects of false test results. This method was used to screen for laboratory error involving digoxin testing.

Methods.—Data were obtained from Medicare Part A and Part B claims for 30,685 digoxin tests performed from 1985 to 1987. The occurrence of death unrelated to heart conditions or digoxin, hospitalization with or without death related to heart conditions or digoxin, or no adverse event within 14 days after digoxin testing was identified by the Medicare diagnostic codes. Patient and laboratory characteristics were analyzed for relationships to the outcomes with logistic regression.

Results.—Death unrelated to heart conditions or digoxin occurred within 14 days after 1,959 digoxin tests. Hospitalization related to heart conditions or digoxin occurred after 3,769 tests. There were no adverse events after 24,957 tests. The risk of an adverse event after digoxin testing was lower in states with stronger laboratory regulations, was greater in association with switching test sites, and was unrelated to testing in low volume physician office laboratories or to the frequency of digoxin testing in a patient in the previous 6 months.

Conclusion.—Adverse patient outcomes after digoxin testing, indicating possible laboratory error, were linked to laboratory characteristics. The downstream event monitoring method of analysis may improve regulatory efforts by identifying proper foci and may improve patient safety.

▶ Wow! You mean that regulation is really good? Whenever someone checks the function of clinical laboratories, some pretty bad outliers turn up. Unfortunately, physicians cannot always tell where the bad laboratories are. That is why it is very important for the states to regulate the laboratories by sending samples around and measuring standard samples or split samples.

M. Weintraub, M.D.

Dietary Vitamin C and β-Carotene and Risk of Death in Middle-aged Men: The Western Electric Study
Pandey DK, Shekelle R, Selwyn BJ, et al (Univ of Texas, Houston; Rush-Presbyterian-St Luke's Med Ctr, Chicago; Northwestern Univ, Chicago)
Am J Epidemiol 142:1269–1278, 1995   1–20

Background.—Dietary antioxidants such as vitamin C and β-carotene have been thought to decrease the risk of many cancers. These antioxidants inhibit the formation of carcinogenic nitrosamines and scavenge and quench reactive oxygen molecules. Thus, DNA is protected from oxidative damages, and immune functions are enhanced. In addition, dietary antioxidants may decrease the risk of coronary heart disease by inhibiting low-density-lipoprotein oxidation. The relationship between dietary vitamin C and β-carotene intake and mortality was investigated in a cohort of middle-aged men.

Methods and Findings.—Data on diet and other factors were obtained in 1958 and 1959 on a cohort of 1,556 Western Electric Company employees. The mean vitamin C intake in the lowest tertile was 66 mg/day and in the highest tertile, 138 mg/day. The mean β-carotene intake in the lowest tertile was 2.3 mg/day and 5.3 mg/day in the highest tertile. During 24 years of follow-up, covering 32,935 person-years, 522 men died. Death was caused by coronary heart disease in 231 men and by cancer in 155. After adjustment for confounding variables, the relative risk of cancer mortality among those in the highest tertile compared with those in the lowest tertile was 0.60; of death from coronary disease, 0.70; and of death from any cause, 0.69.

Conclusions.—In this 24-year follow-up study of middle-aged men, a diet higher in vitamin C equivalent to 1 or 2 oranges a day and higher in β-carotene equivalent to 1 or 2 carrots a day was associated with a 31%

lower risk of death. This correlation persisted after adjustment for several possible confounding variables.

▶ Jeremiah Stamler, one of the authors of this study, has been collecting important epidemiologic data on cardiovascular problems longer than anyone in the United States. He is tough-minded and realistic. This long-standing study sheds light on the possibility that dietary antioxidants such as vitamin C and β-carotene may prevent cancer and coronary heart disease.

A diet higher in vitamin C by 1–2 oranges per day and higher in β-carotene by 1–2 carrots per day was associated with a dramatically lower risk of death from all causes. No alternative explanation is deemed likely. The only caveat is that the associations may result from other nutrients in these fruits and vegetables, and not specifically vitamin C and β-carotene. Nevertheless, the data are mighty impressive. They support the 1989 recommendations of the National Research Council that adults should consume 5 or more servings of fresh fruits and vegetables each day, especially citrus fruits and green and yellow vegetables.

L. Lasagna, M.D.

Treatment of Xerostomia With Polymer-Based Saliva Substitutes in Patients With Sjögren's Syndrome
van der Reijden WA, van der Kwaak H, Vissink A, et al (Academic Centre for Dentistry, Amsterdam, The Netherlands; Univ Hosp, Groningen, The Netherlands)
Arthritis Rheum 39:57–63, 1996   1–21

Objective.—Some patients with Sjögren's syndrome (SS), an autoimmune disease of the exocrine glands, can benefit from using saliva substitutes. Some of the newer products of this type—those containing polyacrylic acid (PAA) and xanthan gum (XG)—have synergistic effects on the elastic or rheologic properties of human saliva, unlike previous products based on porcine gastric mucin. These 3 types of saliva substitutes were compared for their efficacy in reducing oral dryness in patients with SS in a double-blind, placebo-controlled trial.

Methods.—Forty-three patients with primary or secondary SS subjectively rated the 3 different saliva substitutes. In addition, 33 patients compared high- vs. low-viscosity XG-based products. In addition to the subjective ratings, salivary flow rates (SFRs) were compared.

Results.—There was no real difference in effectiveness between the 3 saliva substitutes and placebo, and no difference in patient preference between the 3 products over placebo. Patients who preferred the PAA-based saliva substitute had lower SFRs than those who preferred the porcine mucin–based product. Simulated SFRs were low for patients in whom a low-viscoelastic product reduced oral dryness.

Conclusions.—For patients with SS, the SFR—among other factors— may affect the choice of saliva substitutes for symptomatic treatment of xerostomia. Patients should try various products with different viscoelastic properties to determine which is best for them. Particularly for patients with severe xerostomia, the new polymer-based saliva substitutes, with their varying viscoelastic properties, will aid in the management of oral dryness.

▶ This is the reason for "me-too" drugs. When the doctor does not know which of the large group of medications will be most helpful to his patients, he has to start with one and switch the patient to another, and perhaps another. Of course, what was helpful in this study was the SFR, which may point a doctor in a certain direction in choosing one medication over another. The viscoelasticity of the medication also may determine how much an individual patient likes and will choose a specific medication. It just goes to show you that there is still some room for patient preference.

M. Weintraub, M.D.

2   Drug Action

Folate Synthesized by Bacteria in the Human Upper Small Intestine Is Assimilated by the Host
Camilo E, Zimmerman J, Mason JB, et al (Univ Hosp de Santa Maria, Lisbon Portugal; Hadassah Med School, Jerusalem; Tufts Univ, Boston)
Gastroenterology 110:991–998, 1996   2–1

Introduction.—Humans need exogenous sources of folate to maintain adequate folate status. Some bacteria, including some of those found in the human gastrointestinal (GI) flora, can synthesize folate. Serum folate concentrations are increased in patients with atrophic gastritis, a condition associated with modest bacterial overgrowth in the upper small intestine. However, no studies in humans have directly demonstrated that folate is synthesized in vivo or shown what happens to bacterially synthesized folate. The synthesis of folate by GI flora and its assimilation by the human host were evaluated.

Methods.—Eight healthy men, 2 of whom had atrophic gastritis, were studied before and after 1 week of treatment with omeprazole, 20 mg by mouth twice daily. Each subject had a double-lumen tube placed into the duodenum, through which was perfused ^{3}H-labeled *P*-aminobenzoic acid, a precursor substrate for bacterial folate synthesis. Aspirates from the small intestine and a 48-hour urine collection were analyzed for evidence of folate synthesis and metabolism.

Results.—Duodenal pH and the amount of small intestine microflora were increased in subjects with atrophic gastritis and after omeprazole treatment. The small intestine aspirates showed bacterially synthesized folates. In addition, the urine of patients who had received omeprazole contained increased concentrations of tritiated 5-methyltetrahydrofolate, a major folate metabolite. Comparable increases of this metabolite were noted in the urine of the research subjects with atrophic gastritis.

Conclusions.—Folate is synthesized in the human small intestine in the presence of mild bacterial overgrowth caused by atrophic gastritis and with administration of omeprazole. There is evidence that the host metabolizes some of this bacterially synthesized folate. Its contribution to human nutrition is uncertain, however.

▶ We humans can't synthesize folate, but many bacterial species can, including some that ordinarily live in our GI tract. The reason is that the bugs use a synthetic pathway that is not present in eukaryotes.

It had been assumed that the folate so synthesized by intestinal microflora can be used by host animals (like us), but this study is the first to prove it.

L. Lasagna, M.D.

Acute Tolerance to Subjective But Not Cardiovascular Effects of _d_-Amphetamine in Normal, Healthy Men
Brauer LH, Ambre J, de Wit H (Univ of Chicago; American Med Assoc, Chicago; Duke Univ, Durham, NC)
J Clin Psychopharmacol 16:72–76, 1996   2–2

Background.—Determining the relation between drug concentration and drug effect is important, especially for abused drugs, because it may affect repeated drug administration in a drug-taking episode. Few researchers have studied the relation between plasma levels of _d_-amphetamine and drug effects in healthy volunteers. To extend previous findings, the relation between plasma _d_-amphetamine levels and drug effects was assessed for a longer time (24 hours) and on a wider range of dependent measures in healthy volunteers.

Methods and Findings.—Six men, aged 22 to 31 years, were given single oral doses of 20 mg of _d_-amphetamine on 2 occasions. Plasma levels were found to peak at 4 hours and to remain at detectable concentrations for 24 hours after drug administration. Subjective ratings peaked at 1.5 to 2 hours, returning to baseline values by 3 to 4 hours. Analysis of drug effect vs. drug concentration showed that acute tolerance developed to the subjective but not cardiopressor effects of the drug, suggesting that persons who administer _d_-amphetamine repeatedly to maintain the subjective effects may increase plasma levels and the physiologic effects to a toxic degree.

Conclusions.—As the subjective effects of _d_-amphetamine begin to wane, users of this drug may take additional doses, with potentially dangerous consequences.

▶ Acute tolerance develops to some of the effects of _d_-amphetamine. In fact, the development of tolerance happens with many drugs in a spotty manner. In some cases, this may be very valuable, because the main desired pharmacologic effect is maintained while patients become tolerant to adverse effects.

M. Weintraub, M.D.

Direct Angiotensin Converting Enzyme Inhibitor–mediated Venodilation

Zarnke KB, Feldman RD (Univ of Western Ontario, Canada)
Clin Pharmacol Ther 59:559–568, 1996   2–3

Background.—Angiotensin converting enzyme (ACE) inhibitors are effective in treating patients with hypertension, myocardial infarction, and congestive heart failure, but the mechanisms of their efficacy are unclear. It has been suggested that local effects may mediate ACE vasodilator effects. These local effects were evaluated with linear variable differential transformer (LVDT) measurement of the effects of a local infusion of enalaprilat in dorsal hand veins.

Methods.—Eleven healthy, drug-free, nonsmoking subjects were studied. An LVDT apparatus was used to directly measure changes in the size of small and large dorsal hand veins. Changes in vascular distention in smaller and larger vessels were studied after infusion of enalaprilat with skin temperatures lower than 29°C and higher than 31°C, with or without vasoconstriction with exogenous norepinephrine. The vasodilation effects of insulin and nitroglycerin were also assessed under the same conditions.

Results.—Enalaprilat infusion caused dose-dependent vasodilation in smaller, but not in larger, dorsal hand vessels only when the vessels had been constricted by either temperature or norepinephrine. Enalaprilat mediated vasodilation at an intensity comparable to the effects of insulin, but less than the effects of nitroglycerin. The extent of vasodilation caused by enalaprilat was inversely correlated with the constriction caused by temperature or norepinephrine.

Conclusion.—Enalaprilat mediated vasodilation in dorsal hand veins, with the effects dependent on preconstriction and vessel size. These findings support the idea of the importance of local vasodilator effects in determining the effects of ACE inhibitors.

▶ The technique of infusing drugs into small hand veins is really a very clever technique for establishing the activity of various drugs, not just alone but in combination as well. There have already been important findings from this technique, and I think we are going to see many more.

M. Weintraub, M.D.

H$_1$- and H$_2$-Histamine Receptor-mediated Vasodilation Varies With Aging in Humans

Bedarida G, Bushell E, Blaschke TF, et al (Stanford Univ, Calif; Veterans Affairs Med Ctr, Palo Alto, Calif)
Clin Pharmacol Ther 58:73–80, 1995   2–4

Introduction.—Both structural and functional aging-associated alterations have been noted in the cardiovascular system, including vasodilation. Two major pathways are involved in vasodilation: the cyclic adenosine monophosphate (cAMP)–dependent and the cyclic guanosine mono-phosphate (cGMP)–dependent pathways. Studies have suggested that the β-receptor–mediated cAMP pathway is impaired by aging, which may affect responses to vasoactive drugs. Responses to histamine in hand veins were evaluated in subjects of varying ages to investigate vascular responses to vasoactive drugs with aging.

Methods.—The 16 subjects ranged in age from 21 to 80 years. The dorsal hand vein was preconstricted with phenylephrine, then injected with histamine in various doses. Responses of the vein were measured with a linear variable differential transformer. The dose-response curves were assessed with histamine alone and with histamine after infusions of either the H_2-receptor blocker cimetidine or the H_1-receptor blockers bromphen-iramine or methylene blue.

Results.—Effective vasodilation occurred with histamine in subjects of all ages, without statistically significant age-related variations in response. The infusion of cimetidine had less inhibitory effects on the maximal response to histamine in the elderly than in the young subjects, but the dose that produced half-maximal response was not significantly correlated with age. The residual histamine response was nearly completely abolished with either brompheniramine or methylene blue.

Conclusions.—There is no change in the efficacy or potency of hista-mine-mediated vasodilation with aging. However, elderly subjects demon-strate diminished functioning of the response mediated by the H_2-receptor signal-transduction pathway, whereas the H_1-receptor–mediated pathway is preserved. Aging appears to produce a shift in the balance between the cAMP pathway, which predominates in youth and is blunted in the elderly, and the cGMP pathway, which predominates in the elderly.

▶ Because the study was cross-sectional, the data are a little more difficult to interpret. I would be very nice now to develop a cohort to watch people as they age This is not hard to do, and I think the technique can be standardized and used in the development of this patient group. The thing is, you don't even have to start with all teenagers and wait until they are elderly. One can start with people at all ages and see when the changes develop. This is probably a general principle for many geriatric studies.

M. Weintraub, M.D.

Magnesium Repletion and Its Effect on Potassium Homeostasis in Crit-ically Ill Adults: Results of a Double-Blind, Randomized, Controlled Trial
Hamill-Ruth RJ, McGory R (Univ of Virginia, Charlottesville)
Crit Care Med 24:38–45, 1996   2–5

Objective.—It can be difficult to treat hypokalemia in patients with coexistent hypomagnesemia. Potassium replacement therapy may lead to increased urine potassium excretion and a backward trend in serum po-tassium concentration. The effects of an aggressive magnesium replacement regimen on potassium retention in critically ill patients with hypo-kalemia were evaluated in a prospective, randomized, double-blind, pla-cebo-controlled trial.

Methods.—The subjects were 32 adult surgical ICU patients with cir-culating potassium concentrations of less than 3.5 mmol/L. Patients were assigned to receive active treatment—magnesium sulfate, 2 g in 50 mL of 5% dextrose in water over 30 minutes every 6 hours for 6 doses—or placebo, given by the same schedule. Standard potassium and magnesium replacement therapy continued in both groups, as indicated for a serum potassium concentration of less than 3.5 mmol/L or a serum magnesium concentration of less than 1.8 mg/dL. Colorimetric and potentiometric assays were used to evaluate the serum and urine magnesium and potas-sium concentrations.

Results.—The 2 groups were similar in their baseline serum magnesium and potassium concentrations. Six hours after the start of the study, just 12% of patients in the active treatment group had their test dose withheld because of a magnesium concentration that exceeded 2.8 mg/dL. After 36 and 42 hours, half of the patients had this dose withheld. The 2 groups received similar total amounts of potassium, which included replacement infusions, IV solutions, and parenteral nutrition. However, mean potas-sium excretion in 48 hours was 418 mmol in the control group vs. 173 mmol in the active treatment group. Clinically significant ventricular ec-topy was noted in 3 patients in the active treatment group within the first 12 hours of the study, compared with 5 patients in the control group. None of the patients required treatment for dysrhythmias, and there were no complications of magnesium therapy.

Conclusions.—In the ICU, hypokalemia identifies a group of patients who are likely to have magnesium deficiency. The aggressive magnesium sulfate regimen used in this study safely increases circulating magnesium concentration, enhances magnesium retention, and improves potassium homeostasis.

▶ This study reminds us that there is a relationship between potassium and magnesium balance. It was done in a double-blind, randomized, controlled trial. Congratulations!

M. Weintraub, M.D.

The Role of Antioxidant Vitamins and Enzymes in the Prevention of Exercise-induced Muscle Damage
Dekkers JC, van Doornen LJP, Kemper HCG (Vrije Universiteit, Amsterdam)
Sports Med 21:213–238, 1996   2–6

Introduction.—Tissue damage that occurs after strenuous or unaccus-tomed physical exertion appears to result from not only mechanical forces but also the production of free radicals and the initiation of peroxidation reactions. There is some evidence that elevated oxygen consumption during exercise induces the production of free radicals and other oxidant species and that dietary antioxidants are capable of scavenging peroxyl radicals and preventing muscle damage. The physiology of antioxidants and the findings of rodent and human studies on the effects of exercise on lipid peroxidation are reviewed.

Physiology of Antioxidants.—Because free radical production and lipid peroxidation are positively correlated with increases in skeletal muscle damage, free radicals are likely to be produced to a greater extent during exercise than during rest. With the redistribution of blood during exercise, some tissues may become susceptible to peroxidation. Another factor is the influence of exercise on the reduced nicotinamide–adenine dinucleotide and the reduced nicotinamide–adenine dinucleotide phosphate levels, essential cofactors for activity by some free radical scavenging enzymes. Thus, exercise may disturb the fine balance of the human antioxidant defense system. Identified as protective antioxidants are uric acid, the fat-soluble tocopherol (vitamin E) and β-carotene, and the water-soluble ascorbic acid.

Findings of Rodent and Human Studies.—Exercise to exhaustion leads to an increased hydroperoxide and aldehyde level, indicative of lipid peroxidation, and to significant increases in oxidative and antioxidant enzyme activities. The increased antioxidant activities and antioxidant level counteract lipid peroxidation by scavenging free radicals, thus protecting the muscle from exercise-induced damage. Both the training status of the study participant and the type of muscle examined appear to influence antioxidant enzyme activity. In humans, dietary supplementation with antioxidant vitamins has a beneficial effect on exercise-induced lipid peroxidation. Such supplements can now be recommended to individuals who participate in regular, strenuous exercise. In addition, training leads to increased activity of several major antioxidant enzymes and overall antioxidant status.

▶ The pendulum keeps swinging back and forth in the public literature on the possible health benefits of antioxidant vitamins and enzymes. This review concludes that such antioxidants protect against exercise-induced muscle damage.

L. Lasagna, M.D.

Lack of Effect of Long-term Supplementation With Beta Carotene on the Incidence of Malignant Neoplasms and Cardiovascular Disease
Hennekens CH, Buring JE, Manson JE, et al (Brigham and Women's Hosp, Boston; Harvard Med School, Boston; Harvard School of Public Health, Boston)
N Engl J Med 334:1145–1149, 1996   2–7

Background.—Risks of cancer and cardiovascular disease appear to be somewhat lower in people with a high intake of fruits and vegetables containing beta-carotene. Some plausible mechanisms for this relationship have been suggested by basic science research. The capability of long-term beta-carotene supplementation to prevent cardiovascular disease and malignant neoplasms was studied.

Methods.—The randomized, double-blind trial was conducted as part of the Physicians' Health Study. Beginning in 1982, 22,071 male physicians, aged 40–84 years, were assigned to receive either beta-carotene supplementation, 50 mg on alternate days, or placebo. Eleven percent of the individuals were current smokers and 39% were former smokers at baseline. The trial was scheduled to run through the end of 1995, at which time 99% of the individuals were available for follow-up. Seventy-eight percent of physicians assigned to beta-carotene supplementation were compliant.

Results.—The beta-carotene and placebo groups showed few, if any, differences in the incidence of cardiovascular diseases or malignancies or in mortality. Malignant neoplasms other than nonmelanoma skin cancer developed in 1,273 individuals in the beta-carotene group vs. 1,293 in the placebo group, yielding a relative risk of 0.98. The incidences of lung cancer, death from cancer, death from any cause, and death from cardiovascular disease were also similar in the 2 groups. Neither were there any significant differences in the number of individuals with myocardial infarction, strokes, or any of the previous 3 end points. All of the end points were also comparable among current and former smokers.

Conclusions.—Long-term supplementation with beta-carotene does not appear to reduce the risk of malignant neoplasms, cardiovascular disease, or death in healthy men. Neither was there any evidence that beta-carotene supplementation had a harmful effect. The results provide timely guidance for public health recommendations because the general public has been spending a great deal of money on beta-carotene supplements.

▶ Just remember what your grandmother told you: "Eat your vegetables and pay attention to the policeman on the corner when you cross the street." Actually, you'll probably be better off if you just eat your vegetables rather than take supplements of beta-carotene.

M. Weintraub, M.D.

Cirrhosis and Muscle Cramps: Evidence of a Causal Relationship
Angeli P, Albino G, Carraro P, et al (Univ of Padua, Italy)
Hepatology 23:264–273, 1996   2–8

Introduction.—True muscle cramps reportedly are more prevalent in patients with cirrhosis than in a matched population of noncirrhotic individuals. Some have ascribed muscle cramps to the use of diuretics in cirrhotic patients with ascites.

Objective.—Two protocol studies were carried out to determine the prevalence of muscle cramps in patients with cirrhosis and to explore the underlying pathophysiologic mechanisms. The first study compared 171 patients with cirrhosis and the same number of age- and sex-matched control individuals without evidence of liver disease. A standard questionnaire was used to elicit a history of painful involuntary skeletal muscle contractions. The second study compared the effects of expanding the effective circulating volume by infused human albumin with those of a placebo in 12 cirrhotic patients having more than 3 cramp crises per week.

Results.—Cramps were more prevalent in cirrhotic patients than in matched control individuals. Their occurrence related to both the known duration of cirrhosis and the severity of hepatic dysfunction. Multiple regression analysis showed that cramps were independently associated with the presence of ascites, a low mean arterial pressure, and a high plasma renin activity. In the treatment study, albumin infusion reduced the frequency of cramps compared with the placebo condition. Cramps were eliminated altogether by albumin infusion in 2 of the 12 patients.

Conclusions.—Cirrhotic patients may have muscle cramps because of arterial underfilling. Weekly infusions of human albumin solution help to prevent cramps by increasing the effective circulating volume.

▶ Muscle cramps can be devastating. These involuntary skeletal muscle contractions occur at rest, often (but not invariably) at night, are asymmetric, and affect mostly the calf muscles and small muscles of the foot. (At times they can, however, affect almost any skeletal muscle, including the neck, chest, and hands.) Treatment is usually quinine given prophylactically, although there has also been an over-the-counter (OTC) product that combines quinine with vitamin E. I say "has been" because the FDA has banned OTC quinine (because of rare blood dyscrasias) and, in fact, approves use of this drug only for malaria, despite the abundant clinical evidence that most patients with muscle cramps can take quinine safely and effectively.

This study suggests that cirrhosis of the liver, perhaps via the associated arterial underfilling, may be a cause of muscle cramps and that these cramps are amenable to a new therapeutic approach aimed at increasing circulating blood volume.

L. Lasagna, M.D.

Chili Protects Against Aspirin-induced Gastroduodenal Mucosal Injury in Humans
Yeoh KG, Kang JY, Yap I, et al (Natl Univ, Singapore)
Dig Dis Sci 40:580–583, 1995   2–9

Background.—Chili and its pungent ingredient capsaicin have been shown to protect against injury to the gastric mucosa in experimental animals. No such gastroprotective effect of chili has been demonstrated in humans, although it is hypothesized that it may help explain the differing rates of peptic ulcer disease among racial groups in Singapore. The capability of chili to protect against aspirin-induced acute gastroduodenal mucosal injury in humans was assessed.

Methods.—The study included 18 healthy adults with normal findings on a baseline gastroduodenoscopy. Each participant was studied on 2 occasions, once taking 20 g of chili in 200 mL of water and again taking just water. One half hour after each treatment, the participants took 600 mg of aspirin with another 200 mL of water. Six hours after they took the aspirin, they were reexamined by endoscopy for scoring of gastroduodenal mucosal damage.

Results.—The median gastric lesion score was 1.5 after the participants had taken chili as compared with 4.0 after they had taken water only. Thus, chili pretreatment reduced aspirin-induced gastroduodenal injury. Four individuals were found to have histologic gastritis, the presence and degree of which was not related to the ingestion of chili.

Conclusions.—Chili can protect against gastroduodenal mucosal injury in healthy humans. Chili may aid in mucosal healing and repair by increasing gastric mucosal blood flow. Chili or capsaicin may have therapeutic value in patients with peptic ulcer disease.

▶ In Singapore, Chinese people eat less chili than Malaysians and Southeast Asian Indians and have more peptic ulcer disease per thousand people in the population. However, the authors were struck by a decrease in racial differences in peptic ulcer disease rates over the last 30 years. Therefore, they postulated something in the environment, diet, or something else that might explain the lower incidence of the disease. Because the races have an increasingly similar diet, diet was chosen as the most likely factor for the decrease. Chili might protect against aspirin-induced ulcer disease because of the increased mucosal blood flow caused by capsaicin treatment, as shown in volunteers. Although studies like this require several gastroscopies, they can be repeated in populations such as whites and blacks in the United States to see whether chili powder and its main ingredient, capsaicin, would be protective against the effects of aspirin. One can see the combination therapy now.

M. Weintraub, M.D.

3 Adverse Reactions, Poisoning, and Drug Abuse

Systems Analysis of Adverse Drug Events
Leape LL, for the ADE Prevention Study Group (Harvard Univ, Boston; Brigham and Women's Hosp, Boston; Massachusetts Gen Hosp, Boston; et al)
JAMA 274:35–43, 1995   3–1

Background.—Up to two thirds of unintended injuries resulting from medical therapy may be caused by management errors. Adverse drug events (ADEs) causing injury commonly occur in hospitals. Many medical injuries may result from systems failures, in which an accident is the end result of a chain of events caused by a faulty system design that either induces errors or makes them difficult to detect. Systems analysis methods were used to evaluate the systems failures underlying ADEs and potential ADEs.

Methods.—The analysis included all admissions to 11 medical and surgical units in 2 tertiary care hospitals over a 6-month period. Information on actual and potential drug-related injuries was solicited from unit personnel and by record review. All ADEs and potential ADEs were classified as to whether they were preventable and according to the type of the causative error. The events were ascribed to various stages in the drug-ordering and delivery system by a multidisciplinary panel of physicians, nurses, pharmacists, and systems analysts. The proximal cause, or apparent reason, for each error was classified and the underlying systems failures were identified. Ideas were then generated as to how systems could be redesigned to reduce failures.

Results.—Two hundred sixty-four preventable and potential ADEs were identified as arising from 334 errors. Nearly 80% of the errors occurred in the physician ordering and nurse administration stages. Dosing errors were by far the most common type. Although proximal errors often cut across multiple stages in the drug-ordering and delivery system, lack of knowledge about the drug was the most common cause.

The underlying causes of the errors were 16 major systems failures. Defective dissemination of drug knowledge, especially to physicians, was the most common of these—it accounted for 29% of errors. Eighteen percent of errors involved the unavailability of patient information, such as laboratory results. These and 5 other systems failures—dose and identity checking, order transcription, the allergy defense system, medication order tracking, and interservice communication—were responsible for 78% of errors. All of these systems failures could have been prevented by better information systems.

Conclusions.—Hospital staff willingly participated in the detection and investigation of ADEs. The most frequent types of systems failures were those involving the dissemination of drug knowledge and the availability of drug and patient information. The chances of drug errors will be reduced by systems changes to improve the dissemination and display of drug and patient information.

▶ Errors leading to ADEs are made by physicians, nurses, pharmacists, and system analysts, and not uncommonly. Occasionally, a death or permanent disability hits the news media and efforts are made to decrease the mistakes. Why don't we attack the systems' failures more vigorously?

L. Lasagna, M.D.

An International Collaborative Case-Control Study of Severe Cutaneous Adverse Reactions (SCAR): Design and Methods

Kelly JP, Auquier A, Rzany B, et al (Boston Univ; Institut Gustave-Roussy, Villejuif, France; Univ of Freiburg, Germany; et al)
J Clin Epidemiol 48:1099–1108, 1995   3–2

Objective—An international case-control study was begun in 1990 with the goal of clarifying the cause of Stevens-Johnson syndrome and toxic epidermal necrolysis (TEN). These are among the disorders subsumed under the term "severe cutaneous adverse reactions."

Clinical Aspects.—These reactions are clinically important disorders that range from a mild form with few sequelae to severe involvement producing extensive disfigurement. Accompanying ocular lesions may result in loss of vision. The reported mortality for TEN averages 30% to 50%. The cutaneous manifestations of severe cutaneous adverse reactions may include target-type lesions and purpuric macules. Mucosal lesions such as painful erosions and crusting are present in most patients. Complications resemble those seen in extensively burned patients; they include the loss of large areas of skin, massive edema, and multisystemic problems.

Case Finding.—The estimated incidence of TEN is only about 1 per million per year; Stevens-Johnson Syndrome is somewhat more frequent. The only realistic means of quantifying the risk of such rare disorders is a case-control study, and a very extensive base population is required. The present collaborative study enrolled centers in France, Germany, Italy, and

Portugal. Severe cutaneous adverse reactions may arise both in the ambulatory population and in patients already hospitalized for other reasons.

Present Status.—More than 550 potential cases were accessed by mid-1993, of which 82% were confirmed as definite or probable by a dermatologic review committee. It is anticipated that, at the end of the study, it will be possible to detect, with statistical power of 80%, relative risks of 3.5-fold and greater for drugs used at a weekly prevalence rate as low as 1%. This would include such drugs as aminopenicillins and phenobarbital.

▶ This paper represents something that I have long believed; that is, when you start out to study a subject, it becomes more clearly defined and approachable. One would have to have all of the features of the illness to be counted as having a case of TEN or Stevens-Johnson syndrome to be included in the case-control study. The thing in this case would be the choice of the control group. One might complain that the control group will exclude previous drug use as a cause for hospitalization. The study will rise or fall on this control group, and we have to hope that this is an appropriate selection.

M. Weintraub, M.D.

Probable Adverse Drug Reactions in a Rural Geriatric Nursing Home Population: A Four-year Study

Cooper JW (Univ of Georgia, Athens; Med College of Georgia, Augusta)
J Am Geriatr Soc 44:194–197, 1996   3–3

Background.—Adverse drug reactions (ADRs) within nursing home populations have seldom been studied and have not been studied longitudinally at all. To determine the frequency, severity, and outcomes of ADRs in this population, ADRs were investigated in a long-term resident care population for 2 years in a prospective, longitudinal study.

Methods.—All residents of 2 rural skilled nursing facilities for more than 30 days were followed prospectively. The drug regimens were reviewed with a problem-oriented approach by a consultant pharmacist, using an algorithmic approach to identify probable ADRs and to rate their severity. All ADRs were confirmed with chart review and/or patient assessment.

Results.—Over the 2-year period, there were 444 probable ADRs that occurred in 217 of the 332 residents studied. These residents had a mean of 1.9 probable ADRs. Compared with the other residents, those with ADRs were prescribed more drugs per patient. There were no other statistically significant differences between the patient groups. The most commonly involved organ system in the ADRs was cardiovascular, followed by the CNS, gastrointestinal, endocrine, immune, hematologic, pulmonary, and renal systems. The most commonly involved drugs were diuretics, followed by antipsychotics, anxiolytics, potassium supplements, digoxin, nonsteroidal anti-inflammatory drugs (NSAIDs), insulin, theophylline, H_2-receptor antagonists, anti-infectives, anticonvulsants, and thyroid supplements. Thirty-four patients had 39 multiple drug interaction ADRs. Central nervous system depressants were the drug class most commonly involved in these multiple drug interaction ADRs, followed by antihypertensives, potassium-altering therapy, and NSAIDs. Repetitions of the same ADR in the same patient were common.

Conclusions.—Adverse drug reactions occur commonly in the nursing home population, particularly in those treated with multiple drugs. Inadequate attention to patient history and unrealistic therapeutic expectations may contribute to the incidence of ADRs in this population.

▶ Does an ADR represent the patient's having more problems and being sicker or does it represent an intrinsic property of the medication? Of course, there are mixtures of both types in this paper. However, the patients who had a probable drug reaction were older, more likely to be female, and taking more drugs than those who did not have an adverse drug reaction. Readers have to look over the drugs their patients take and make a judgement as to whether they are really needed, or whether they could be stopped.

M. Weintraub, M.D.

Hospitalisation for Adverse Events Related to Drug Therapy: Incidence, Avoidability and Costs
Dartnell JG, Anderson RP, Chohan V, et al (Royal Melbourne Hosp, Parkville, Australia)
Med J Aust 164:659–662, 1996   3–4

Introduction.—Previous studies have reported widely varying rates of drug-related hospitalizations. The incidence of drug-related admissions (DRAs) was determined, and their avoidability and costs were investigated.

Methods.—All admissions via the emergency department and resulting in a hospital stay of at least 24 hours during a 1-month period were reviewed. Cases of DRAs, excluding intentional overdose, were identified. Avoidability was classified as definitely, possibly, or not avoidable. The cause of the DRAs was also classified as prescribing factors, patient noncompliance, or adverse drug reactions.

Results.—Of the 965 total admissions, 55 (5.7%) were DRAs. The DRAs were classified as definitely avoidable in 5.5%, possibly avoidable in 60%, and not avoidable in 34.5%. The causes were identified as prescribing factors in 26%, patient noncompliance in 27%, and adverse drug reactions in 47%. There were 83 drugs involved in DRAs, with drugs prescribed for cardiovascular disease most commonly involved. The estimated annual cost of DRAs was $3,496,956, including $1,629,494 for unavoidable DRAs, $1,673,245 for possibly avoidable DRAs, and $194,217 for definitely avoidable DRAs.

Conclusions.—The incidence of DRAs was 5.7%. Few of the DRAs were definitely avoidable, suggesting that there is little clearly improper use of prescribed drugs. However, a substantial number of DRAs were possibly avoidable. These admissions are costly. Strategies for reducing DRAs may include improving patient compliance, improving communication between hospital and community pharmacies, and increasing recognition of adverse drug reactions and their possible causes.

▶ Many studies have attemped to quantify the incidence of hospital admissions for adverse events related to drug therapy. The numbers vary a lot, in part because linking an adverse event to 1 or more drugs is often difficult, because untoward events that are never seen in the absence of drug exposure are almost unheard of. The challenge is to avoid as many adverse drug reactions as *can* be avoided. As this paper reports, many of the adverse events resulting in hospitalization are only "possibly avoidable."

L. Lasagna, M.D.

The Poisoned Patient With Altered Consciousness: Controversies in the Use of a 'Coma Cocktail'
Hoffman RS, Goldfrank LR (New York Univ; Bellevue Hosp, New York; New York City Dept of Health)
JAMA 274:562–569, 1995   3–5

Introduction.—Nearly 2 million Americans are reportedly exposed each year to drugs and toxins. When a potentially poisoned patient presents with altered consciousness, the focus is on the first 5 minutes of management. The overall results of management are excellent, but the use of a so-called coma cocktail, which consists of hypertonic dextrose, thiamine, and naloxone, remains controversial.

Objective.—A MEDLINE search was made for English-language publications from 1966 to 1994 that dealt with the use of a coma cocktail. Analysis of diagnostic usefulness and efficacy were limited to large trials, but smaller trials and case reports were reviewed to identify adverse effects.

Consensus Findings.—Some physicians believe that routine use of 50% dextrose solution is warranted because as many as 1 in 12 patients with altered mental status may be hypoglycemic. There is a risk of hyperkalemia from glucose loading. The literature review supports the empirical use of both hypertonic dextrose and thiamine for patients whose consciousness is altered. Rapid reagent strips may be used, but they may fail to detect clinical hypoglycemia that does not correspond to "numerical" hypoglycemia. Thiamine is used to treat Wernicke's encephalopathy—a rare cause of altered mental status—and to prevent administered carbohydrate from precipitating encephalopathy when nutritional stores are limited. The use of naloxone should be limited to patients with clinically evident opioid intoxication. Flumazenil is used to reverse sedation that results from treatment and also in the rare case of benzodiazepine overdose.

▶ In general, we don't put many review articles in the YEAR BOOK OF DRUG THERAPY. However, some of them are important enough to include because of their careful review of the literature and suggestions for therapy based on review of the data. The authors' analysis recommends a "cocktail" of hypertonic dextrose and thiamine hydrochloride to the patients whose consciousness s altered. This sounds a lot like the Blockley cocktail of years ago. The Blockley is no more, but the cocktail lives forever.

M. Weintraub, M.D.

Digitalis-induced Visual Disturbances With Therapeutic Serum Digitalis Concentrations
Butler VP Jr, Odel JG, Rath E, et al (Columbia–Presbyterian Med Ctr, New York; Univ of Iowa, Iowa City; Veterans Affairs Hosp, Iowa City)
Ann Intern Med 123:676–680, 1995 3–6

Background.—Visual abnormalities are the most frequent symptoms of digitalis intoxication. They occur often in patients with high serum digitalis concentrations and typically resolve after a dosage decrease. However, 6 patients with therapeutic or subtherapeutic serum digitalis levels and no other signs of digitalis toxicity had typical digitalis-associated visual disturbances.

Methods.—Five elderly patients with photopsia and 1 with decreased visual acuity were referred for ophthalmologic evaluation. Their serum digoxin concentrations were measured, and electroretinography was performed.

Results.—The serum digoxin concentrations were within or below the therapeutic range in all 6 patients. None of the patients had cardiac or gastrointestinal signs of digitalis intoxication. When digoxin therapy was discontinued in 5 patients, all of them experienced a gradual resolution of their symptoms and a normalization within 1–2 weeks. In 1 patient, digoxin therapy was re-instituted, leading to recurrent photopsia within 4 days, which again resolved after the drug was discontinued. Of the 5 patients who underwent cone electroretinographic studies, 4 had prolonged b-wave implicit times, which normalized in the 3 patients who discontinued digoxin therapy. In the fifth patient, the b-wave implicit times were in the normal range during digoxin therapy but shortened after digoxin was discontinued. No patients had evidence of permanent retinal damage after discontinuation of digoxin.

Conclusions.—Digitalis intoxication should be suspected in patients experiencing new visual symptoms even if their serum digitalis levels are within or below the normal therapeutic range. The effects of digitalis may be monitored with changes in the b-wave implicit time on cone electroretinography, which should be measured before and during digitalis therapy.

▶ These patients had of a variety of visual abnormalities, including flashing lights, yellow and white dancing sparks, flickering, glare, "snow on grass and trees," and decreased visual acuity and color discrimination. Sometimes the troubles occurred only in the light with the eyes open, but sometimes with the eyes closed as well.

An important lesson here is that elderly patients (and others as well) can have digitalis-induced visual disturbances in the absence of other adverse reactions and with serum digitalis levels generally conceded to be within or below the "therapeutic" range.

L. Lasagna, M.D.

Allergic Reactions to Penicillins: A Changing World?
Blanca M (Carlos Haya Hosp, Malaga, Spain)
Allergy 50:777–782, 1995   3–7

Objective.—Certain new phenomena related to allergic reactions to β-lactam antibiotics have been found in recent years. These include immediate reactions that are selective for certain semisynthetic penicillins, a type of serum sickness induced by cefaclor, and delayed reactions to aminopenicillins in the presence of good tolerance to benzylpenicillin. Current trends in the incidence and types of allergic reactions to penicillins and other β-lactams were studied.

Reactions to β-lactams.—The total amount of β-lactams prescribed—especially amoxicillin—has increased significantly in recent years. There are few data on adverse reactions to different β-lactams or changes in selectivity to β-lactams over time. Recent studies suggest that minor determinants of amoxicillin, ampicillin-, or both make a much greater contribution to skin-test positivity than they previously did. Study of the IgE response to β-lactams has been facilitated by the development of methods to quantify IgE antibodies to penicillin in vitro. It is unknown why some patients respond to different penicillin determinants whereas others have a selective response to amoxicillin, but it may be related to the increased use of the latter drug. A wide range of "nonimmediate" reactions to penicillin derivatives has been reported, including contact dermatides; severe desquamative lesions and rash, exanthema, or both. In most such cases, there appears to be a cell-mediated immune reaction or some as-yet-unidentified idiosyncratic mechanism. As with immediate reactions, the increasing frequency of delayed reactions seems to be related to the growing use of amoxicillin. The use of cephalosporins is increasing as well. Although some allergic reactions to cephalosporins result from cross-reactivity to penicillins, others represent a selective reaction. Cefaclor-induced serum sickness has been reported from many countries.

Discussion.—Over the past decade or more, patients have come to be exposed to many different, potentially haptenic—and thus potentially allergenic—antibiotic chemical structures. As a result, allergic reactions to β-lactams are no longer restricted to penicillins and first-generation cephalosporins. More data on the use of penicillins around the world will help in understanding the varying patterns of their appearance. In vitro IgE assays, although less sensitive than skin tests, are still useful in defining specificities. Advances in diagnostic testing should consider that the side-chain of β-lactam antibodies makes an important contribution to IgE recognition.

▶ This author has summarized a lot of material about the changing patterns of antibiotic use as penicillin has largely been replaced by such β-lactams as ampicillin, amoxicillin, cloxacillin, and cephalosporins. Whether allergic reactions are more or less frequent as a consequence is hard to say.

L. Lasagna, M.D.

Massive Overdose of Sustained-release Verapamil: A Case Report and Review of Literature
Ashraf M, Chaudhary K, Nelson J, et al (Univ of Tennessee, Knoxville)
Am J Med Sci 310:258–263, 1995   3–8

Objective.—Overdose of sustained-release verapamil may result in hypotension, bradycardia, metabolic acidosis, and hyperglycemia. There is no specific antidote for verapamil toxicity. A case of massive overdose and a literature review are presented.

   Case Report.—Woman, 45, was brought to the emergency department 10 hours after ingesting 100 capsules of 240-mg sustained release verapamil. She received intravenous naloxone, glucose, atropine, and thiamine en route. Her pulse and heartbeat were irregular. Gastric lavage was performed. She received intravenous dopamine and calcium gluconate when her blood pressure dropped. Her ECG showed QRS widening, type 1 atrioventricular block, and left bundle branch block. Intravenous drugs were continued and she was placed on mechanical ventilation. She became hypotensive and was given intravenous dopamine, epinephrine, and insulin in addition to the other regimens. She received clindamycin for aspiration pneumonia. She was gradually weaned from drug therapy and mechanical ventilation as her condition improved. She was discharged on day 28 taking sertraline hydrochloride and trazodone.

Discussion.—Twenty cases of sustained-release verapamil toxicity were reviewed. Hypotension, rhythm disturbances, decreased mental status, and hyperglycemia were commonly reported. Six deaths occurred (30%). The primary therapy was supportive, including gastric lavage with charcoal administration. The use of ipecac was not recommended. Calcium infusion could reverse shock and conduction abnormalities. Atropine was not effective, whereas dopamine and epinephrine may have had some effect. Isoproterenol, amrinone, and glucagon led to improvement.

Conclusion.—Patients with verapamil toxicity receive mainly supportive treatment. Inotropic drugs, glucagon, calcium, and cardiac pacing therapy may be effective in other than severe cases. Calcium and glucagon infusions were very beneficial to the patient in the case discussed.

▶ The described case reminds us that we have to remember to carry out standard lifesaving measures; in this case, gastric lavage and charcoal. The use of calcium and glucagon was helpful, but one should be ready to use transvenous pacing in verapamil toxicity, particularly with such a large overdose. Fortunately, this patient survived.

M. Weintraub, M.D.

Rolaids-Yogurt Syndrome: A 1990s Version of Milk-Alkali Syndrome
Muldowney WP, Mazbar SA (Kaiser Permanente Med Ctr, Santa Clara, Calif)
Am J Kidney Dis 27:270–272, 1996   3–9

Background.—The milk-alkali syndrome consists of hypercalcemia, systemic alkalosis, and renal insufficiency in a patient with a history of taking calcium carbonate and consuming milk products. This condition is not seen as often as in the past, because H2 blockers, rather than antacids, are increasingly used to treat disorders of acid secretion. Now, drug companies are marketing their antacids as calcium supplements to prevent osteoporosis. A case of milk-alkali syndrome associated with this use of antacids is reported.

> *Case Report.*—Woman, 35, with a long history of anorexia–bulimia came to the emergency department with severe fatigue and nausea. She was taking an antacid containing calcium carbonate—four 500-mg tablets per day—in an attempt to prevent osteoporosis. She did not drink milk, but she ate at least two 8-ounce cups of yogurt per day. The patient was confused and constipated and had demonstrable muscle weakness in the extremities. Laboratory tests showed alkalosis, hypercalcemia (serum calcium level, 16 mg/dL), and renal failure (serum creatinine level, 3.6 mg/dL). Management included IV infusion of normal saline along with cessation of antacid and yogurt consumption. Renal function returned slowly, which suggested that hypercalcemia rather than volume depletion was responsible for the patient's renal insufficiency.

Discussion.—The use of antacids as calcium supplements may be implicated in patients with milk-alkali syndrome, a potentially dangerous but usually reversible metabolic disorder. Reversal depends on prompt recognition of concurrent hypercalcemia and alkalosis and cessation of calcium carbonate use. Patients with renal insufficiency and chronic vomiting should avoid taking calcium-containing antacid products and an excessive calcium intake.

▶ The milk-alkali syndrome, consisting of hypercalcemia, renal insufficiency, and systemic alkalosis, was much more common in the past, when people treated themselves with calcium-containing antacids and milk for peptic ulcer disease. Now you can get H2 blockers that effectively treat the symptoms of ulcer disease and antibiotics and omeprazole for *Helicobacter pylori*, the main bacterial cause of many cases of peptic ulcer disease. However, many people still take calcium-containing antacids in an attempt to raise serum calcium for the prevention or treatment of osteoporosis and even for hypertension. This case report is really quite interesting and should be read in the original for use in the differential diagnosis of multiple myeloma, rhabdomyolysis, and excess ingestion of vitamin D. This is a 1990s case of a sort of yuppy milk-alkali syndrome.

M. Weintraub, M.D.

Pattern of Neurobehavioral Deficits Associated With Interferon Alfa Therapy for Leukemia
Pavol MA, Meyers CA, Rexer JL, et al (Univ of Texas MD Anderson Cancer Ctr, Houston)
Neurology 45:947–950, 1995   3–10

Objective—Interferon causes a wide range of neurologic side effects when used to treat cancer, and these often prove to be the dose-limiting factor. The cognitive and emotional status of patients with chronic myelogenous leukemia who were treated with interferon alfa (IFN-α) was studied.

Patients and Treatment.—Fifteen men and 10 women, 24–70 years of age, were studied; their mean age was 15 years. The patients tended to be well educated, and many were professionals. The mean time since leukemia was diagnosed was 33 months, and patients had received IFN-α for 26 months on average. Treatment was given subcutaneously, usually on a daily basis, in an average weekly dose of 51 million IU. Sixteen leukemic patients not given IFN-α served as a control group.

Findings.—An unexpectedly large number of interferon-treated patients had scored below expectations on tests of verbal memory, delayed visual memory, verbal fluency, visual sequencing, and motor dexterity. Both verbal memory and graphomotor performance on the Digit Symbol test correlated with the time since diagnosis. About half the study patients had increased Minnesota Multiphasic Personality Inventory scores for hypochondriasis, depression, and hysteria, but scores did not correlate with the time since diagnosis.

Conclusion.—These findings suggest frontal-subcortical dysfunction in many leukemic patients who are treated with IFN-α.

▶ There are a number of ways of approaching the problem uncovered by this survey of patients who received IFN-α. First, leukemia cells in the spleen and bone marrow could be directly targeted. Second, a large group could be hooked to the drug that would effectively keep it out of the CNS. Third, it might be possible to use 1 or more medications to protect the CNS. Finally, one could avoid giving the medication. Certainly the pattern and appearance of the deficits noted in treatment make it necessary to do a risk-benefit analysis. We must be certain that the effectiveness merits the risk of serious side effects. We can't forget Woody Allan's comment that his brain was his second favorite organ.

M. Weintraub, M.D.

Neurotoxicity Related to the Use of Topical Tretinoin (Retin-A)
Bernstein AL, Leventhal-Rochon JL (Kaiser Permanente Med Ctr, Hayward, Calif)
Ann Intern Med 124:227–228, 1996   3–11

Introduction.—Acne vulgaris is often treated with topical tretinoin, a vitamin A analogue. Although neurologic complications have been associated with oral vitamin-A supplementation, topical forms of vitamin A are believed to allow only minimal systemic absorption and have not been associated with neurotoxicity. However, a patient who used large amounts of topical tretinoin experienced treatment-associated neurologic and psychiatric symptoms.

> *Case Report.*—Woman, 39, was healthy except for a mild, untreated depression and chronic hepatitis C. She had begun using topical tretinoin to treat her acne 6–8 weeks earlier. She acquired the topical tretinoin from a friend, and did not initially report her use of it when she visited the neurology department with complaints of headache, memory loss, and unsteadiness. She had truncal ataxia (which required her to use a walker), mild dysarthria, and finger-to-nose ataxia, although she had normal motor and sensory test results. Her anxiety and depression had worsened during the previous 6 weeks. She was treated with doxepine hydrochloride, which brought temporary improvement, but recurrent symptoms. At this point, she reported use of large amounts of topical tretinoin. Use of the drug was discontinued for 4 weeks, then restarted to treat worsening acne. Discontinuation brought improvement in the patient's symptoms, which recurred when the medication was restarted. The use of topical tretinoin was again discontinued. The patient's symptoms completely resolved within 4 weeks and did not recur with 8 months of follow-up.

Discussion.—Patients with preexistent hepatic dysfunction may experience neurotoxicity with retinoic acid treatment because they may be unable to conjugate retinoic acid to an excretable form or may produce reduced retinol-binding proteins, and thus prevent effective transport. Therefore, topical retinoids should be avoided or prescribed with caution for patients with established or potential hepatic dysfunction.

▶ Even topical drugs can be absorbed from the skin. Topical medications so absorbed can have serious adverse effects. This patient did not get her medication from a physician and did not receive any of the critical teaching that one expects with tretinoin. She did not report tretinoin ingestion to the physicians who worked her up for neuropathy. However, its use was very closely related to the adverse effects. This patient may have been more sensitive to the neurologic effects resulting from her long-standing hepatic injury.

M. Weintraub, M.D.

Piperazine Neurotoxicity: Worm Wobble Revisited
Conners GF (Children's Natl Med Ctr, Washington, DC)
J Emerg Med 13:341–343, 1995   3–12

Introduction.—Piperazine salts are widely used in countries where roundworm and pinworm infestations are common, but they are not frequently prescribed in the United States. Piperazine-related ataxia usually is a result of overdose or renal insufficiency. The term worm wobble has been proposed for this complication, which was encountered in an otherwise-healthy American child.

> *Case Report.*—Boy, 9 years, who had previously been healthy, was seen for incoordination, frequent dropping of objects, and regular falling. He had complained of abdominal pain several days before and his mother—a pediatric nurse—began giving him a "worm syrup" that contained piperazine citrate. The boy had taken 5 mg of the syrup per kilogram each morning for 1 week up to the day before he appeared at the hospital. The pain had rapidly subsided. The boy walked with a broad-based gait and performed very poorly on the finger-to-nose and heel-to-shin tests. These abnormalities resolved over 24 hours, and the patient has since been well.

Discussion.—In the United States, piperazine is legally available only by prescription, but it is readily available in nonprescription forms elsewhere. A wide range of neurotoxic effects are described, including seizures, hypotonia, vertigo, hallucinations, and depersonalization. The possibility of drug toxicity should be considered when an otherwise-healthy child with recent abdominal pain becomes ataxic.

▶ This paper reminds us that we have to do a number of things when looking at potential adverse reactions. First, do not be misled by the profession of the child's parents, in this case a pediatric nurse who had incorrectly treated her child. Second, look at the issue of over-the-counter drugs, in this case an illegal over-the-counter drug containing a medication that is usually a prescription medication. Third, remember that drugs can cause almost any type of adverse effect.

M. Weintraub, M.D.

Diclofenac-associated Hepatotoxicity: Analysis of 180 Cases Reported to the Food and Drug Administration as Adverse Reactions
Banks AT, Zimmerman HJ, Ishak KG, et al (George Washington Univ, Washington, DC; Armed Forces Inst of Pathology, Washington, DC)
Hepatology 22:820–827, 1995   3–13

Introduction.—Nonsteroidal anti-inflammatory drugs appear to differ in the character and severity of hepatic injury they may provoke. Diclofenac, approved in the United States in 1988 for the treatment of osteoarthritis, rheumatoid arthritis, and ankylosing spondylitis, is reported in the medical literature to have caused approximately 60 cases of hepatic injury, primarily acute hepatocellular injury. A retrospective analysis of cases reported to the Food and Drug Administration from November 1988 through June 1991 considered the clinical, biochemical, and histologic features and possible mechanisms of diclofenac-associated hepatotoxicity.

Methods and Patients.—The FDA received 434 reports of diclofenac-associated hepatic injury during the review period. After 254 cases were eliminated because of duplicate reporting, inadequate data, foreign sources, or other possible causes for liver enzyme abnormalities, 180 cases remained for study. The pattern of injury was classified as hepatocellular, cholestatic, mixed, or indeterminate, and the mechanism of injury as immunologic idiosyncrasy or metabolic idiosyncrasy. The patient group included 142 women and 38 men, 68% of whom were older than 60 years.

Results.—Osteoarthritis was the indication for diclofenac in 139 patients and rheumatoid arthritis in 22 patients. The ratio of females to males among cases of hepatic injury compared with the male-to-female ratio of users of the nonsteroidal anti-inflammatory drug yielded a relative risk of 2.0 for females. Two thirds of the patients had signs or symptoms, and one third were identified by increased levels of aspartate transaminase and alanine transaminase, noted incidentally or by monitoring. Jaundice was present in 50% of patients overall and in 75% of patients with symptoms. Seven of the 90 icteric patients died. In two thirds of cases the biochemical pattern of injury was hepatocellular or mixed hepatocellular. A pattern of cholestatic injury was present in 8% and an indeterminate pattern in 24%. Sections of liver, available for 21 cases, showed hepatic injury 1 month after starting diclofenac treatment in 24%, by 3 months in 63%, and by 6 months in 85%. No patient had evidence of hypersensitivity such as rash, fever, or eosinophilia, suggesting that metabolic idiosyncrasy was the probable mechanism.

Conclusions.—The hepatic injury induced by diclofenac is mainly hepatocellular, and the mechanism of injury appears to be metabolic idiosyncrasy. Most affected patients were women with osteoarthritis. Because half of all cases were detected in the first 2 months, physicians should consider possible hepatic toxicity when jaundice, nausea, or vomiting occur early after starting treatment with the drug.

▶ This paper is a wonderful example of the possibility of interaction between the academy and the FDA to use the data sources of the latter to approach and describe important adverse effects.

M. Weintraub, M.D.

Variability in Risk of Gastrointestinal Complications With Individual Non-steroidal Anti-inflammatory Drugs: Results of a Collaborative Meta-analysis
Henry D, Lim LL-Y, Rodriguez LAG, et al (Univ of Newcastle, NSW, Australia; Universidad Complutense de Madrid; Pharmacoepidemiology Research, Ciba-Geigy SA, Barcelona; et al)
BMJ 312:1563–1566, 1996   3–14

Introduction.—It is difficult to compare data on comparative risk of gastrointestinal complications with individual non-steroidal anti-inflammatory drugs (NSAIDs) because reports vary in methods used for analysis. The range of relative risks of serious gastrointestinal complications reported with individual NSAIDs was investigated using a meta-analytic method.

Methods.—A MEDLINE search was conducted for relevant reports from 1985–1994. Authors of relevant reports were contacted and asked to update their published reports and were questioned about their knowledge of other relevant trials. For each report, the relative risk of gastrointestinal complications was calculated for each drug listed. Drugs were ranked according to relative risk. Relative risks for drug dosages were calculated, using ibuprofen as reference.

Results.—Twelve investigations were amenable to meta-analysis. Of these, 11 provided comparative data on ibuprofen and other agents. Fourteen NSAIDs were included. The lowest relative risk was associated with ibuprofen use, then diclofenac. Indomethacin, naproxen, sulindac, and aspirin were associated with moderate risk. Azapropazone, tolmetin, ketoprofen, and piroxicam were correlated with the highest risk. The higher doses of ibuprofen were associated with relative risks similar to those of naproxen and indomethacin use.

Conclusion.—Ibuprofen was associated with the lowest relative risk of severe gastrointestinal toxicity. The low relative risk of ibuprofen was attributed to the low doses used in clinical practice. It is possible that the advantages of low-risk drugs could be lost if doses were increased. The use of NSAIDs associated with low risk may help reduce morbidity and mortality.

▶ I don't have to tell you how much I do not like meta-analyses unless they support my preconceived notions of what is correct. Well, what do you know, this one does. It indicates that ibuprofen is the drug least likely to cause gastrointestinal adverse effects.

M. Weintraub, M.D.

Reversible Membranous Nephropathy Associated With the Use of Non-steroidal Anti-inflammatory Drugs
Radford MG Jr, Holley KE, Grande JP, et al (Mayo Clinic and Mayo Found, Rochester, Minn)
JAMA 276:466–469, 1996   3–15

Introduction.—The association between nonsteroidal anti-inflammatory drug (NSAID) use and minimal-change glomerulopathy is well known, but that membranous nephropathy (MN) can be caused by NSAIDs is less recognized. A retrospective chart review of patients diagnosed with stage I or early stage II MN by renal biopsy was conducted to determine the frequency of MN associated with NSAID use.

Methods.—Between January 1975 and May 1995, 125 patients who underwent renal biopsy were diagnosed with stage I or early stage II MN. Twenty-nine of these patients were taking NSAIDs when nephrotic syndrome developed, and 13 met criteria for NSAID-associated MN: onset of nephrotic symptoms while taking routine doses of an NSAID, no other causes of MN identified, and a rapid remission of nephrotic syndrome after withdrawal of the NSAID. The records of these patients were reviewed for clinical characteristics, treatment and outcome.

Results.—Patients had a mean age of 55 years and had taken NSAIDs for a median of 43 weeks before symptom onset. Drugs involved were diclofenac, fenoprofen, ibuprofen, tolmetin, and nabumetone. Onset of symptoms was usually rapid. In most cases (92%), patients were admitted with nephrotic syndrome; mean proteinuria was 10.2 g/d. Decreases in proteinuria occurred after NSAIDs were discontinued. At follow-up, which ranged from 5 months to 13 years, none of the patients exhibited evidence of renal insufficiency or significant proteinuria.

Discussion.—Because MN is the most common cause of nephrotic syndrome in adults and NSAID use is widespread, the problem of NSAID-associated MN is likely to be underrecognized. Only 8 additional case reports were found in a MEDLINE search from 1966 through July 1995. Use of NSAIDs should be considered in the differential diagnosis of MN and excluc ed in patients who enroll in trials that assess the treatment of MN.

▶ The poir t here may be that physicians should be more attuned to finding out whether or not their patients have nephrotic syndrome when they are taking NSAIDs. Even more important will be the reversal of the nephrotic syndrome when the NSAIDs are stopped. Why do we put up with so many adverse effects from these medications? The answer may be that they work very well fcr some of the indications for which they are prescribed. In truth, however, if somebody came up with something safer, I think the market would rapidly decrease for some of the NSAIDs, except for their use as simple analgesics in lower doses and when taken intermittently.

M. Weintraub, M.D.

Signs and Symptoms of Carbamazepine Overdose
Schmidt S, Schmitz-Buhl M (Abteilung Neurologie, Bonn, Germany; Forschungsstelle für Gesundheitserziehung, Cologne, Germany)
J Neurol 242:169–173, 1995   3–16

Introduction.—Treatment of seizures and other conditions with carbamazepine (CBZ) has been associated with a wide range of side effects, including neurologic, cardiovascular, hepatic, hematologic, and cutaneous reactions.

Objective.—Adverse reactions and their correlates were studied in 427 patients recorded from 1966 to 1992 as having CBZ overdose. The average age was 23 years, and the average dose of CBZ in 271 cases was 10.8 g.

Findings.—Mortality in 307 evaluable patients was 13%. Half of all patients attempted suicide. Neurologic dysfunction was the most common manifestation of acute overdose. Five of 16 patients who also ingested alcohol diec. The average dose of CBZ in patients who died was 24 g, and the average plasma CBZ level in 8 patients was 37 µg/mL. Both patients with cardiac arrest died, as did 2 of 5 patients who had acute renal failure, and 7 of 16 with acute respiratory insufficiency. Patients younger than 15 years of age had lower mortality than older patients.

Summary.—Carbamazepine overdose appears to follow a less-threatening course in patients younger than 15 years. A dose greater than 24 g is associated with increased mortality risk.

▶ This paper comes from Germany; however, there is no reason to suspect that the overdose picture is different from that seen in the United States. Large case series such as this allow us to look at the features of a medication in overdose. The fatality rate of 13% is relatively high, and the only thing that predicted it was the size of the dose exceeding 24 g. As usual, young patients seem to have less trouble with the overdose. This may be because of their physiologic resistance or a lower dose ingested. Another important factor was that the group who died seemed to include men to a much greater extent than women, although the overdosing pattern was similar. This does go along with the notion that when men attempt a suicide, they really mean it.

M. Weintraub, M.D.

Peripheral Neuropathy Associated With Simvastatin
Phan T, McLeod JG, Pollard JD, et al (Univ of Sydney, Australia; Concord Hosp, Sydney, Australia; Westmead Hosp, Sydney, Australia; et al)
J Neurol Neurosurg Psychiatry 58:625–628, 1995   3–17

Background.—Simvastatin, a cholesterol-lowering drug that inhibits hydroxymethylglutaryl co-enzyme A, may cause several adverse neurologic effects. However, peripheral neuropathy has not, to date, been associated with simvastatin use. Four patients with this reaction were studied.

Series.—The patients were 3 women and 1 man, aged 39 to 66 years. Sensorimotor neuropathy developed in all patients during simvastatin treatment and completely or partially resolved when treatment was stopped. In 1 patient, the onset of sensorimotor neuropathy occurred within days of beginning therapy. In another 2 patients, however, symptoms did not develop for 2 years. The neuropathy had the electrophysiologic and pathologic features of axonal degeneration. Clinical findings included proximal and distal weakness and muscle fasciculations as well as persistent abnormalities of sensory conduction after recovery, suggesting that toxic damage may have occurred to anterior horn cells and dorsal root ganglia.

Conclusions.—Simvastatin should be considered among the causes of peripheral neuropathy. If muscle weakness or sensory disturbances develop in patients receiving simvastatin, the drug should be withdrawn.

▶ Unfortunately, we are not told about potential causative factors for the development of peripheral neuropathy of the sensorimotor type. Nor are we told about the features that led to resolution in some patients and no resolution in others. In 1 case, it was clear that the patient's condition was rapidly worsening and warranted an investigation of her medications. I hope this paper will cause us all to look at patients receiving simvastatin and assess them for beginnings of neuropathy. Just as an aside, although 1 patient had familial hypercholesterolemia and 1 patient had hyperlipidemia, the actual cholesterol levels were not given.

M. Weintraub, M.D.

Is Cimetidine Associated With Neutropenia?
Strom BL, Carson JL, Schinnar R, et al (Univ of Pennsylvania, Philadelphia; UMDNJ-Robert Wood Johnson Med School, New Brunswick, NJ; Health Information Designs Inc, Arlington, Va)
Am J Med 99:282–290, 1995   3–18

Background.—Cimetidine is believed to be safe enough for over-the-counter use. However, there is still some concern about cimetidine-induced neutropenia.

Methods.—Medicaid databases from 6 states were used to investigate the association between cimetidine and neutropenia in a population-based, case-control study. The patients studied were discharged from the hospital and had a diagnosis of neutropenia. Four randomly chosen controls were matched to each patient for age, sex, state, and year of diagnosis.

Findings.—After adjustment for potentially confounding variables, cimetidine use was associated with an odds ratio of 1.2 for the development of neutropenia. No dose- or duration-response relationship was evident. Hospitalization because of neutropenia or agranulocytosis from cimetidine use was estimated to occur no more often than once in every 116,000 patients and no more than once in every 573,000 patients receiving a 6-week course of this drug.

Conclusions.—Patients using cimetidine are apparently not at increased risk of neutropenia. If there is an association between cimetidine and neutropenia, it is very small. The sporadic cases of agranulocytosis reported in the literature are probably coincidences, cases occurring in a small subgroup of patients at unique risk, or indicators of an effect smaller than can be detected in the current study.

▶ How far has pharmacoepidemiology gone! We have new databases, we have new statistical tests, we have new relationships for a drug and the duration of time or dose, and we have better ways of examining the data. If only we were smarter about choosing our drugs and interpreting the information resulting from our studies.

M. Weintraub, M.D.

Eosinophilia Associated With Bupropion
Malesker MA, Soori GS, Malone PM, et al (Creighton Univ, Omaha, Neb; Univ of Minnesota, Minneapolis)
Ann Pharmacother 29:867–869, 1995   3–19

Background.—The antidepressant bupropion is chemically unrelated to tricyclic, tetracyclic, or other known antidepressant drugs. The side effects commonly associated with bupropion include agitation, dry mouth, insomnia, headache or migraine, nausea or vomiting, constipation, and tremor. The first reported case of eosinophilia associated with orally administered bupropion treatment was studied.

Case Report.—Woman, 72, was hospitalized for assessment of chest pain. Five days earlier, the patient had started bupropion treatment. While she was in the hospital, her eosinophil count increased to 0.6 fraction of 1.00. The absolute eosinophil count was $6,693 \times 10^6$/L. Her white blood cell count was 18.5×10^9/L. Bupropion was concluded to be the precipitating agent in this case of eosinophilia because of the temporal sequencing of events and the rapid decline of the eosinophil count after the medication was stopped. Other potential causes of this patient's eosinophilia were thoroughly reviewed and ruled out.

Conclusions.—No previous cases of eosinophilia associated with bupropion therapy have been reported in the literature. Eosinophilia can be caused by parasitic infections and allergic disease as well as medication use. In the patient described here, other possible causes were considered and excluded.

▶ The most important aspect of this study was that the physicians stopped all medications and restarted some of them in an effort to rule out the causative agent. Luckily, the patient was not receiving any medications that could not be stopped transiently and restarted. One point not mentioned in the write-up was that this patient had had a number of drug-related allergies. It is possible that allergic patients will have more allergies.

M. Weintraub, M.D.

Photosensitivity From Pyridoxine Hydrochloride (Vitamin B₆)
Morimoto K, Kawada A, Hiruma M, et al (Natl Defense Med College, Saitama, Japan)
J Am Acad Dermatol 35:304–305, 1996   3–20

Objective.—Vitamin B_6, one form of which is pyridoxine, is a widely used over-the-counter vitamin. The case of a patient with photosensitivity caused by pyridoxine hydrochloride was reported.

Case Report.—Woman, 35, had a 3-month history of pruritic edema on sun-exposed areas (Fig 1). She had been taking pyridoxine hydrochloride, 200 mg/day, as part of a multivitamin supplement, for 4 months. An oral photochallenge test performed after the patient took the vitamins showed a normal minimum erythema dose, but erythema was produced by 6.75 J/cm^2 of ultraviolet A irradiation. Patch and photopatch testing with the various ingredients contained in the supplements showed a positive response only with 10% and 1% pyridoxine hydrochloride (Fig 2). No such reaction was produced by pyridoxine testing in healthy controls.

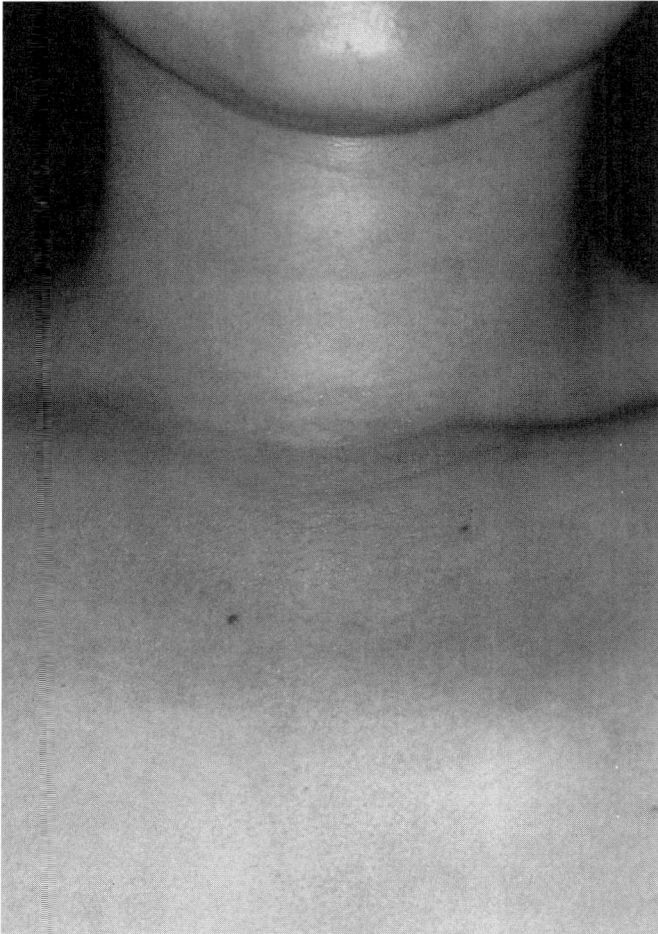

FIGURE 1.—Erythema on neck. (Courtesy of Morimoto K, Kawada A, Hiruma M, et al: Photosensitivity from pyridoxine hydrochloride (vitamin B$_6$). *J Am Acad Dermatol* 35:304–305, 1996.)

Discussion.—The patient in this report was taking 200 mg/day of pyridoxine hydrochloride, compared with a recommended dietary allowance of 1.6 mg/day. The photosensitivity in this case may have resulted from a transient high concentration of vitamin B$_6$ in the patient's blood after she took this high dose of pyridoxine.

▶ Vitamin B$_6$ is present in many multivitamin preparations available over the counter. This seems to be the first report of photosensitivity from pyridoxine, although a letter appeared in a dermatology journal in 1984 that described a

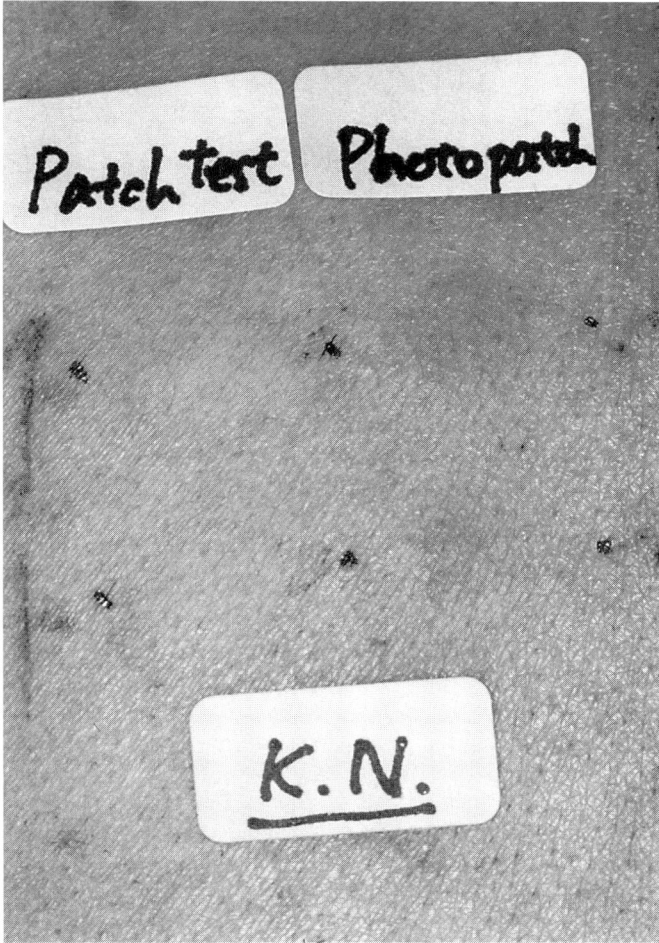

FIGURE 2.—Positive photopatch test with 10% and 1% pyridoxine hydrochloride in petrolatum 24 hours after ultraviolet A irradiation. (Courtesy of Morimoto K, Kawada A, Hiruma M, et al: Photosensitivity from pyridoxine hydrochloride (vitamin B$_6$). *J Am Acad Dermatol* 35:304–305, 1996.)

patient with skin changes, probably caused by B$_6$, and suggested that sunlight might be involved.[1]

L. Lasagna, M.D.

Reference

1. Baer RL, Stillman MA: Cutaneous skin changes probably due to pyridoxine abuse (letter). *J Am Acad Dermatol* 10:527–528, 1984.

Pituitary Apoplexy After Leuprolide Administration for Carcinoma of the Prostate

Morsi A, Jamal S, Silverberg JDH (Univ of Toronto)
Clin Endocrinol (Oxf) 44:121–124, 1996   3–21

Objective.—A case of sudden pituitary apoplexy in a patient being treated for prostate cancer with leuprolide was reported.

> *Case Report.*—Man, 74, with headache, dizziness, weakness, and vomiting 15 minutes after receiving an intramuscular injection of leuprolide, 7.5 mg, had a large pituitary adenoma diagnosed. An MRI scan revealed a large pituitary mass and hemorrhage. On day 3 the mass was surgically decompressed, and 12 days later he died of cardiac arrest. A pulmonary adenoma was found at autopsy.

Discussion.—Because leuprolide, a gonadotropin-releasing hormone (GnRH) analogue, initially stimulates production of luteinizing hormone (LH) and testosterone, it probably increased the metabolic activity of the tumor, which led to hypoxia and infarction.

Conclusion.—Because the frequency of pituitary tumors is as high as 20% in the general population and approximately one fourth of these are gonadotropinomas, endocrine and confrontational visual testing should be performed before leuprolide is administered to men.

▶ Pituitary apoplexy can be dramatic and usually occurs in adenomatous glands, although it has been reported in normal pituitaries. A variety of drugs have been incriminated as possible causes—anticoagulants, isosorbide dinitrate, chlorpromazine, and bromocriptine. This case is the first to be reported after leuprolide, but because it is an analogue of GnRH, in a sense it's not a first because GnRH has been previously implicated. The mechanism for the apoplexy remains a mystery.

L. Lasagna, M.D.

Hyperkalemia in Hospitalized Patients Treated With Trimethoprim-Sulfamethoxazole

Alappan R, Perazella MA, Buller GK (St Mary's Hosp, Waterbury, Conn; Yale Univ, New Haven, Conn)
Ann Intern Med 124:316–320, 1996   3–22

Background.—Hyperkalemia has been widely reported as a complication of high-dose trimethoprim treatment in patients with AIDS. The effect of standard-dose trimethoprim-sulfamethoxazole on serum potassium concentrations was studied in patients hospitalized for various infectious diseases.

Methods.—Eighty patients treated for at least 5 days with oral or IV trimethoprim-sulfamethoxazole at doses of no more than 320 mg/day of trimethoprim and 1,600 mg/day of sulfamethoxazole and 25 control patients treated for at least 5 days with other antibiotic agents not affecting potassium homeostasis were studied prospectively in the hospital. Serum potassium, sodium, and chloride concentrations; serum carbon dioxide content; anion gap; blood urea nitrogen concentration; and serum creatinine concentrations were measured daily before and during treatment in both groups.

Results.—The 2 groups were similar for pretreatment potassium values, types of infection, and previous medication with agents that could alter potassium homeostasis. The serum potassium concentration increased significantly in the treatment group but not in the control group, with significant differences between the groups on days 4 and 5. After treatment discontinuation and/or a potassium-lowering intervention, the potassium concentration decreased. The highest peak potassium concentrations were found in patients with a baseline serum creatinine concentration of 106 µmol/L or greater. There was no significant association between the peak potassium concentration and diabetes or age.

Conclusion.—Hyperkalemia is common among patients treated with trimethoprim-sulfamethoxazole at standard doses, especially on the fourth or fifth day of treatment. Renal insufficiency increases the risk of more severe hyperkalemia in these patients.

▶ In patients with AIDS, hyperkalemia develops when patients take trimethoprim. In addition, patients, in general, have an increase in serum potassium values with trimethoprim. The purpose of this study was to investigate the serum potassium levels of patients receiving trimethoprim-sulfamethoxazole. Even after a drug has been on the market for many years, new side effects can be seen. Often, investigators attempt to measure something new, as opposed to standard things that can go wrong. The authors of this study tried to pinpoint various factors that might raise the serum potassium levels of certain types of patients. They weren't able to tease them apart, but they did show that at least during hospitalization, hyperkalemia did not develop in patients treated with other antibiotics.

M. Weintraub, M.D.

Minocycline Induced Autoimmune Hepatitis and Systemic Lupus Erythematosus-like Syndrome
Gough A, Chapman S, Wagstaff K, et al (Harrogate District Hosp, England; Keele Univ, Staffordshire, England; Selly Oak Hosp, Birmingham, England; et al)
BMJ 312:169–172, 1996
3–23

Background.—Minocycline is commonly prescribed for acne, not only because it may be taken only once or twice per day, but also because there are no reports of resistance. As of early 1994, there were 11 reports of minocycline-induced systemic lupus erythematosus and 16 reports of hepatitis. Information on patients who have had severe adverse reactions to minocycline was studied.

Methods—The cases of the 11 patients with systemic lupus erythematosus, the 16 patients with hepatitis, and 7 additional patients who had severe adverse reactions to minocycline were reviewed.

Results.—While taking minocycline for acne, 2 patients died, 1 of severe hepatitis and coma, and 1 of pancytopenia. One patient required a liver transplantation. Although acne can cause arthritis and is associated with autoimmune liver disease, a drug reaction is indicated in these patients because their symptoms resolved after the drug was discontinued, even though their acne worsened. Symptoms recurred in 5 patients after they began taking minocycline again. Other reactions included polyarthritis or polyarthralgia of the small joints of the hands and wrists, fever, and hepatitis.

Conclusions.—These findings should make practitioners more aware of the reactions to minocycline that can occur. It is important to recognize these reactions early because they can be severe. In this way, it may be possible to improve recovery and avoid invasive treatment and procedures, such as immunosuppressants and liver biopsies. Caution is advised when prescribing minocycline, and safer alternatives should be considered.

▶ This tetracycline antibiotic has been on the market for almost a quarter of a century and is well absorbed, convenient to take, and widely prescribed in the United Kingdom for acne. Unfortunately, its use sometimes leads to severe liver disease, as does the use of other drugs in this antibiotic class. It also belongs on the list of agents capable of inducing systemic lupus erythematosus-like syndromes. These syndromes resolve when minocycline is discontinued.

L. Lasagna, M.D.

Scalp Hair Loss Caused by Octreotide in a Patient With Acromegaly: A Case Report
Nakauchi Y, Kumon Y, Yamasaki H, et al (Kochi Med School, Japan)
Endocr J 42 385–389, 1995   3–24

Introduction.—Octreotide, a somatostatin analogue, is widely used to treat acromegaly. Its commonly reported adverse effects include pain at the injection site, cholecystolithiasis, and gastrointestinal symptoms. Another rare adverse effect was seen in a patient with acromegaly, who was successfully treated with octreotide but had drug-related hair loss that necessitated drug discontinuation.

Case Report.—Woman, 71, was admitted to a hospital with acromegalic facial features and high serum levels of growth hor-

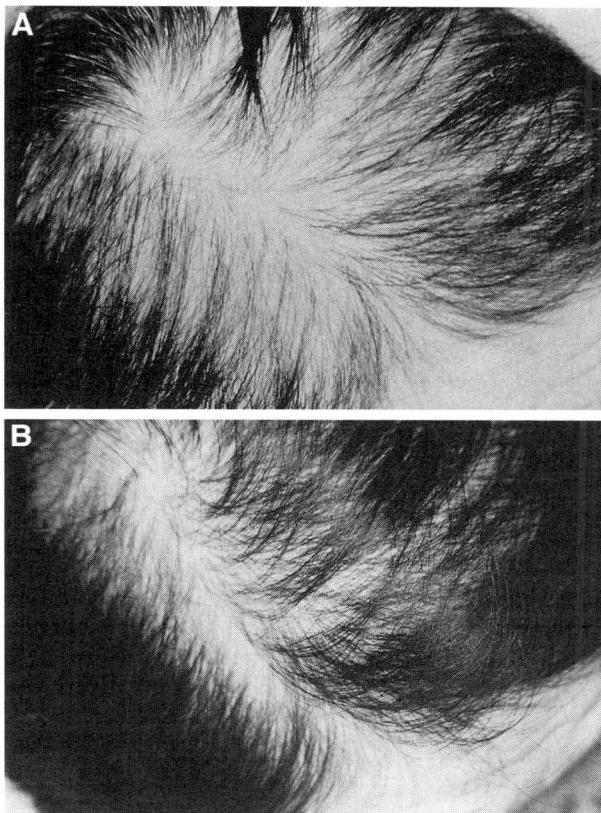

FIGURE 4.—Scalp hair (clinical course). **A,** after 5 months of treatment with octreotide, diffuse scalp hair loss occurred. **B,** 5 months after the cessation of octreotide, hair growth resumed. (Courtesy of Nakauchi Y, Kumon Y, Yamasaki H, et al: Scalp hair loss caused by octreotide in a patient with acromegaly: A case report. *Endocr J* 42:385–389, 1995.)

mone (GH) and IGF-1. She had a 20-year history of conservatively treated spondylosis deformans. Laboratory tests and brain MRI confirmed the diagnosis of acromegaly associated with a GH-producing pituitary adenoma. The patient was treated with 200 µg/day of octreotide via self-injection. She responded to treatment with reduced serum GH and IGF-1 levels and reduction of the adenoma. However, she experienced hair loss within 6 months of the initiation of octreotide treatment. Therefore, the octreotide was discontinued and replaced with bromocriptine therapy, which was ineffective. After the serum GH and IGF-1 levels rose again and the pituitary adenoma increased in size, the patient was treated definitively with a transsphenoidal pituitary adenectomy. Six months after octreotide was discontinued, her hair had resumed its growth (Fig 4).

Discussion.—Hair loss is a rare side effect of octreotide treatment, but it should be considered in patients treated with this drug. The mechanisms involved in octreotide-related hair loss are not known, but the loss may be caused by the acute and complete suppression of GH and IGF-1 or by a direct effect of the drug on hair follicle cells.

▶ Octreotide can reduce the size of pituitary adenomas in patients with acromegaly and often is attended by complaints about pain at the site of injection and a variety of gastrointestinal symptoms (abdominal cramps, nausea, bloating, flatulence, diarrhea, and steatorrhea). Hair loss as a consequence of its use is rare.[1]

L. Lasagna, M.D.

Reference

1. Jönsson A: Octreotide and loss of scalp hair. *Ann Intern Med* 115:913, 1991.

The Prismatic Case of Creutzfeldt-Jakob Disease Associated With Pituitary Growth Hormone Treatment
Hintz RL (Stanford Univ, Calif)
J Clin Endocrinol Metab 80:2298–2301, 1995   3–25

Introduction.—Sixty cases of Creutzfeldt-Jakob disease (CJD) have been reported worldwide in association with treatment with growth hormone (GH) purified from pituitaries. The index case is described, as well as the resulting withdrawal of pituitary GH use.

Case Report.—Man, 20, was referred for ataxia. In his infancy, diagnoses of decreased growth rate, secondary hypothyroidism, and insulin-dependent diabetes mellitus were established. He had been treated with daily GH in large doses since the age of 3 years. Shortly after the ataxia occurred, severe dementia developed in the patient. Rapid deterioration resulted in hospitalization, and the patient died within 6 months of the onset of ataxia. Spongiform encephalopathy characteristic of CJD was discovered on autopsy.

Subsequent Cases.—Subsequently, 60 cases of CJD have been reported in patients treated with pituitary GH, including 15 patients in the United States. Evidence from these patients and from animal studies have suggested that the pituitary GH supplies were contaminated with the CJD infectious agent. In addition, the affected patients may have had a genetic susceptibility to CJD, an allelic homozygosity at codon 129 of the chromosome 20 amyloid gene. There were latency periods of 16–34 years between the initiation of treatment with pituitary GH and the onset of symptoms of CJD among the first 9 patients, suggesting that there may be many more cases reported in the future.

Consequences.—The therapeutic use of human pituitary GH has been ended worldwide. Synthetic GH has been approved for use in the United States and has been associated with very few complications. However, GH is a potent biological agent, requiring constant and careful surveillance for rare but serious complications.

▶ This sentinel case ultimately led to the cessation of therapeutic use of human pituitary GH after 30 years of use. Creutzfeldt-Jakob disease resulting from transmission of its infectious agent has been identified in patients in the United States, United Kingdom, and France, and at least 60 cases have occurred to date. Because of the long incubation period, others may eventually be added to this tragic list.

Recombinant synthetic GH has made it possible to achieve the benefits of treatment without the risk of CJD, but the widening use of GH around the world requires us to keep on our guard for possible rare adverse events from this potent biological agent.

L. Lasagna, M.D.

Royal Jelly–induced Asthma and Anaphylaxis: Clinical Characteristics and Immunologic Correlations
Leung R, Thien FCK, Baldo B, et al (Alfred Hosp, Victoria, Australia; Royal North Shore Hosp, St Leonards, Australia)
J Allergy Clin Immunol 96:1004–1007, 1995   3–26

Background.—Royal jelly, a honeybee secretion, is commonly used as a health tonic. Five patients with asthma and anaphylaxis induced by royal jelly were recently reported. Further clinical and immunologic details on these 5 patients were presented along with those of 2 new patients.

Patients and Methods.—The patients were 6 women and 1 man aged 19 to 66 years. Four had taken royal jelly previously. Reactions ranged from an acute life-threatening asthma attack, anaphylaxis, and respiratory arrest to acute wheezing. Sera from all 7 patients showed increased levels of anti-IgE antibody uptake by nitrocellulose disks with adsorbed royal jelly proteins. Five serum samples had levels at least 10 times greater than those of nonallergic control subjects. Thirty-eight percent to 52% of sera from patients known to be allergic to bee venom and other allergic subjects, respectively, showed uptake of anti-IgE at least twice that of nonallergic control subjects.

Conclusion.—Persons with clinical sensitivity to royal jelly have serum IgE antibodies to a number of royal jelly components. Although antibody-binding patterns were heterogeneous, 2 proteins of molecular weights of 55 and 47 kd were recognized by sera from all patients, suggesting that these components may be the major allergenic proteins in royal jelly. The recognition of these proteins by sera from a number of patients with bee

60 / Drug Therapy

venom sensitivity and other common allergies suggests that there may be "sensitized" individuals at risk for adverse reactions on exposure to royal jelly.

▶ One could say that royal jelly is all toxicity with no beneficial effect. It really does depend on your faith in the collection of material from honey bees. Fortunately, given its high use, there really are very few adverse reactions, but one has to remember that the benefit is really quite low, as well.

M. Weintraub, M.D.

Agranulocytosis and Near Fatal Sepsis Due to 'Mexican Aspirin' (Dipyrone)
Dorr VJ, Cook J (Univ of Kansas, Kansas City)
South Med J 89:612–614, 1996   3–27

Background.—Unconventional medical therapy is widely used but rarely reported to physicians. A case of near fatal sepsis and agranulocytosis related to the use of dipyrone is reported. Dipyrone is an analgesic and antipyretic agent that has been banned in the United States but is available in Mexico.

> *Case Report.*—Woman, 51, was admitted with a 3-day history of fever, chills, headache, tinnitus, nausea, vomiting, diarrhea, arthralgia, and myalgia. She had been taking aspirin (Dolo-Tiaminol) from Mexico for the previous 2 years. She had a low hemoglobin value and elevated white blood cell count. Her bone marrow biopsy revealed hypocellularity and no myelopoiesis, but with normal erythroid and megakaryocytic production. She was treated with antibiotics and granulocyte colony-stimulating factor (G-CSF) but remained febrile, and splenomegaly and a diffuse rash eventually developed. She had negative tests for HIV, rheumatoid factor, antinuclear antibody, hepatitis, Epstein-Barr virus, cytomegalovirus, herpes simplex virus, parvovirus B19, *Ehrlichia* sp., Lyme disease, Rocky Mountain spotted fever, and all bacteria. After 15 days of hospitalization, the patient had acute septic shock, requiring emergency intubation. She was managed with aggressive antibiotic and pulmonary intervention, which brought eventual improvement. The Dolo-Tiaminol contained 250 mg of dipyrone, which appeared to be the cause of the agranulocytosis.

Discussion.—Dipyrone has been commonly associated with agranulocytosis. Initially patients typically appear to have a febrile oropharyngeal infection. The white blood cell count usually normalizes within approximately 1 week, but may occur within 2 days to 1 month. Management is primarily supportive along with antibiotic therapy. Mortality occurs in

24% to 32% of the patients. It is thought that dipyrone induces agranulocytosis through an immune reaction. The lack of a therapeutic effect of G-CSF in the patient described supports this theory. It may be important to inquire about alternative drug therapy in patients with unusual or unexpected health problems.

▶ Dipyrone is a "relative" of aminopyrine, both of which are associated with agranulocytosis. Dipyrone is banned in the United States, Canada, and some European countries. Obviously "Mexican aspirin" can (rarely) be seriously toxic, as can other alternative remedies purchased in other countries.

L. Lasagna, M.D.

Liver Injuries Induced by Herbal Medicine, Syo-saiko-to (Xiao-chai-hu-tang)
Itoh S, Marutani K, Nishijima T, et al (Saitama Med School, Japan)
Dig Dis Sci 40:1845–1848, 1995   3–28

Background.—Syo-saiko-to is an herbal medicine that has been used for centuries to treat patients with common cold symptoms or abdominal discomfort and nausea. More recently, it has been used in Japan to treat liver diseases, especially chronic viral hepatitis. However, 4 patients treated with syo-saiko-to experienced liver injuries associated with the drug.

Methods.—Four women, aged 42–58 years, were admitted to a hospital with evidence of liver disease. All were treated with 7.5 g of syo-saiko-to per day. Liver tests were performed during and after treatment. Syo-saiko-to was administered a second time in 2 patients and as a challenge in 2 patients. The laboratory changes associated with these administrations were noted. Liver biopsy was performed in all 4 patients.

Results.—In all 4 patients, the serum glutamic oxaloacetic transaminase and serum pyruvic transaminase levels rose substantially within 1.5–3 months after syo-saiko-to therapy was initiated. The levels then decreased to nearly normal within 10 days to 1 month after the withdrawal of the drug. In all patients, after syo-saiko-to was prescribed again or administered as a drug challenge, the levels of serum glutamic oxaloacetic transaminase and serum glutamate pyrovic transaminase rose sharply. The liver biopsy specimens revealed portal tract fibrosis and inflammation in all patients, with necrosis seen in various degrees in 3 patients. The parenchymal hepatocytes had microvesicular fatty changes, and centrilobular areas had bile thrombi.

Conclusions.—The histologic changes seen in patients treated with syo-saiko-to were consistent with a diagnosis of drug-induced acute liver injury or cholestasis. These changes occurred after a latent period of 1.5–3 months.

▶ On my first visit to China, in 1974, I was repeatedly told that traditional herbal medicines were devoid of toxicity. For a Westerner accustomed to the puritanical notion that everything desirable in this world carries a downside, or a price of some sort (such as drug toxicity), this was hard to swallow (pun not intended).

Since that time, at least 12 articles have appeared reporting adverse effects of herbal medicine on the liver. This paper indicts as a hepatotoxin an herbal medicine used in both China and Japan.

L. Lasagna, M.D.

Hepatitis After the Use of Germander, a Herbal Remedy
Laliberté L, Villeneuve J-P (Hôpital Saint-Luc, Montreal)
Can Med Assoc J 154:1689–1692, 1996   3–29

Introduction.—Phytotherapy, the treatment of diseases with herbal remedies, is becoming increasingly popular in industrialized nations. The potential toxicity of herbal medicine is often unknown. In France, several cases of hepatitis associated with the use of germander (*Teucrium chamaedrys*) have been reported, and germander has been banned. An aromatic plant of the mint family, germander is ingested as an herbal tea with alleged choleretic and antiseptic properties. Recently, germander has been marketed for use in weight control, with recommended dosages ranging from 600 to 1,600 mg/day. Two cases of acute hepatitis associated with germander ingestion have been reported in Canada, where this drug is sold in local pharmacies.

> *Case 1.*—Woman, 55, had been taking 1,600 mg/day of germander for the treatment of hypercholesterolemia. After 6 months, she was admitted to the hospital with asthenia, jaundice, nausea, and vomiting. A liver biopsy showed bridging necrosis and collapse, mild portal-tract fibrosis, and lobular and portal-tract inflammatory infiltration with polymorphonuclear and mononuclear cells. After germander therapy was stopped, liver function test results improved over the next 2 months.
> *Case 2.*—Woman, 45, had been ingesting germander, 260 mg/day to lose weight for 6 months. She had jaundice, but her use of germander initially was not noticed. However, she stopped taking the medication on her own because she felt sick. Her liver function test results gradually improved. She felt better after 4 months, and again began taking germander. Hepatitis and asthenia recurred 1 week later. After she stopped taking germander, she showed progressive improvement.

Conclusion.—Acute cytolytic hepatitis has been linked with germander in France, where 26 cases of acute hepatitis resulting from the ingestion of either germander capsules or germander tea have been reported. In general, after 9 weeks of ingestion of germander, hepatic toxic effects appear, characterized by jaundice and high aspartate and alanine aminotransferase levels. Cases of hepatitis in which the cause remains unknown should alert physicians to the possibility that the patients may be ingesting herbal remedies.

▶ The lesson that we are supposed to learn from this particular paper is that we must ask our patients whether they are taking any herbal remedies or food supplements in addition to over-the-counter and prescription medications. A full drug history will frequently reveal the symptoms of very rare or otherwise undiagnosable conditions.

M. Weintraub, M.D.

Renal Infarction Secondary to Nasal Insufflation of Cocaine
Goodman PE, Rennie WP (East Carolina Univ, Greenville, NC; Long Island Jewish Med Ctr, New Hyde Park, NY)
Am J Emerg Med 13:421–423, 1995   3–30

Background.—Cocaine abuse is associated with many complications, primarily cardiac or cerebrovascular. Renal infarction—a lesser known complication of cocaine abuse—was studied.

> *Case Report.*—Man, 37, was seen in an emergency department with a 4-hour history of right-sided abdominal pain, nausea, and diarrhea. He admitted to insufflating cocaine powder about 2 hours before the onset of abdominal pain. Abdominal CT scans were obtained with IV and intraluminal contrast (Fig 2). Low attenuation of the anterior, medial, and lateral aspects of the middle and lower thirds of the right kidney was consistent with failure of uptake secondary to infarction. The patient's symptoms resolved over several hours with hydration only. After discharge, the patient was seen by a nephrologist, who found no evidence of renal insufficiency or renovascular hypertension.

Conclusions.—Renal infarction should be included in the differential diagnosis of patients with atypical flank or abdominal pain after cocaine abuse. Computed tomography with intraluminal and IV contrast is useful to establish this diagnosis and to help exclude other possible diagnoses.

▶ Add renal infarction to all the other risks of cocaine abuse.

L. Lasagna, M.D.

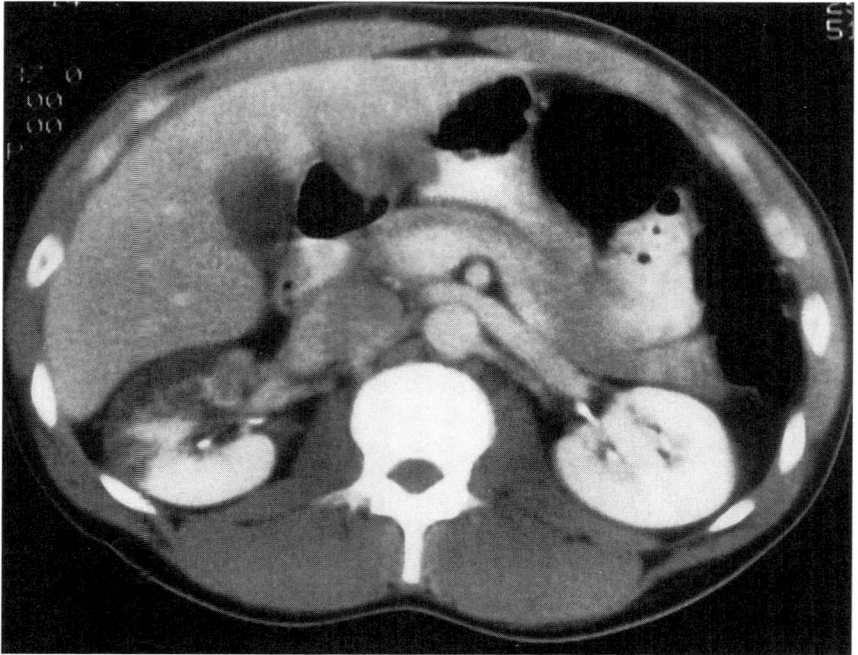

FIGURE 2.— Computed tomography shows greatly decreased, heterogeneous uptake of contrast media by anterolateral aspects of the right kidney, with normal uptake posteriorly. No occlusion of the right renal artery is noted. Normal uptake of contrast media by the left kidney is noted. (Courtesy of Goodman PE, Rennie WP: Renal infarction secondary to nasal insufflation of cocaine. *Am J Emerg Med* 13:421–423, 1995.)

Lead Poisoning From an Intra-articular Shotgun Pellet in the Knee Treated With Arthroscopic Extraction and Chelation Therapy: A Case Report

Bolanos AA, Demizio JP Jr, Vigorita VJ, et al (Kingsbrook Jewish Med Ctr, Brooklyn, NY Lutheran Med Ctr, Brooklyn, NY)
J Bone Joint Surg Am 78–A:422–426, 1996   3–31

Introduction.—Although rare, gunshot injuries are a well-documented cause of lead intoxication. A patient with plumbism secondary to gunshot injuries to the knees, whose treatment included arthroscopic removal of the lead pellet and chelation therapy, is discussed.

Case Report.—Woman, 41, arrived at the emergency department with acute exacerbation of long-standing pain in her right knee. She had been shot in both knees 23 years before and had been treated operatively. She had slipped and abducted her right lower extremity and subsequently had increased pain and effusion. She reported a 12-year history of progressively severe headaches. Radiographic studies showed multiple shotgun pellets in the right knee area. She had increased lead concentrations in the serum, urine, and synovial fluid. She underwent arthroscopic surgery to remove a shotgun pellet and several fragments. In addition, synovectomy and débridement was done arthroscopically. Examination of the removed fragments confirmed that they were lead. She was treated postoperatively with oral chelation therapy, which was continued for 2 weeks on an outpatient basis. Her headaches and knee pain were completely resolved, and her serum lead concentrations decreased progressively.

Discussion.—Early lead poisoning may have minor, nonspecific signs and symptoms. In this patient, lead poisoning was discovered incidentally. The treatment of lead intoxication secondary to gunshot injuries has traditionally consisted of open surgical removal of the fragments and IV chelation therapy. However, for this patient, arthroscopic removal of lead and oral chelation therapy (administered on an outpatient basis) was successful. This approach is recommended for the treatment of lead in the intra-articular space.

▶ Most lead poisoning in the past has been related to the ingestion of lead-based paint by children, but occupational exposure (in painters, lead miners, battery factory workers, etc.) and contaminated "moonshine" are also causative.

Lead intoxication from gunshot injuries is rare but well documented, especially when the lead is exposed to synovial fluid, which seems to dissolve lead more effectively than either serum or water.

L. Lasagna, M.D.

4 AIDS

A Short-term Study of the Safety, Pharmacokinetics, and Efficacy of Ritonavir, an Inhibitor of HIV-1 Protease
Danner SA, for the European-Australian Collaborative Ritonavir Study Group (Academic Med Ctr, Amsterdam; St Vincent's Hosp, Sydney, Australia; Abbott Labs, Abbott Park, Ill; et al)
N Engl J Med 333:1528–1533, 1995   4–1

Background.—Ritonavir, a novel HIV-1 protease inhibitor with both good oral bioavailability and significant in vitro anti-HIV properties, may prove to be more clinically effective against HIV-1 than reverse-transcriptase inhibitors. The antiviral activity and safety of ritonavir was evaluated in this double-blind, randomized, placebo-controlled phase 1 and 2 study.

Patients and Methods.—Eighty-four patients, aged 18 years or older, with confirmed HIV-1 infection and a CD4+ lymphocyte counts greater than 50 cells/mm³ were studied. A 4-week, placebo-controlled phase and a subsequent drug maintenance phase were carried out. Patients were randomly assigned to receive 1 of 4 regimens of ritonavir (300 mg, 400 mg, 500 mg, or 600 mg twice daily) or matching placebo. After the first study phase was completed, all patients continued to the maintenance phase. Patients initially receiving placebo were again randomly assigned in a double-blind fashion to one of the ritonavir dosages used in their treatment group. Clinical efficacy was determined by evaluating CD4+ lymphocyte count and plasma concentrations of HIV-1 p24 antigen and viral RNA.

Results.—Demographic features, HIV risk factors, body weight, and Karnofsky performance scores were comparable between treatment groups. Patients in all 4 dosage groups showed comparable increases in CD4+ lymphocyte counts and decreases in the log number of copies of HIV-1 RNA per millimeter of plasma during the first 4 weeks. Returns to baseline levels were noted in the 3 lower-dosage groups by 16 weeks, however. The 7 patients receiving 600 mg of ritonavir showed a mean increase from baseline in the CD4+ lymphocyte count of 230 cells mm³ after 32 weeks. The mean decrease in the plasma concentration of HIV-1 RNA, determined using a branched-chain DNA assay, was 0.81 in this highest-dosage group. A polymerase chain reaction–based assay also was used to measure RNA in a subgroup of 17 patients in the 2 higher-dosage groups. After 8 weeks of treatment, a mean maximal reduction in viral

RNA of 1.54 log was noted. Treatment-related side effects included nausea, circumoral paresthesia, increased hepatic aminotransferase levels, and elevated triglyceride levels. Ten patients withdrew from the study because of treatment-related effects.

Conclusions.—Early findings indicate that ritonavir has significant antiviral and immunostimulatory effects, although specific clinical advantages associated with this agent have not yet been determined. Additional studies are encouraged.

A Preliminary Study of Ritonavir, an Inhibitor of HIV-1 Protease, to Treat HIV-1 Infection
Markowitz M, Saag M, Powderly WG, et al (New York Univ; Univ of Alabama, Birmingham; Washington Univ, St Louis, Mo; et al)
N Engl J Med 333:1534–1539, 1995   4–2

Background.—Human immunodeficiency virus type 1 (HIV-1) protease is needed for virions to develop and become infective. Preliminary pharmacokinetic studies have shown that ritonavir, an HIV-1 protease inhibitor, is well absorbed in humans, with plasma concentrations that are considerably higher than inhibitory concentrations achieved in vitro. To evaluate the safety and clinical efficacy of this agent, a phase 1 and 2 clinical trial was performed.

Patients and Methods.—Sixty-two patients with viral loads of 25,000 or more copies of HIV-1 RNA per millimeter of plasma and CD4 counts of 50–500 cells per cubic millimeter were enrolled in the study. All patients had discontinued all antiviral therapy and concomitant medications, with the exception of prophylaxis against *Pneumocystis carinii*. Over 12 weeks, a 4-week placebo-controlled, double-blinded trial was performed, after which an 8-week dose-blinded phase was done. One of 4 dosages of ritonavir (200 or 300 mg 3 times daily, or 200 or 300 mg 4 times daily) or placebo were administered during the first 4 weeks. Patients initially given placebo were then randomly assigned to either 200 or 300 mg of ritonavir in their group during the subsequent 8-week period. Serial plasma viremia measurements and serial CD4 cell counts were done to evaluate patient response.

Results.—Fifty-two patients completed the entire study. The most frequently observed adverse effects were diarrhea and nausea. Reversible elevations in serum triglycerides and γ-glutamyltransferase levels were the most commonly noted laboratory anomalies. A prompt antiviral effect was found with use of ritonavir. Among the 4 dosage groups, the mean maximal reduction in the number of copies of HIV-1 RNA per millimeter of plasma ranged between 0.86 and 1.18 log. A partial maintenance of the antiviral effect was noted after 12 weeks of therapy, with a mean reduction of 0.5 log observed.

A more sensitive assay for HIV-1 RNA also was used in a subgroup of 20 patients. Results showed that plasma viremia was reduced by a mean of

1.7 log. At 12 weeks, the antiviral effect was partially maintained, with a mean decrease of nearly 1.1 log noted. At week 4 of ritonavir treatment, CD4 counts had increased to a median of 74 cells per cubic millimeter. At week 12, a median increase of 83 CD4 cells per cubic millimeter was observed.

Conclusions.—Ritonavir is a safe and well tolerated agent, with substantial antiviral effects. The evident lack of overlapping toxicity with existing treatments for AIDS and the novel mechanism of action suggest that ritonavir is suitable for combined therapy with HIV-1 reverse transcriptase inhibitors. Additional clinical studies are needed to determine how this drug can be integrated with existing antiretroviral treatment strategies.

▶ These 2 studies (Abstracts 4–1 and 4–2) involve a member of a new class of marketed HIV protease inhibitors. Such inhibitors lead to the production of noninfectious particles and represent an interesting alternative to the inhibition of reverse transcriptase in the treatment of HIV infection, or possibly an adjunct to the latter type of anti-HIV treatment in combination regimens.

The early work in this field was hampered by the poor oral bioavailability of members of the class, but ritonavir has shown very good oral bioavailability in dogs and monkeys.

It seems clear that this agent can affect surrogate end points (CD4 cell counts and plasma viremia), but only future studies will tell us whether AIDS can be prevented or delayed by this agent, and survival time increased.

L. Lasagna, M.D.

Delta: A Randomised Double-blind Controlled Trial Comparing Combinations of Zidovudine Plus Didanosine or Zalcitabine With Zidovudine Alone in HIV-infected Individuals

Delta Coordinating Committee (Mortimer Market Centre, London; INSERM SC10, Villejuif, France)

Lancet 348:283–291, 1996   4–3

Background.—Although zidovudine (AZT) has benefits for patients infected with HIV, these benefits are small and tend to last only briefly. The Delta trial was designed to test whether the combination of AZT with other available drugs might be advantageous in delaying disease progression or extending survival.

Methods.—Combinations of AZT (600 mg/day) with didanosine (ddI, 400 mg/d) or zalcitabine (ddC, 2.25 mg/day) were compared with the use of AZT alone. Patients were infected with HIV and had either a CD4 count of less than 350×10^6/L or symptoms of HIV disease (those with AIDS had a CD4 count greater than 50×10^6/L). The randomized, double-blind study marked the first use of AZT for 2,124 participants; 1,083 participants had been receiving AZT for 3 months or more.

Results.—Death occurred in 699 participants and 936 of the 2,765 participants without AIDS either saw the development of AIDS or died during the 30-month median follow-up period. Regardless of their disease stage at entry, patients who had not received AZT before showed substantial benefit from both combination regimens in terms of survival. The use of AZT plus ddI resulted in a 42% reduction in mortality over the use of AZT alone; AZT plus ddC reduced mortality by 32%. Significant improvement in the survival of patients who had previously taken AZT occurred with the addition of ddI (relative reduction 23%) but not ddC (relative reduction 9%). Overall, the addition of ddI resulted in a relative reduction in mortality of 33% compared to AZT alone; for the addition of ddC, the reduction was 21%. Patients not previously treated with AZT also showed benefit in terms of disease progression. Toxicity was within the expected limits.

Conclusions.—Combinations of AZT with ddI or ddC produce a substantial reduction in mortality over the use of AZT alone in patients infected with HIV. Combinations with other drugs under investigation, such as the protease inhibitors, might be expected to produce even greater clinical benefits.

▶ The problem with AIDS trials is that when the investigators publish them, they are already out of date. The fact that new drugs are appearing all the time, and that now even new classes of AIDS drugs are coming along, is really a problem for the practitioner who may have to get this information from the newspaper. Certainly, with some of the newer AIDS drugs coming out, we will expect to see more extended survival with drug therapy. Unfortunately, the cost of these therapies may be more than the average patient with AIDS can spend and more than the insurance company will be willing to spend.

M. Weintraub, M.D.

Study of the Role of Vitamin B$_{12}$ and Folinic Acid Supplementation in Preventing Hematologic Toxicity of Zidovudine

Falguera M, Perez-Mur J, Puig T, et al (Arnau de Vilanova Hosp, Lleida, Spain)
Eur J Haematol 55:97–102, 1995   4–4

Background.—Zidovudine and other antiretroviral drugs can aggravate the hematopoietic dysfunction caused by HIV infection. The mechanism of zidovudine's bone marrow toxicity may involve subnormal levels of vitamin B$_{12}$ and folate. Vitamin B$_{12}$ and folinic acid supplementation were studied for their capability to prevent zidovudine-induced bone marrow suppression.

Methods.—The prospective, randomized trial included 75 adults seropositive for HIV with CD4+ cells counts of less than 500/mm^3 who had not previously been treated with zidovudine. All patients received zidovudine in a dose of 500 mg/day. Those assigned to group I received zidovudine alone, and those in group II also received folinic acid, 15 mg/day, and IM vitamin B_{12}, 1,000 µg/month. The patients were followed up to see whether severe myelotoxicity, defined as a hemoglobin level of less than 8 g/dL or a neutrophil count of less than 1,000/mm³, developed.

Results.—Sixty patients completed the study, and 14 others were excluded for noncompliance. The 2 groups were comparable at baseline. During treatment, the group II patients had significantly increased vitamin B_{12} and folate levels. Hemoglobin; hematocrit; mean corpuscular volume; and white cell, neutrophil, and platelet counts, however, were similar throughout follow-up. Thirteen percent of patients in group I and 24% of patients in group II had severe hematologic toxicity. Vitamin B_{12} and folate levels were unrelated to the occurrence of myelosuppression.

Conclusions.—For the overall population of patients with HIV infection treated with zidovudine, vitamin B_{12} and folinic acid supplementation do not appear to help prevent treatment-related myelotoxicity. Such supplementation could still be beneficial in certain patient subgroups, however, such as those who have deficiencies of these vitamins or who have more advanced HIV disease.

▶ Patients infected with HIV often suffer from anemia, leukopenia, and granulocytopenia even without taking zidovudine (AZT), but this therapy can worsen the hematologic toxicity. Because such patients often have subnormal blood levels of vitamin B_{12} and folate, it was not unreasonable to see if augmenting the intake of these nutrients could diminish the myelosuppression. This study suggests that these substances probably aren't terribly important in general in this situation, but before we forget about the possibility, the study should be repeated, using only patients that seem deficient.

L. Lasagna, M.D.

Role of Zidovudine Antiretroviral Therapy in the Pathogenesis of Acquired Immunodeficiency Syndrome–related Lymphoma
Levine AM, Bernstein L, Sullivan-Halley J, et al (Univ of Southern California, Los Angeles)
Blood 86:4612–4616, 1995   4–5

Introduction.—Lymphoma is an AIDS-defining condition and a major cause of mortality in patients with AIDS. The etiology of AIDS-related lymphomas is uncertain; it has been suggested that zidovudine and other antiretroviral agents may play a pathogenetic role. The impact of antiretroviral treatment in the development of AIDS-related lymphoma was evaluated in a population-based, case-control study.

Methods.—The study included HIV-seropositive patients with biopsy specimen–confirmed intermediate- or high-grade lymphoma. These patients and their controls were interviewed about their use of zidovudine and other antiretroviral drugs. A total of 112 HIV-infected homosexual or bisexual men with lymphoma and the same number of asymptomatic

HIV-positive controls were studied. In addition, 49 of the patients who had lymphoma were matched to 49 patients who had AIDS but did not have lymphoma.

Results.—About 40% of each group had used zidovudine. Zidovudine treatment had continued for a mean of 19 months in the patients with lymphoma, 23 months in the asymptomatic controls, and 11 months for the AIDS controls. When comparing the AIDS patients with lymphoma and their AIDS controls without lymphoma, the matched relative odds of lymphoma associated with previous zidovudine use was 0.43. When comparing all lymphoma cases with the nonlymphoma AIDS controls, the unmatched relative odds of zidovudine-associated lymphoma was 0.93.

Conclusions.—In HIV-positive homosexual or bisexual men, previous treatment with zidovudine does not appear to increase the risk of lymphoma. It seems more likely that antiretroviral treatment prolongs survival, thus providing more time for AIDS-related lymphoma to develop.

▶ Patients with AIDS are prey to a spectrum of infections and neoplasms. Lymphoma is the first AIDS-defining condition in 3% of these patients in the United States and its incidence increases with time, causing death in 12% to 15% of patients with AIDS. All groups seem at risk for this complication, as opposed to Kaposi's sarcoma, which occurs primarily in homosexual or bisexual males.

This case-control study addressed the concern that zidovudine (AZT) might actually cause lymphomas; the findings do not support this hypothesis.

L. Lasagna, M.D.

Identification of Levels of Maternal HIV-1 RNA Associated With Risk of Perinatal Transmission: Effect of Maternal Zidovudine Treatment on Viral Load

Dickover RE, Garratty EM, Herman SA, et al (Univ of California, Los Angeles; Roche Molecular Systems, Somerville, NJ; Long Beach Mem Med Ctr, Los Angeles)

JAMA 275:599–605, 1996   4–6

Background.—The quantity of HIV in the mother's blood at delivery is an important risk factor in mother-to-infant transmission of HIV. In asymptomatic women with HIV infection, zidovudine can cut the risk of perinatal HIV transmission by two thirds. It is important to find out whether there is some critical threshold or pattern of HIV replication in maternal blood that predicts perinatal transmission to the fetus. Associations between the mother's HIV-1 level during gestation and at delivery, zidovudine treatment of the mother, and risk of perinatal HIV transmission were examined using prospectively collected data.

Methods.—The analysis included 97 neonates of 92 HIV-1-seropositive mothers prospectively followed in a larger study of maternal-fetal HIV-1 transmission. In this nonrandomized study, 42 mothers in 43 pregnancies received zidovudine during pregnancy, labor and delivery, or both. In addition, 11 neonates received zidovudine prophylactically for their first 6 weeks of life. Polymerase chain reaction was used to quantitate HIV-1 DNA in peripheral blood mononuclear cells. Logistic regression was used to determine the value of virologic and immunologic markers in predicting HIV-1 transmission. The variables analyzed were viral load, CD4+ cell count, and zidovudine use.

Results.—Twenty-two percent of the neonates were infected with HIV-1. Seventy-five percent of the mothers who transmitted HIV-1 to their offspring had plasma HIV-1 RNA levels at delivery of greater than 50,000 copies per milliliter, compared with 5% of those who did not transmit HIV-1. When the HIV-1 RNA level was less than 20,000 copies per milliliter, viral transmission never occurred. In a subgroup of 50 mothers followed through gestation, 7 had increasing HIV-1 replication over time, 29 had a decreasing viral load, and 14 had a stable viral load.

Receiving zidovudine during gestation produced a median eightfold decrease in plasma RNA levels, from 43,043 to 4,238 copies per milliliter at delivery. None of the 22 women receiving this treatment transmitted HIV-1 to their offspring. In comparison, 4 of 4 women with high HIV-1 levels who were treated with zidovudine transmitted the virus to their offspring. This occurred despite the in vitro sensitivity of the virus to zidovudine.

Conclusions.—The risk of perinatal transmission of HIV-1 depends heavily on the mother's HIV-1 RNA levels. Viral thresholds during late gestation or labor and delivery are associated with a high and a low risk of transmission. Zidovudine treatment can reduce the mother's HIV-1 RNA level before delivery and thus help to protect against transmission of the infection. New preventive approaches are needed for mothers with high or increasing levels of virus or those whose virus does not respond to zidovudine.

▶ The law talks about "victimless crimes," but AIDS has "blameless victims," such as patients with hemophilia or patients with hemophilia who received contaminated blood products or babies born of infected mothers.

This study challenges us to come up with ways to reduce the risk of perinatal HIV transmission by decreasing maternal viral levels.

L. Lasagna, M.D.

N-Acetyltransferase 2 Polymorphism in Patients Infected With Human Immunodeficiency Virus

Kaufmann GR, Wenk M, Taeschner W, et al (Univ Hosp Basel, Switzerland; Univ of Basel, Switzerland)
Clin Pharmacol Ther 60:62–67, 1996   4–7

Background.—Variability of drug metabolism is partly dependent on the functioning of 2 enzymes responsible for most of the hepatic acetylation activity: N-acetyltransferase 1 (NAT1) and N-acetyltransferase 2 (NAT2). At least 7 mutations of the *NAT2* gene have been found to cause a slow acetylation phenotype. A previous study reported that the slow acetylator phenotype was more common in patients with AIDS than in asymptomatic patients with HIV infection and healthy control subjects. The association of slow acetylation with genetic determination and with advancing stages of HIV infection was investigated.

Methods.—Fifty consecutive HIV-infected patients without current acute opportunistic infections were classified by infection stage. The *NAT2* phenotype was determined in each patient by measuring the urinary metabolic ratio of caffeine metabolites after oral caffeine administration. The *NAT2* genotype was determined with polymerase chain reaction and restriction fragment length polymorphism.

Results.—Of the 50 patients, HIV infection was at stage A in 10 patients, stage B in 20, and stage C in 20. The acetylation phenotype was slow in 32 patients and rapid in 18 patients. There was complete concordance between phenotype and genotype in all but 2 patients. There was no increase in the incidence of slow acetylation in the advancing stages of HIV infection. There was also no correlation between the CD4 cell count and NAT2 activity.

Conclusion.—Impaired N-acetylation is determined genetically and is not related to the stage of HIV infection. Because slow acetylation may have an impact on individual metabolic capacity, knowledge of the patient's acetylation phenotype or genotype may be clinically important in treatment planning and monitoring.

▶ Some years ago a friend of mine told me about the change in phenotype of AIDS patients. This was such a striking alteration of a condition caused by the AIDS virus that I was actually struck dumb. It seemed to me that it was more likely a question of drug-drug interactions, or immunosuppression, or some effect on the liver caused by either the virus or other therapy. Well, the abstracted study says that it's OK; we can rest easy, sleep again at night, and know that the AIDS infection isn't really changing the phenotypic expression of, at least, acetyltransferase in AIDS patients.

M. Weintraub, M.D.

5 Asthma

Model for Outcomes Assessment of Antihistamine Use for Seasonal Allergic Rhinitis

Harvey RP, Comer C, Sanders B, et al (Kaiser-Permanente System, Denver; Presbyterian/St Lukes, Denver; Pharmatec Inc, Denver)
J Allergy Clin Immunol 97:1233–1241, 1996   5–1

Background.—Although first-generation antihistamines are an inexpensive mainstay of therapy for seasonal allergic rhinitis, they can produce side effects such as sedation and impairment of motor activity that may be more severe than the patient realizes. Formulary medication choices within managed care organizations may be based exclusively on efficacy, safety, and cost. The multiattribute utility theory (MAUT) integrates diverse outcomes into the decision-making process by prioritizing the advantages and disadvantages of treatments. The MAUT was used in conjunction with a rhinitis quality-of-life questionnaire and efficacy, safety, and cost data to analyze the outcome of the use of cetirizine, chlorpheniramine, and terfenadine to simulate formulary decision-making processes.

Methods.—Patients received 1 of the 3 randomly assigned drugs for 2 weeks, after which they could either continue with that drug or, if dissatisfied, receive another randomly assigned drug. Patients kept daily diaries of symptoms and cost, and completed validated questionnaires. The antihistamines were ranked using the MAUT. Patients were not blind as to treatment, mimicking the clinical situation.

Results.—Cetirizine and chlorpheniramine were ranked more effective than terfenadine by patient and physician assessment. After the first 2-week period, 69.4% of patients treated with cetirizine, 50% of patients treated with terfenadine, and 28.9% of patients treated with chlorpheniramine were satisfied with the therapy and did not wish to change medications. Treatment with cetirizine resulted in the greatest improvement in quality of life score; treatment with terfenadine, the least. The incidence of sedation was least for terfenadine and greatest with chlorpheniramine.

Conclusions.—The selection of an antihistamine is best made with an MAUT approach that considers quality of life. Patients and physicians most favored cetirizine, then chlorpheniramine, then terfenadine.

▶ This study was done in a managed care setting. Theoretically, the managed care people should be interested in balancing the adverse effects and costs of various medications. One of the drugs, chlorpheniramine, caused a 40% sedation rate in the first 2 weeks of the study, which fell to 17%, compared to much lower rates (6.7% and 5.1%) for terfenadine. Chlorpheniramine costs much less. These authors use a kind of special term, "multi-attribute evaluation," which is a way of saying that many features of a medication's effect are measured. What has happened is that a new medication, which is a metabolite of terfenadine, is now on the market. It does not have the torsades de pointes adverse effect of terfenadine. I do not know much about the cost of this new medication, but one imagines that it will be significantly more than chlorpheniramine. We will have to see how its multiattribute evaluation turns out.

M. Weintraub, M.D.

Protocol Therapy for Acute Asthma: Therapeutic Benefits and Cost Savings
McFadden ER Jr, Elsanadi N, Dixon L, et al (Case Western Reserve Univ, Cleveland, Ohio)
Am J Med 99:651–661, 1995   5–2

Objective.—The treatment of acute asthma is not standardized; this is a major impediment to lowered morbidity in patients with acute asthma. An interactive-care protocol that was based on systematic use of standard medication and employed decision algorithms derived from sequential measures of patients' progress was examined.

Methods.—Asthmatic patients, 16 years of age or older, who were admitted to the hospital for emergency treatment for an acute exacerbation received clinical and physiologic evaluations and were treated with albuterol by nebulizer for 3 doses 20 minutes apart. At 1 hour after admission, evaluations were repeated. Asymptomatic patients were discharged. Symptomatic patients were treated with theophylline and methyl prednisone intravenously after 1 hour. After reassessment, asymptomatic patients were discharged. Symptomatic patients were either admitted to the medical ICU (MICU) or treated with aminophylline and steroids and reassessed. Asymptomatic patients were discharged, and symptomatic patients were admitted to MICU (Fig 1).

Results.—In the 8 months before the protocol was used, 429 cases of exacerbation of asthma were treated. Patients were treated with 1–6 doses of nebulized albuterol at various intervals; a combination of aerosolized and/or injected sympathomimetrics was administered 33 times, 92 patients received a methylxanthine, 172 received glucocorticoids and sympathomimetrics, and 58 patients received all 3. Peak expiratory flow rate measurements were not performed systematically and in relation to the physiologic measures. During the first year of the protocol period, 404 of the 526 patients treated were discharged and 122 were admitted. Peak expiratory flow rate measurements improved significantly in both groups. In a period of physician turnover, both preprotocol and protocol approaches were used. Medications were prescribed according to physician experience,

Asthma Protocol — ED

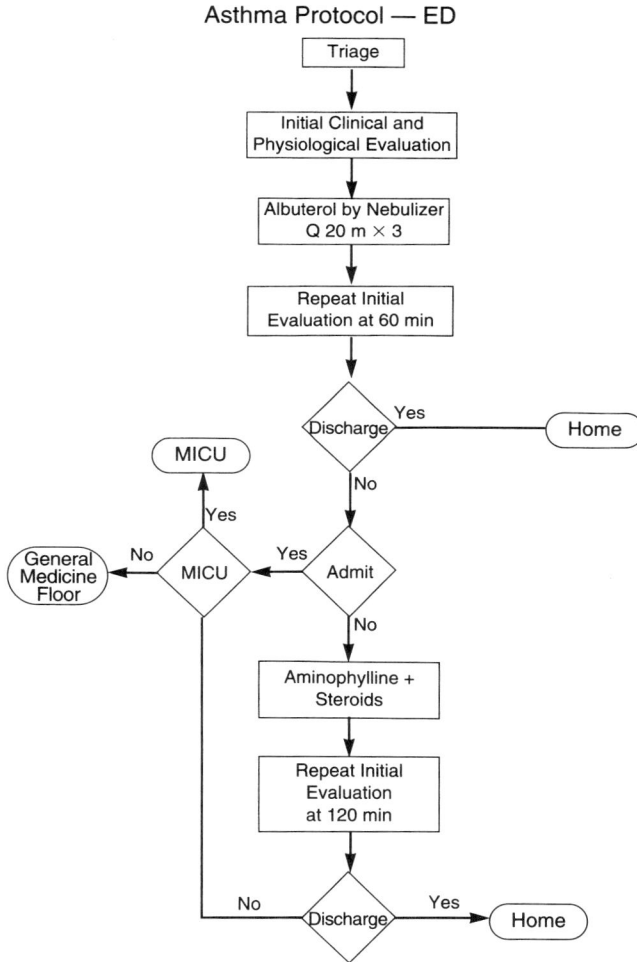

FIGURE 1.—Emergency department care path and decision algorithms. The *rectangles* contain the instructions, the *triangles* represent decision points, and the *elliptical symbols* indicate the final dispositions. *Abbreviations: ED*, emergency department; *MICU*, medical ICU. (Reprinted by permission of the publisher from McFadden ER Jr, Elsanadi N, Dixon L, et al: Protocol therapy for acute asthma: Therapeutic benefits and cost savings. *AMERICAN JOURNAL OF MEDICINE* 99:651–661. Copyright 1995 by Excerpta Medica, Inc.)

criteria were not applied uniformly, and the number of admissions increased.

Conclusion.—Protocol use significantly shortened the time the patient spent in the emergency room and resulted in longer periods of remission. There was a significant cost benefit that accompanied these clinical benefits.

▶ The medical care for asthma and chronic obstructive pulmonary disease is expensive. In 1 study that measured the cost in 1989, the authors calculated $500 million for the total expenditure, of which 30% was spent on drugs. Actually, this is quite interesting because in most cases drug costs are 10%, but let's accept their figures. One way to reduce cost and maintain quality is to devise a therapeutic plan for, in this case, the emergency room. In the best of these protocols, the patient care and decisions about that are paramount in the analysis. Although money is not a primary measure, there can be significant savings with application of the guidelines.

I have one small nit to pick with the authors of this study. In the graph of the asthma protocol (see Fig 1), the arrow between MICU and discharge should, I think, have 2 arrowheads; 1 that goes back to MICU, the other to discharge. That is a small thing, however, in the larger and more important picture for this protocol.

M. Weintraub, M.D.

Compliance With Inhaled Asthma Medication in Preschool Children
Gibson NA, Ferguson AE, Aitchison TC, et al (Royal Hosp for Sick Children, Glasgow, Scotland; Univ of Glasgow, Scotland)
Thorax 50:1274–1279, 1995   5–3

Background.—Many young children with asthma are using large-volume spacers. School-age children have poor compliance with inhaled prophylactic asthma therapy, particularly when more than 2 daily doses are prescribed. Asthmatic preschool children differ from older children in that their parents either administer their asthma therapy directly or supervise it closely. The impact of parental supervision of drug administration on compliance in children with asthma was assessed.

Methods.—Twenty-nine asthmatic children, aged 15 months to 5 years, who were using a metered-dose inhaler with a large-volume spacer for prophylactic asthma medication were studied. The children were receiving various drug regimens. For each drug administration through the inhaler, the date and time were recorded by an electronic timer. The parents were asked to record the child's symptoms and medication compliance using diary cards.

Results.—The median percentage of study days on which the patient was fully compliant with asthma medication was only 50%. A median of 77% of prescribed doses was administered. Compliance was worse for children in day care. There was no relationship between the prescribed frequency of medication and the children's symptom scores. Compliance was not significantly different for children on 2-, 3-, or 4-times daily regimens.

Conclusions.—Asthmatic preschool children have low levels of compliance with prophylactic inhaled medication, even though their parents supervise their therapy closely. The compliance programs probably play a key role in the difficulty of controlling asthmatic symptoms in preschool children. Further studies should specifically examine drug compliance in preschool children and the factors influencing it.

▶ Failure of an anti-asthmatic medication to relieve symptoms is unwelcome and frustrating when the fault lies in the drug or the inhaler, but failure resulting from poor compliance on the part of the patient or relatives is maddening.

L. Lasagna, M.D.

How Patients Determine When to Replace Their Metered-dose Inhalers
Ogren RA, Baldwin JL, Simon RA (Scripps Clinic and Research Found, La Jolla, Calif)
Ann Allergy Asthma Immunol 75:485–489, 1995   5–4

Introduction.—The rates of asthma morbidity and mortality are increasing. The use of metered-dose inhalers beyond their specified maximum number of actuations has been proposed as a contributing factor in this trend. To examine this potential factor, patients with asthma were surveyed regarding their awareness of the manufacturers' specifications and methods of determining when to replace their inhalers.

Methods.—During a 1-year period, 63 patients with asthma between the ages of 10 and 84 years were surveyed. All of the surveyed patients were using at least 1 metered-dose inhaler. The survey addressed their awareness of the specified maximum number of actuations and their methods of determining when to replace their inhaler. In addition, various metered-dose inhalers were tested to determine the number of actuations contained beyond the specified maximum number of actuations and the flotation status of fully actuated canisters.

Results.—Fewer than half (46%) of the patients were aware of the manufacturer's specified maximum number of doses in their canisters. Most (73%) used physical methods (assessing weight, force, or taste) to determine when to replace their inhaler. The flotation method was used by only 8%. Only 8% counted the number of actuations and replaced the inhaler when the recommended maximum actuations were used. In 11%, a backup inhaler was kept and used when the expected response from the first inhaler dose did not occur.

The flotation method was not an accurate method of determining that the maximum number of actuations had been reached. There was great variation in the number of actuations possible in the inhalers beyond the recommended maximum.

Conclusions.—Most of the surveyed patients used inaccurate and potentially dangerous methods of determining when to replace their metered-dose inhaler. These common practices may contribute to the increased risk of asthma morbidity and mortality and warrant further study.

▶ Many patients use aerosol inhalers badly. It is hard to be helped by an inhaler with an exhausted drug supply.

L. Lasagna, M.D.

Outpatient Treatment of Adult Asthma

Kleerup EC Tashkin DP (Univ of California, Los Angeles)
West J Med 163:49–63, 1995   5–5

Background.—Asthma is a common disease that carries a major cost in terms of restricted activity. The morbidity and mortality of asthma appear to have been increasing, whether because of changes in the disease, environment, or population; unrecognized effects of the drugs used for asthma; or failure to adopt treatment recommendations. Most asthma management takes place on an outpatient basis under the direction of primary care physicians. Recent recommendations for asthma therapy were reviewed to develop a stepped approach to the outpatient management of adult asthma.

Asthma and Asthma Treatment.—The mechanisms of asthma are complex and incompletely understood, involving interactions between respiratory, inflammatory, and neural cells and their mediators. Asthma therapy seeks to prevent or relieve symptoms, to permit normal activities of daily living and exercise, to restore or maintain pulmonary function, to avoid adverse treatment effects, and to minimize inconvenience and cost to the patient. The principles by which these goals are achieved are patient education, assessment and monitoring of asthma severity, avoidance or control of factors that trigger asthmatic attacks, establishment of a plan for routine and exacerbation management, and regular follow-up care.

Stepped Approach.—Therapy is initially tailored to the severity of the patient's symptoms, then increased or decreased as indicated. Decisions about anti-inflammatory therapy are based on the patient's signs, symptoms, or lung function abnormalities. Patients with moderate-to-severe disease should receive initial treatment for acute exacerbation, followed by aggressive maintenance therapy with subsequent increments or reductions in therapy. Low-dose maintenance therapy is indicated for patients with milder asthma, who may also use a short-acting β_2-agonist before exercise or exposure to triggering factors. Some patients with severe asthma may need 24-hour-a-day bronchodilator therapy. All patients should have medications to treat acute exacerbations, usually a short-acting β_2-agonist and oral prednisone. Asthma is a lifelong disease for many patients, and close attention is needed to recognize situations in which disease control is deteriorating or there is a chance to reduce drug therapy.

Summary.—A stepped approach to therapy is recommended for the outpatient management of asthma in adults, emphasizing the use of anti-inflammatory therapy, such as inhaled corticosteroids, cromolyn sodium, and nedocromil sodium. Acute exacerbations, complicating factors, asthma in pregnancy, preparation for surgery, and times when to refer to a specialist also need to be considered.

▶ This thorough review is impossible to abstract properly. Read the original in its entirety

L. Lasagna, M.D.

Inadequate Outpatient Medical Therapy for Patients With Asthma Admitted to Two Urban Hospitals

Hartert TV, Windom HH, Peebles RS Jr, et al (Johns Hopkins Univ, Baltimore, Md)
Am J Med 100:386–394, 1996   5–6

Introduction.—In the United States, the incidence and mortality of asthma have increased. Those who reside in the inner cities, particularly the poorer populations, are at high risk for asthma morbidity and the prevalence is higher among blacks than whites. Factors contributing to the increase in asthma among urban populations may include overcrowded living environments, deteriorated dwelling facilities, indoor allergens, and dysfunctional families. The National Asthma Education Program Expert Panel sponsored by the National Heart, Lung, and Blood Institute published guidelines in 1991 to help physicians and patients in managing asthma. A survey was conducted 1 year later to determine whether management of asthma followed these guidelines.

Methods.—The cross-sectional survey included 101 patients with asthma who were admitted to a hospital with an asthma exacerbation. Within 48 hours of admission, the patients were surveyed with a validated questionnaire about their chronic outpatient medical management and the measures that were taken to alleviate the asthma symptoms that led to their hospitalization.

Results.—For this group of patients, the average asthma admission rate was 2.5, which was indicative of moderate to severe disease. Inhaled anti-inflammatory therapy was prescribed for less than half these patients. Only 11% of the patients who had been shown the metered-dose inhaler technique by a health care professional could perform this technique correctly. A physician had outlined an action plan in the event of an acute exacerbation for only 28% of the patients. No changes were made in the treatment regimen for 60% of the patients who contacted their physician during the exacerbation that preceded admission. The average β-agonist metered-dose inhaler use during the 24 hours before admission for those whose exacerbation lasted at least 24 hours was 44.8±7.8 puffs. The most significant correlates of inhaled β-agonist use during this period were older age, current smoking, and black race.

Conclusion.—In this population of inner-city patients, asthma management was marked by underuse of anti-inflammatory therapy, inadequate communication between patient and physician regarding an action plan, inability to use the inhalation device properly, and inadequate physician intervention. The guidelines must be addressed more carefully by physicians to reduce asthma morbidity in the urban United States.

▶ This study helps in understanding why asthma therapy is not efficacious, particularly in blacks, and why the mortality rate is increasing. The components of the National Asthma Education Program (NAEP) are really very important, and also very achievable. However, only 11% of the patients in this study administered a multidose inhaler correctly on all 5 components. Another problem was the use of β-agonists rather than steroids or cromolyn in appropriate patients. Importantly, there was no action plan discussed by the patients and physicians. Aggressive treatment by doctors for exacerbations also was not provided. Unfortunately, physicians are not following the NAEP guidelines, and that may be one factor involved in the care of these poorly educated inner-city patients. A group of colleagues, in discussing the NAEP guidelines, said it was not a matter of deciding what was the optimal therapy, but getting the patients to physicians who could teach and monitor them. We do not teach those skills in medical school. Doctors really do have to pick them up on their own, and I am not sure they can.

M. Weintraub, M.D.

Budesonide Inhaled via Turbuhaler: A More Effective Treatment for Asthma Then Beclomethasone Dipropionate via Rotahaler

Tjwa MKT (De Wever Hosp, Heerlen, The Netherlands)
Ann Allergy Asthma Immunol 75:107–111, 1995   5–7

Background.—Chlorofluorocarbon-propelled metered dose inhalers are being replaced by dry powder inhalers as agents used in the treatment of asthma. The effects of 2 inhaled glucocorticosteroids in dry powder inhalers—budesonide, delivered by Turbuhaler, and beclomethasone dipropionate (BDP), delivered by Rotahaler—were compared.

Methods.—Sixteen adults with moderately severe asthma were enrolled in the randomized, crossover study that consisted of 2 8-week treatment periods. Inhaled steroid treatment was stopped for 4 weeks at the end of the study. Before the study, treatment consisted of inhaled steroids at a median dose of 0.60 mg/day. During the study, treatment consisted of 0.20 mg twice a day. Peak expiratory flow rate was determined twice a day; lung function, every 4 weeks; and airway responsiveness, before and after each treatment period.

Findings.—A significant deterioration of lung function, airway responsiveness, and symptoms occurred during the steroid-free washout period in the 12 patients who completed the study. This period had to be shortened for 5 patients. The mean morning peak expiratory flow during budesonide therapy was significantly higher than during BDP therapy. Airway responsiveness improved 1.1 doubling concentrations after budesonide, but declined 0.3 doubling concentrations after BDP. The difference between values after the 2 treatments was 1.4 doubling concentrations. The improvement in forced expiratory flow in 1 second was slightly greater during budesonide than BDP therapy; the difference was 4.3% predicted. Most patients said that the budesonide Turbuhaler was more effective and easier to use than the BDP Rotahaler (Fig 1).

Conclusions.—Budesonide delivered by Turbuhaler appears to be more effective than BDP delivered by Rotahaler. The local potency of budes-

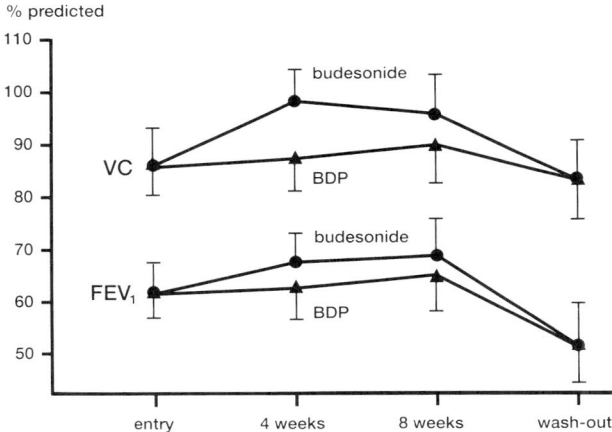

FIGURE 1.—Forced expiratory vital capacity and forced expiratory volume in 1 second, as percentage of predicted before and after 4 and 8 weeks treatment with budesonide via Turbuhaler (*circles*) and beclomethasone dipropionate via Rotahaler (*triangles*), and after a 4-week washout period (mean ± SEM). *Abbreviations:* VC, vital capacity; FEV_1, forced expiratory volume in 1 second, BDP, beclomethasone. (Courtesy of Tjwa MKT: Budesonide inhaled via Turbuhaler: A more effective treatment for asthma than beclomethasone dipropionate via Rotahaler. *Ann Allergy Asthma Immunol* 75:107–111, 1995.)

onide is greater than that of BDP, and the Turbuhaler deposits more drug particles in the lung than Rotahaler.

▶ The Pulmocort Turbuhaler is scheduled for FDA approval in 1996 and should be a boon for patients with asthma in the United States. (European asthmatics have benefitted from its virtues for some years.)

The advantage seems to lie less on the steroid present than on the delivery system, which is actuated by breaths rather than relying on the right timing of breath and drug delivery from pressurized metered-dose inhalers. As a result, the Turbuhaler deposits more drug particles in the lung. It's not surprising that the patients in the trial overwhelmingly preferred the Turbuhaler.

L. Lasagna, M.D.

Eosinophil Activity Reflects Clinical Status in Patients With Asthma Before and During a Prednisolone Course

Skedinger M, Halldén G, Lundahl J, et al (Karolinska Hosp, Stockholm)
Ann Allergy Asthma Immunol 75:250–255, 1995   5–8

Rationale.—Asthma is becoming increasingly common in the Western world. Either excessive or insufficient treatment may cause harm. A simple means of evaluating the current activity of asthma would be therapeutically useful. Because asthmatic inflammation typically involves eosinophils, it seems logical to monitor eosinophil activity. A technique of cell membrane permeabilization now is available for use in conjunction with flow cytometry to estimate eosinophil activity.

Objective and Methods.—Asthmatic symptoms were correlated with eosinophil activity in 9 patients whose asthma had become worse and was believed to warrant a course of orally administered steroid therapy. Twenty-two healthy nonallergic individuals also were studied. Serum levels of eosinophilic cationic protein (ECP) were measured by radioimmunosorbent assay. The expression of intracellular ECP was determined by cell flow cytometry using a monoclonal antibody against activated ECP.

Findings.—Initially, 4 patients had more than 6% eosinophils in the peripheral blood, and 5 had elevated serum ECP levels. Seven of the 9 patients had increased intracellular ECP. During prednisolone treatment, the percentage of eosinophils decreased in all patients but 1. Only 1 patient continued to have an elevated serum ECP level, and intracellular ECP values did not differ from those in controls. All patients were less symptomatic during steroid treatment. In particular, nocturnal symptoms were less prominent. Several patients had higher peak expiratory flow values when restudied during treatment.

Conclusion.—Monitoring eosinophilic activity may well prove useful in estimating the value of asthma treatment.

▶ It seems clear that inhaled corticosteroids are better for asthmatics than are oral steroids, but some patients seem to need "topping off" with oral steroids during exacerbations.

To avoid or decrease toxicity, it would be desirable to give "enough" steroid by mouth but not "too much." As airway inflammation is now generally thought to lead to deterioration in asthma control, we could use a simple test to measure airway inflammation. Because eosinophilic granulocytes characterize asthmatic inflammation, and it is well accepted that the eosinophil level in peripheral blood correlates with the severity of asthma, and secreted ECP in serum has been reported to correlate as well (although denied by others), this research makes a lot of sense. I hope others will study this approach.

L. Lasagna, M.D.

Beta-2 Agonists in Asthma
The Thoracic Society of Australia and New Zealand (Alfred Hosp, Melbourne, Australia; Concord Hosp, Sydney, Australia; Royal Children's Hosp, Melbourne, Australia)
Aust N Z J Med 25:358–361, 1995   5–9

Purpose.—The results of recent epidemiologic studies have raised controversy about the role and safety of β-agonist treatment for patients with asthma. Results showing a higher incidence of asthma mortality and poorer disease control in patients using fenoterol have led to questions about a possible class effect for all β-agonists and about the use of the new, longer-acting preparations. Toward making clear recommendations regarding the use of β-agonists in asthma, the available data on this topic were reviewed.

Recommendations.—On the basis of the literature, a number of recommendations for the reasonable use of β-agonists in asthma can be made. Patients who are using their β-agonist metered-dose inhalers with increasing frequency may be experiencing a change in disease severity. As such, they should receive a thorough review of their treatment. Because high-dose β-agonist therapy carries significant risks, including both adverse reactions and theoretical risks, the β-agonist dose should be kept as low as possible to maintain symptom control. For patients with stable asthma, appropriate bronchodilation can be achieved using metered-dose inhalers with spacer devices or dry powder inhalers. Thus nebulized β-agonists should be used only in case of emergency, or in patients with unstable asthma. Most patients will achieve better control of asthma with "on-demand" rather than regular use of β-agonists.

The available data suggest that nonselective β-agonists should not be used, even in reduced doses. The only indication for epinephrine and other such agents is to avoid potential cardiac stimulation in life-threatening asthma or asthma caused by anaphylaxis. The new long-acting β-agonists warrant careful postmarking surveillance to ensure that any adverse impact on morbidity or mortality is identified. These new agents should not be given as monotherapy, and the patients who use them should receive regular follow-up with a respiratory physician.

Discussion.—All recommendations in this study meet the suggested guidelines for asthma treatment of the American, British, and Australian Thoracic Societies. Controlled trials are needed to establish the role of short- and long-acting regular β-agonists in the treatment of patients with chronic stable asthma.

▶ This position paper by the Thoracic Society of Australia and New Zealand is a wise primer and provides advice similar to that given by thoracic societies in the United Kingdom and the United States.

L. Lasagna, M.D.

Theophylline: Potential Antiinflammatory Effects in Nocturnal Asthma
Kraft M, Torvik JA, Trudeau JB, et al (Univ of Colorado, Denver)
J Allergy Clin Immunol 97:1242–1246, 1996   5–10

Introduction.—Theophylline may have an antiinflammatory role in the treatment of asthma. Animal trials have shown that theophylline is able to block cellular influx into the lungs and alter cellular activity. Worsening of nocturnal asthma has been associated with increased cellular influx into the lungs and cellular activation. The potential antiinflammatory effect of theophylline was prospectively evaluated in 8 patients with nocturnal asthma.

Methods.—Theophylline was administered once daily at 7:00 PM using a randomized, double-blind, placebo-controlled, crossover design. Treatment periods were 2 weeks each and were separated by a 1-week washout period. At the end of each treatment period, patients underwent spirometry at 3:30 AM and bronchoscopy with bronchoalveolar lavage (BAL) at 4:00 AM.

Results.—At completion of the placebo period, the mean awakening decrement in FEV_1 was 26.6%. With theophylline, the mean percent fall in overnight FEV_1 was significantly improved to a mean awakening decrement in FEV_1 of 10.4%. There was also a significant and inverse correlation between 4:00 AM theophylline level and overnight fall in FEV_1. There were no significant between-group differences in 4:00 AM BAL cell count in regard to total white blood cell count or percentages of macrophages, lymphocytes, or eosinophils. Seven of 8 patients receiving theophylline had a significant greater than 10% decrease in the neutrophil infiltrate into the lavage fluid, compared to placebo. There was a significant correlation between decrement in BAL neutrophils and serum theophylline concentration. Leukotriene B_4 (LTB_4) levels from macrophages obtained from BAL fluid fell significantly with theophylline, compared to placebo. The theophylline-induced change in LTB_4 was significantly correlated with a decrease in BAL granulocytes. There were no significant between-group changes in thromboxane β_2 levels.

Conclusion.—Overnight lung function in asthma was improved with theophylline administration. This improvement was associated with suppressed alveolar macrophage LTB_4 production, decrement in BAL neutrophils, and correlation between theophylline-induced decreases in LTB_4 and decrement in BAL granulocytes.

▶ When a colleague of mine mentioned some years ago that he felt that theophylline had antiinflammatory effects, I remember saying "Mmm-hmm" and then going home and thinking about it. He said that somebody should study the drug on nocturnal asthma, particularly cough, which patients with asthma have, particularly at night. Well, somebody has done that. You can judge for yourself how far the field has advanced in the years since this colleague of mine mentioned the effects of theophylline on inflammation.

M. Weintraub, M.D.

Bone Mineral Density and the Risk of Fracture in Patients Receiving Long-term Inhaled Steroid Therapy for Asthma
Toogood JH, Baskerville JC, Markov AE, et al (Victoria Hosp, London, Ont, Canada; Univ of Western Ontario, London, Ont, Canada; Inst of Phthisiatry and Pulmonology, Kiev, Ukraine; et al)
J Allergy Clin Immunol 96:157–166, 1995   5–11

Introduction.—For moderate or severe asthma, the current treatment of choice is inhaled steroid therapy. However, there are concerns about the safety of this therapy. Long-term orally administered steroid therapy has been associated with a high incidence of osteoporosis. Inhaled steroids have been shown to have an adverse effect on bone turnover, but the clinical importance of these metabolic changes is not established. Therefore, the effects of inhaled and orally administered steroid treatment on bone density were studied in a cross-section survey of patients with asthma representing a wide range of drug exposures.

Methods.—Data on drug usage were obtained from the clinical records of a nonrandom sample of 69 patients with asthma, selected to represent patients with low, medium, and high exposures to both inhaled and orally administered steroid drugs. Bone density was measured at the lumbar spine with dual-energy x-ray absorptiometry or dual-energy photon absorptiometry and was reported in absolute densities and as z scores (standard deviations from the normal predicted bone density determined for age and sex). Evidence of vertebral fracture or nonosseous clinical stigmata of hypercortisonism was also determined.

Results.—Both nonosseous stigmata of chronic hypercortisonism and vertebral wedge fracture with biconcave deformity were significantly associated with reduced lumbar bone mineral density and low lumbar bone mineral density z scores (LBMD-Z). Significant decreases in LMBD-Z were seen in association with the duration of past orally administered steroid therapy and with the current daily dose of inhaled steroid. However, the LBMD-Z value increased in association with a higher cumulative lifetime dose of inhaled steroid, greater physical activity, age, female sex, and years of estrogen therapy.

Conclusions.—Long-term use of inhaled steroid drugs is associated with normal or nearly normal bone density and minimal increase in the risk of fracture. Therefore, long-term inhaled steroid therapy may increase bone density and reduce the risk of fracture in patients with prednisone-dependent asthma, even those with a long history of orally administered steroid use, current high daily doses of inhaled steroids, or both. Supplemental estrogen therapy may also preserve normal bone density in postmenopausal women, even with prolonged exposure to orally administered and inhaled steroid therapy.

▶ This paper reinforces the belief that inhaled corticosteroids are safer than oral steroids, as one might expect on the "magic bullet" vs. the "buckshot" approach to asthma. On the other hand, the inhalation route is not free of trouble, so that the daily dose should be kept as low as possible. Most patients in this study seemed to be well controlled by steroid doses less than 2 mg/day.

L. Lasagna, M.D.

Dose-related Decrease in Bone Density Among Asthmatic Patients Treated With Inhaled Corticosteroids

Hanania NA, Chapman KR, Sturtridge WC, et al (Univ of Toronto)
J Allergy Clin Immunol 96:571–579, 1995   5–12

Introduction.—Anti-inflammatory medications, primarily inhaled corticosteroids, are increasingly being used as the initial treatment of symptomatic asthma. However, because most patients with asthma require long-term therapy, there are concerns about systemic absorption and side effects. To assess possible side effects of long-term inhaled corticosteroid therapy, bone density and biochemical markers of bone turnover and adrenal function were compared in 2 groups of patients with asthma.

Methods.—Thirty-six patients with asthma in 2 age- and sex-matched groups were studied. Group A included patients who had been using inhaled steroid therapy for at least 1 year. Group B included patients who had never been treated with either inhaled or orally administered steroid medication. Serum osteocalcin, calcium, phosphate, and alkaline phosphatase levels were measured. Bone mineral density was measured with dual-energy x-ray absorptiometry at the lumbar spine, the left femoral neck, and Ward's triangle. A cosyntropin test was used to assess adrenal function.

Results.—Group A had significantly lower levels of serum osteocalcin. No significant differences were found in the other biochemical markers of bone turnover. Suppressed baseline serum cortisol levels were found in 4 patients and decreased serum cortisol levels were found after stimulation with adrenocorticotropic hormone in 3 patients, all in group A, whereas all patients in group B had normal baseline and stimulated cortisol levels. Bone density measurements were significantly reduced in group A for the femoral neck but not for the lumbar spine or Ward's triangle. In group A only, there were significant correlations between baseline and stimulated serum cortisol levels and the bone density at all 3 sites.

Conclusions.—Patients with asthma who are managed with long-term inhaled corticosteroid therapy may have reduced bone density and adrenal suppression, suggesting that these drugs are absorbed systemically. The reduced serum osteocalcin levels in these patients suggests that suppression of osteoblast function may play a role in the reduction of bone density. Further study is needed to evaluate the potential of serum cortisol measurement as a marker for susceptibility to decreased bone density after inhaled steroid therapy.

▶ Here's another study on inhaled corticosteroids and bone density. This one, too, found a dose-related effect on bone density.

L. Lasagna, M.D.

6   Blood Disorders

Aspirin Therapy: Optimized Platelet Inhibition With Different Loading and Maintenance Doses
Buerke M, Pittroff W, Meyer J, et al (Johannes Gutenberg-Univ, Mainz, Germany)
Am Heart J 130:465–472, 1995   6–1

Background.—Low doses of aspirin inhibit platelet thromboxane formation, but high doses are associated with an increased risk of gastrointestinal bleeding. Some clinical situations, such as unstable angina or myocardial infarction, benefit from a high aspirin loading dose and rapid platelet aggregation. Sixty-four healthy men took part in a study designed to determine the precise effect of loading doses and maintenance doses of aspirin.

Methods.—The volunteer participants had a mean age of 28 years. None had a history of aspirin sensitivity or any abnormal findings from physical examination or blood tests. Participants were randomized into 8 groups receiving either placebo or aspirin (40, 100, 300, or 500 mg) as a loading dose for the first day. During the remaining 14 days of the study period, the men took either placebo or 40 or 100 mg/day of aspirin. Blood samples were obtained at baseline and at 5 additional times to assess the effects of aspirin on platelet aggregation, bleeding time, and thromboxane synthesis.

Results.—All volunteers completed the study without experiencing aspirin-related side effects or other complications. The bleeding time was prolonged significantly 2 hours after administration of the 2 highest loading doses of aspirin. The entire group had a mean initial bleeding time of 6.1 minutes; this increased at 2 hours to 10.1 minutes in the 300-mg group and to 11.3 minutes in the 500-mg group. The bleeding time was also prolonged at 24 hours with loading doses of 100, 300, and 500 mg but not with 40 mg of aspirin. Collagen-induced platelet aggregation was significantly inhibited 2 hours after the first administration of 100, 300, and 500 mg aspirin; the 300- and 500-mg loading doses inhibited serum thromboxane B_2 synthesis by more than 99% at 2 hours. Blood samples obtained at 14 days showed significant prolongation of bleeding times and significant inhibition of collagen-induced platelet aggregation and serum thromboxane B_2 synthesis for the various aspirin dose combinations.

Conclusions.—The combination of a 300-mg loading dose of aspirin and a 40-mg daily maintenance dose significantly reduced platelet thromboxane synthesis and effectively inhibited platelet aggregation during a 14-day period. Higher loading or maintenance doses offered no additional advantage, whereas the lower dose regimens failed to rapidly and effectively inhibit platelet aggregation. The 300/40-mg combination should help in avoiding aspirin-related side effects.

Transdermal Modification of Platelet Function: An Aspirin Patch System Results in Marked Suppression of Platelet Cyclooxygenase
McAdam B, Keimowitz RM, Maher M, et al (Royal College of Surgeons, Dublin)
J Pharmacol Exp Ther 277:559–564, 1996   6–2

Background.—Aspirin is an effective antithrombotic, inhibiting platelet cyclooxygenase and preventing thromboxane A_2 production. However, it may induce gastrointestinal (GI) toxicity, even at low doses. The feasibility of delivering aspirin transdermally was investigated.

Methods.—Two patch systems were investigated, 1 without (type A) and 1 with (type B) the permeation enhancer limonene. In 1 investigation, 2 type A patches were applied daily for 14 days to 10 healthy volunteers (6 men and 4 women), aged 23 to 59 years. In another investigation, 1 type B patch was applied daily for 14 days to 9 men, aged 22 to 61 years. In 4 of these men, patch application was extended to 21 days.

Findings.—Daily application of 2 type A patches with a total surface area of 100 cm^2 containing 84 mg per patch reduced serum thromboxane B_2 (TXB_2) in the 6 men by day 14. In the women, serum TXB_2 suppression was less pronounced. An analysis of the residual drug in the patch demonstrated that each patch delivered 18 mg on day 1 and 17 mg on day 14, comparable in women and men. In the 9 men studied in the second investigation, daily application of a single patch B with a 50-cm^2 surface area and containing 120 mg of aspirin resulted in 60% suppression of serum TXB_2 by day 14 and 84% by day 21. Patch B delivered 33 mg of aspirin daily. Analysis of aspirin and salicylate in plasma detected no aspirin. Plasma salicylate by day 14 was 157 ng/mL with patch A and 133 ng/mL with patch B. In an analysis of aspirin applied by patch to the skin in 3 subjects, marked hydrolysis to the inactive product, salicylic acid, was demonstrated.

Conclusions.—A platelet cyclooxygenase-suppressing dose of aspirin can be delivered transdermally by patch. The rate of delivery is low, reflecting hydrolysis of the drug in the skin. The permeation enhancer limonene improves delivery. This novel route of delivery may minimize the risk of GI toxicity and be applicable to other antithrombotic agents.

▶ The first paper shows the importance of a loading dose with aspirin to rapidly achieve a biochemical effect. The 40-mg loading dose was really quite ineffective, whereas a 100-mg or 300-mg dose was more effective in achieving suppression of platelet cyclooxygenase. However, the Dutch TIA Trial Study had a 0.9% fatal bleeding result using 30 mg of aspirin.[1] That is why the second group of investigators attempted to give the aspirin transdermally at very low doses. And, in fact, they were able to suppress platelet cyclooxygenase. They also wanted to separate COX-1 and COX-2 on the basis of the low dose. COX-1 is an enzyme located in platelets, in endothelium, and in the stomach and duodenum, where it may account for toxicity. COX-2 may be located in the joints and be associated with the effect on pathology (i.e., arthritis). It is great to realize that almost a century after the discovery of aspirin, so much interesting work is still being done to determine the appropriate doses for various beneficial clinical effects.

M. Weintraub, M.D.

Reference

1. The Dutch TIA Trial Study Group: A comparison of two doses of aspirin (30 mg vs. 283 mg a day) in patients after a transient ischemic attack or minor ischemic stroke. *N Engl J Med* 325:1261–1266, 1991.

Danazol Relieves Refractory Pruritus Associated With Myeloproliferative Disorders and Other Diseases
Kolodny L, Horstman LL, Sevin B-U, et al (Univ of Miami, Fla)
Am J Hematol 51:112–116, 1996   6–3

Background.—Patients with myeloproliferative disorders (MPDs) and other systemic immunologic, dermatologic, and neoplastic disorders frequently experience severe pruritus. Numerous treatments have been used to bring relief, including antihistamines, epinephrine, cimetidine, tricyclic antidepressants, β-adrenergic blockers, and glucocorticoids. However, some patients have refractory pruritus. The promising results achieved in these patients with danazol therapy are reported.

Methods.—Twenty-two patients with chronic pruritus refractory to conventional therapies were studied. The patients included 8 with MPDs, 7 with autoimmune disorders, and 7 with skin diseases. The application of danazol at 400 to 800 mg/day was added to the previous medications for itching. On response, the other medications for itching were tapered and discontinued. After a sustained response, a trial of dosage reduction or discontinuance of danazol was attempted, with the dosage increased or resumed if there was a relapse. The need for long-term therapy was evaluated by discontinuing danazol therapy after a year or more of treatment. Side effects were monitored closely.

Results.—Twelve of the 22 patients (54%) had a response to danazol therapy, including 5 of the 8 patients with MPDs, 3 of the 7 patients with autoimmune disorders, and 4 of the 7 patients with skin disorders. Symptomatic improvement occurred in a mean of 22 days. A trial withdrawal resulted in a relapse in 9 responders, with relief after retreatment with danazol. Similarly, dosage reduction resulted in a relapse in 7 responders, with repeated response after a dosage increase. After at least 1 year of treatment, the patients had sustained remission after danazol was discontinued. Most of the patients tolerated danazol therapy well. Three patients had serious side effects: reduced liver function, skin rash, and both skin rash and worsened liver function test results.

Conclusions.—Danazol appears to be a safe and effective therapy for patients with refractory pruritus associated with many systemic disorders. Larger, controlled, prospective studies are warranted to verify these findings.

▶ It is really remarkable how often doctors who can treat dry mouth, urinary incontinence, dry eyes, thrombosed hemorrhoids, and other minor symptoms can make a patient's quality of life so much better. This is another situation just like those described above in which a new intervention can take over the treatment of pruritus that is refractory to antihistamines, epinephrine, tricyclic antidepressants, glucocorticoids, all the measures for keeping the skin hydrated and soft and smooth, and cooling measures. Close medical follow-up will be required because danazol is an androgen, which may lead to some serious adverse effects. Fortunately, none were seen in the study abstracted here.

M. Weintraub, M.D.

Recombinant Erythropoietin Improves Cognitive Function in Patients Maintained on Chronic Ambulatory Peritoneal Dialysis

Temple RM, Deary IJ, Winney RJ (Royal Infirmary of Edinburgh, Scotland; Univ of Edinburgh, Scotland)
Nephrol Dial Transplant 10:1733–1738, 1995   6–4

Background.—The encephalopathy and intellectual declines observed in patients receiving hemodialysis often are ascribed to hypertension and arteriosclerosis, but uremia and other factors also may contribute. Recent studies of recombinant human erythropoietin (r-HuEPO) treatment in patients receiving hemodialysis have suggested that chronic severe anemia makes a significant but reversible contribution to cognitive dysfunction. Cognitive function, as measured by standard psychometric tests, has been shown to improve in patients receiving hemodialysis who are treated with r-HuEPO. A similar study was performed in patients receiving maintenance chronic ambulatory peritoneal dialysis (CAPD).

Methods.—The study included 17 patients receiving CAPD, 9 of whom received r-HuEPO and 8 of whom did not. The patients in the r-HuEPO group underwent psychometric testing before and after r-HuEPO treatment; their mean hemoglobin level was 9.0 g/dL before treatment and 7.7 g/dL after treatment. The other 8 patients, whose mean hemoglobin level was 7.7 g/dL, were assessed with the same battery of tests. The 2 groups were matched for age, duration of dialysis, and social class. Another test was used to estimate the patients' premorbid IQ.

Results.—After starting r-HuEPO treatment, the current IQ of patients in the treatment group increased by a mean of 7.2 points, approaching the patients' premorbid cognitive function. In contrast, the control group showed a nonsignificant improvement of 0.3 point in current IQ. The r-HuEPO group also showed improvement on a test of concentration and speed of information processing. Memory also tended to improve with r-HuEPO treatment, but the only significant improvement was in delayed recall. No apparent changes were found on a test of attention, ability to sequence, and ability to shift cognitive set.

Conclusions.—In patients receiving CAPD, as in those receiving hemodialysis, anemia appears to make a measurable but reversible contribution to cognitive dysfunction. Treatment with r-HuEPO is followed by improvements in brain electrophysiologic and psychometric variables. With r-HuEPO, uremic cognitive dysfunction may be reversed to near premorbid levels.

▶ We've known for over 150 years about brain dysfunction in uremic patients, but the mechanisms are still elusive. It looks as though anemia is at least a contributing factor and (praise God) is a reversible contributor.

L. Lasagna, M.D.

Angiotensin-converting Enzyme Inhibitors and Higher Erythropoietin Requirement in Chronic Haemodialysis Patients
Dhondt AW, Vanholder RC, Ringoir SMG (Univ Hosp, Gent, Belgium)
Nephrol Dial Transplant 10:2107–2109, 1995   6–5

Purpose.—In patients with chronic renal failure who are not receiving recombinant human erythropoietin (r-HuEPO), circulating erythrocyte counts fall with angiotensin-converting enzyme (ACE) inhibitor treatment. Less is known about the erythropoietic effects of ACE inhibitor treatment on patients undergoing chronic hemodialysis who are receiving exogenous r-HuEPO. Patients receiving chronic hemodialysis were studied to see whether the amount of r-HuEPO they received was related to ACE inhibitor treatment.

Methods.—The cross-section study included 49 patients undergoing hemodialysis who had been receiving r-HuEPO for more than 6 months. Twenty-two patients were receiving antihypertensive treatment with an ACE inhibitor, most commonly lisinopril. Patients who were and were not receiving an ACE inhibitor were compared for dose of administered r-HuEPO, along with other factors.

Results.—Mean r-HuEPO dosage was 56 IU per kilogram per dialysis session in the patients who were receiving ACE inhibitor treatment vs. 36 IU per kilogram per dialysis session in those not receiving ACE. None of the other factors investigated differed between the 2 groups, including hematocrit, ferritin, and transferrin saturation. Hematocrit and r-HuEPO dose at 3 months before the study were not significantly different from the study values.

Conclusions.—Patients undergoing chronic hemodialysis who take an ACE inhibitor need significantly higher doses of r-HuEPO to achieve the same mean hematocrit. It may be that ACE inhibitor treatment reduces responsiveness to erythropoietin, or that the patients' remaining endogenous erythropoietin production is decreased. Whatever the cause, the influence of ACE inhibitors on r-HuEPO activity could have a considerable economic impact.

▶ These data certainly suggest that ACE inhibitors lead to a need for higher doses of EPO in patients on chronic hemodialysis. As this involves added expense (EPO is not cheap), one should ask whether ACE inhibitors are better in some way than other antihypertensives in these patients.

L. Lasagna, M.D.

A Randomized Placebo-controlled Study of Enalapril in the Treatment of Erythrocytosis After Renal Transplantation

Beckingham IJ, Woodrow G, Hinwood M, et al (City Hosp, Nottingham, England; Univ Hosp, Nottingham, England)
Nephrol Dial Transplant 10:2316–2320, 1995   6–6

Background.—Erythrocytosis is a common complication of renal transplantation and is associated with an increased occurrence of thromboembolic events. It is thought that excessive erythropoietin production may be involved in the erythrocytosis, but the exact mechanisms are unknown. The use of angiotensin-converting enzyme inhibitors (ACEIs) has been associated with reduced hematocrit in other settings. The use of ACEIs in patients with erythrocytosis after renal transplantation was evaluated in a randomized, double-blind trial of low-dose enalapril.

Methods.—Twenty-five patients received either 2.5 mg daily of enalapril or placebo for 4 months. There were no serious side effects throughout the study period.

Results.—Hematocrit fell throughout the study in the treatment group and was unchanged in the placebo group. The difference at 4 months between these 2 groups was highly significant. There was no change in serum erythropoietin in either group during this study.

Conclusions.—Low-dose ACEIs are a safe, effective, and noninvasive therapy for erythrocytosis occurring after renal transplantation. The mechanism of action remains unknown.

▶ Erythrocytosis occurs in up to 17% of renal transplant recipients, although, in this study, the total was 7%. The mechanism of action has not been determined for ACEIs and erythrocytosis. However, it remains very interesting to anyone because the discovery of an active chemical, one with biological effects, can open up a whole host of interesting possibilities, including new drug development. In addition, enalapril, through another of its potential mechanisms of action, may prevent pulmonary thromboembolic disease.

M. Weintraub, M.D.

7 Cardiovascular Disorders

Clinicians and Patients With Hypertension: Unsettled Issues About Compliance
Rudd P (Stanford Univ, Calif)
Am Heart J 130:572–579, 1995   7–1

Introduction.—Arterial hypertension in patients who are ambulatory is currently managed most with long-term, orally administered medications. Therefore, maintaining optimal adherence to therapeutic regimens is crucial. There may be several barriers to patient compliance, which may vary over time. These factors and strategies to optimize patient compliance were studied.

Interpreting the Failure to Achieve Blood Pressure Goals.—The prescription of drugs for hypertension is still largely an empirical process. Therefore, when patients fail to achieve their therapeutic goals, it is important to identify the reasons for this failure. The possible reasons include behavioral factors (patient adherence to the regimen), biological factors (related to the disease process), pharmacologic factors (related to pharmacokinetic and pharmacodynamic variances), and combinations. Clinicians will frequently escalate the regimen without accurately determining patient adherence, which could expose the patient to dangerously excessive dosages if the patient is hospitalized or if patient compliance improves.

Frequency of Dosing.—Studies have shown that patient compliance is higher with once-daily dosing than with multiple daily dosing. However, patients who miss a once-daily dose may experience subtherapeutic drug concentrations. In addition, abrupt changes in drug concentrations in patients with poor compliance could result in special toxicities.

Realistic Interventions.—Successful interventions to improve patient compliance should include 3 features: individualization, multifactorial components, and continual or periodic reinforcement. Empirical trials have shown that fear tactics and education about the pathophysiologic course of hypertension or treatment mechanics are ineffective. In contrast, successful strategies include simplifying the regimen, tailoring the regimen to the patient's routines with links to daily tasks, providing increased supervision, setting explicit goals, and providing feedback.

Conclusions.—Physicians treating patients with hypertension with long-term medications given orally must consider patient compliance when prescribing or adjusting regimens, because treatment success largely depends on the patient's adherence to the prescribed regimen.

▶ Peter Rudd is one of the leaders in the coterie of scientists who have addressed the generic issue of compliance with prescription directions as well as the deleterious effects of the all-too-common failure of patients to follow directions.

Treating hypertension is especially troublesome because the disease is often asymptomatic (until you start taking drugs for it), and treatment needs to be for life to forestall cardiovascular damage well in the future.

Probably half of the diagnosed and treated patients with hypertension in the United States take their drugs properly, a small percentage are terrible at compliance, and more than one third seem to vacillate between perfect compliance and treatment lapses that may last for days. This paper discusses at length some of the intervention options to ameliorate this sorry state of affairs.

L. Lasagna, M.D.

Low-dose Thiazides in the Treatment of Hypertension: Benefits and Risks in Perspective

Silverberg DS, Rotmensch HH, Iaina A (Ichilov Hosp, Tel-Aviv, Israel; Maccabi Health Fund, Tel-Aviv, Israel)
J Hum Hypertens 9:869–873, 1995   7–2

Introduction.—During the past 15 years, because of the variety of newly introduced medications and concerns about the lack of cardioprotective properties, the use of diuretics has declined in the treatment of hypertension. However, recent research has confirmed the efficacy of low-dose thiazides against hypertension and shown their cardioprotective effects.

Effects of Thiazide Therapy.—Low doses of thiazides produce an antihypertensive effect comparable to that of other therapeutic drugs, including angiotensin-converting enzyme (ACE) inhibitors and calcium blockers, with no pseudotolerant reactions. Diuretics are superior to most other drugs in controlling hypertension in patients who are elderly or of African descent or have systolic hypertension. Diuretics have been found to be cardioprotective because they prevent coronary heart disease as well as strokes.

Adverse Effects.—Although higher doses of thiazides can induce peripheral and hepatic insulin resistance or impotence, these effects are rarely seen with lower doses. The low doses also are rarely associated with hypokalemia, hyponatremia, and hypomagnesemia. Although the mean fasting blood sugar may increase slightly, the risk of new-onset diabetes is low. However, patients with established diabetes should be treated first with ACE inhibitors. There may be diuretic-induced hyperuricemia, but deteriorating renal function has not been reported in association with this condition, and gout is a very rare complication. The subjective side effects are dose-related and occur with a similar incidence as those associated with other antihypertensives. No serious adverse reactions or threats to quality of life, mood, or cognitive function are associated with diuretic therapy.

Conclusions.—Properly selected patients with hypertension can be safely and effectively treated with low-dose diuretics, with adequate follow-up, including measurements of blood urea and electrolyte levels. Contraindications include baseline azotemia or diabetes, a history of gout, and concurrent use of ACE inhibitors.

▶ Recommendations about first-line therapy for hypertension vary from year to year and from country to country. Now that we have learned that lower doses of diuretics are just as effective in lowering blood pressure as the higher ones we believed necessary in the old days, and safer, it seems appropriate to consider them as the treatment of choice for many patients, and as probably the most cost-effective antihypertensive remedies.

L. Lasagna, M.D.

Combination Therapy for Systemic Hypertension
Kaplan NM (Univ of Texas, Dallas)
Am J Cardiol 76:595–597, 1995   7–3

Background.—In most patients with hypertension, a single drug in relatively low doses is sufficient initial therapy. In more than one third of these patients, however, initial doses must be increased or a second drug added to control the hypertension. Combination therapy for systemic hypertension was investigated.

Types of Combinations.—When a second drug must be added, it is logical to use a drug from a different class. A diuretic, if not used initially, often will be the drug added, because a diuretic will probably enhance the efficacy of all other classes of antihypertensive drugs. A diuretic may be especially beneficial when volume expansion is a major feature of the hypertension, as in patients with renal insufficiency; when volume expansion is secondary to the reactive sodium retention that may follow the use of many antihypertensive agents, especially centrally acting α-agonists such as clonidine; and in patients whose hypertension is resistant to multiple vasodilatory medications because the dilated vascular bed is refilled with increased volume and the expected decline in blood pressure does not occur. The use of diuretics as the first or second drug of choice, however, has been associated with several problems, including adverse effects on known coronary risk factors. Some of these effects occur only with fairly large doses of diuretics.

Effects of Treatment on Overall Risk Status.—Optimal treatment of patients with hypertension must include an evaluation of concomitant risk factors and the selection of pharmacologic and nonpharmacologic antihypertensive treatment that improves these factors. Both diuretics and β-blockers can adversely affect coronary risk factors.

Combinations Without a Diuretic.—For patients with more significant hypertension, many studies have demonstrated the efficacy of drug combinations that do not include a diuretic. The combined α- and β-receptor blocker labetalol is an effective nondiuretic available as a single molecule. Some combinations are not appropriate, such as a β-blocker with verapamil or diltiazem—calcium antagonists that slow atrioventricular conduction. An especially attractive combination being prescribed today is that of an angiotensin-converting enzyme inhibitor and a calcium antagonist. The combination of an angiotensin-converting enzyme inhibitor and a nondihydropyridine calcium-channel blocker may be especially advantageous for patients with hypertension and diabetic nephropathy and for those with left ventricular hypertrophy.

▶ This paper is not a clinical trial. It is a consideration of a treatment decision by a thoughtful practitioner. It is worth reading in its entirety, but the abstract does it justice.

M. Weintraub, M.D.

Effects of Dietary Calcium Supplementation on Blood Pressure: A Meta-analysis of Randomized Controlled Trials
Bucher HC, Cook RJ, Guyatt GH, et al (McMaster Univ, Hamilton, Ontario, Canada; Univ of Waterloo, Kitchener, Ontario, Canada)
JAMA 275:1016–1022, 1996   7–4

Introduction.—Several lines of evidence suggest an inverse relationship between calcium intake and blood pressure, although observational studies of the effect of calcium on blood pressure have had inconsistent findings. In a systematic overview of the question, randomized controlled trials of the effects of calcium supplementation on systolic and diastolic blood pressure in nonpregnant, normotensive, and hypertensive individuals were analyzed.

Methods.—Trials were identified through a search of Medical Literature Analysis and Retrival System On-Line (MEDLINE) and Excerpta Medica Database (EMBASE) from 1966 to May 1994. Complete texts of these studies were examined for eligibility, and the first authors were contacted for additional data. Participants were required to have been randomized to calcium supplementation or placebo and to have blood pressure measured for at least 2 weeks. Thirty-three articles involving 2,412 patients were eligible for analysis.

Results.—Most of the studies evaluated patients for 4–14 weeks, and 5 had an intervention period of more than 6 months. Pooled analysis revealed statistically significant reductions in systolic (mean, −1.27 mm Hg) and diastolic (mean, −0.24 mm Hg) blood pressure. Differences in treatment effects could not be attributed to any of the possible mediators of blood pressure reduction, nor did it appear that variations were explained by baseline blood pressure. The pooled analysis found statistically significant heterogeneity for the pooled estimate of diastolic blood pressure but not for the estimate of systolic blood pressure.

Conclusion.—Overall, calcium supplementation (1,000–2,000 mg daily) appears to lead to a small reduction in systolic blood pressure. Specific subpopulations, such as pregnant women, may experience more important effects on blood pressure. At present, calcium supplementation would not appear to be useful for patients with mild hypertension.

▶ For more than a decade, it has been repeatedly suggested that dietary calcium affects the blood pressure in an inverse relationship. If true, we need to do something about calcium intake because at least some of our citizens at high risk for hypertension have an inadequate intake of this cation.

L. Lasagna, M.D.

Left Ventricular Systolic Function After Marked Reduction of Ventricular Hypertrophy Induced by 5 Years' Enalapril Treatment
González-Juanatey JR, Reino AP, Acuña JMG, et al (Clínico Universitario, Santiago de Compostela, Spain)
Eur Heart J 16:1981–1987, 1995   7–5

Background.—Chronic hypertension typically leads to left ventricular hypertrophy or myocardial remodelling. However, drug-related reductions in blood pressure do not correlate with regression of hypertrophy, and there has been little study of changes in left ventricular systolic function in relation to antihypertensive treatment. Therefore, the effects of long-term treatment with an angiotensin-converting enzyme inhibitor on left ventricular mass and function were studied prospectively in patients with essential hypertension.

Methods.—Twenty-eight previously untreated patients with essential arterial hypertension received treatment with enalapril for 5 years. Echocardiography was done and blood pressure was measured at rest and during exercise before treatment; after 8 weeks and 1, 3, and 5 years of treatment; and 8 weeks after treatment was stopped.

Results.—Blood pressure, both at rest and during exercise, decreased significantly by 8 weeks after treatment began, after which time there were no further statistically significant changes during treatment. Blood pressure then increased to baseline levels by 8 weeks after treatment was stopped. The left ventricular mass index decreased progressively during treatment, whereas fractional fiber shortening and ejection fraction increased progressively during 5 years of treatment. These results were maintained 8 weeks after treatment was stopped.

Conclusions.—Treatment of essential hypertension with enalapril for 5 years resulted in regression of left ventricular hypertrophy and improvement in left ventricular systolic function. These improvements were maintained after treatment was stopped, even after blood pressure values increased to pretreatment measurements.

▶ Although left ventricular hypertrophy is at first a rational attempt by the body to cope with hypertension, the hypertrophy eventually leads to heart failure, myocardial ischemia, arrhythmias, and sudden death.

Enalapril seems not only to decrease blood pressure, but also to progressively reduce left ventricular hypertrophy with some actual improvement in left ventricular systolic function. The provocative additional finding in this study is the maintenance of these improvements during 8 weeks without treatment despite a return of blood pressure to pretreatment values. Fascinating!

L. Lasagna, M.D.

The Efficacy and Tolerability of Enalapril in a Formulation With a Very Low Dose of Hydrochlorothiazide in Hypertensive Patients Resistant to Enalapril Monotherapy
Guul SJ, Os I, Jounela AJ (Vejle Hosp, Denmark; Ullevål Univ, Oslo, Norway; Deaconess Hosp, Oulu, Finland)
Am J Hypertens 8:727–731, 1995   7–6

Introduction.—The combination of an angiotensin converting enzyme inhibitor with low-dose hydrochlorothiazide (HCTZ) appears to reduce the adverse metabolic effects caused by HCTZ as it enhances the antihypertensive qualities of the inhibitor. A multicenter study of patients with essential hypertension not adequately controlled with enalapril alone was designed to determine the lowest tolerable and effective dose of HCTZ in combination with enalapril.

Methods.—The study recruited 402 patients from 29 centers in Denmark, Finland, and Norway. Those who entered the double-blind phase of the trial had persistent supine diastolic blood pressure (DBP) of 95 mm Hg or higher after an 8-week course of enalapril (20 mg once daily). Nonresponders were randomized to 20 mg enalapril/placebo (98 patients), 20 mg enalapril/6 mg HCTZ (99 patients), or 20 mg enalapril/12.5 mg HCTZ (99 patients) for another 8-week period. Data recorded during follow-up included heart rate, blood pressure, and the results of blood tests and urinalysis.

Results.—All 3 treatment groups exhibited significant reductions in supine DBP during the 8-week period. At all timepoints, the mean reductions were significantly larger for the HCTZ groups than for the enalapril monotherapy group. No significant differences were noted between the 6 mg and 12.5 mg HCTZ groups. Analysis of reductions in supine systolic blood pressure and standing blood pressure yielded similar results. Upon completion of the study, the rate of response was 55% for enalapril alone, 69% for enalapril/6 mg HCTZ, and 73% for enalapril/12.5 mg HCTZ.

Response was defined as supine DBP of lower than 95 mm Hg or a reduction of 5 mm Hg or more. With systolic blood pressure of lower than 95 mm Hg or a reduction of 10 mg Hg or more, response rates for the 3 treatment groups were 42%, 61%, and 62%, respectively. No serious laboratory or clinical adverse events were attributed to treatment.

Conclusion.—A very low daily dose of HCTZ (6 mg) given in conjunction with enalapril (20 mg daily) significantly reduced blood pressure in patients with essential hypertension who had failed to respond to enalapril monotherapy. Neither dose of HCTZ caused adverse metabolic effects, but the smaller dose adequately enhanced blood pressure control.

▶ The best thing about this study is the demonstration that low doses of hydrochlorothiazide are effective without metabolic consequences. The dose of hydrochlorothiazide is really quite interesting. It started off relatively high at 100 mg and later at 50 mg, but then was lowered to 25 mg and then lowered again to 12.5 mg and lowered again to 6 mg. It may even have an effect at doses lower than that.

M. Weintraub, M.D.

Short Acting Dihydropyridine (Vasodilating) Calcium Channel Blockers for Hypertension: Is There a Risk?
Beevers DG, Sleight P (City Hosp, Birmingham, England; John Radcliffe Hosp, Oxford, England)
BMJ 312:1143–1145, 1996   7–7

Background.—Properly randomized and blinded trials involving patients with hypertension were conducted to show that thiazide diuretics and beta-blockers prevent myocardial infarction and stroke, and reduce mortality. However, newer medications such as the calcium channel blockers and angiotensin-converting enzyme inhibitors have not been so tested because of the considerable difficulty, expense, and ethical dilemmas involved. Instead, studies involving these drugs have used surrogate end points such as reduction of blood pressure or left ventricular hypertrophy, or reduction of microproteinuria or macroproteinuria. Surrogate end points should not be relied on, however, when surveillance or case-control studies throw up evidence of possible harm; mortality data from randomized trials must be sought.

Dilemma.—Disturbing data were released after a retrospective case-control study of patients with hypertension: patients treated with calcium channel blockers had more heart attacks than those treated with beta blockers. Furthermore, the risk of myocardial infarction increased with higher doses of calcium channel blockers. Data from 3 observational reports prompted the United States National Heart, Lung, and Blood Institute to issue a warning statement to physicians (1995) stating that short-acting nifedipine should be used with caution, if at all. Later, an advisory committee to the Food and Drug Administration declared most calcium channel blockers to be safe for use in patients with hypertension, but indicated that short-acting nifedipine should not be used in patients with unstable angina or hypertension.

Outlook.—Calcium channel blockers differ considerably from each other; trials involving patients with ischemic heart disease suggest that if left ventricular dysfunction is absent and if a calcium channel blocker is needed nonacutely, verapamil and diltiazem are the preferred choices. Avoiding the use of short-acting formulations such as nifedipine in high doses appears sensible. Urgent need exists for proper large-scale trials of calcium channel blockers in hypertension.

▶ This paper reports a worrisome member of the series of epidemiologic evaluations of short-acting calcium channel blockers (CCBs). Caplan and Gifford[1] reviewed the importance of the initial therapy choice in hypertension. They recommend that individualization of therapy should be encouraged to provide the greatest benefit with the fewest adverse events at the lowest cost. The FDA has made a judgment that the short-acting CCBs should not be taken off the market despite the results of the first round of these studies. The FDA faced a difficult problem because the fact that there is a wide range of medications for hypertension means that patients will have a greater choice and that physicians can choose the most appropriate drug for each patient. I do not know how this one is going to play out. We all need to stay tuned.

M. Weintraub, M.D.

Reference

1. Caplan NM, Gifford RW: Choice of initial therapy for hypertension. *JAMA* 275:1577–1580, 1996.

Discordance Between Meta-analyses and Large-scale Randomized, Controlled Trials: Examples From the Management of Acute Myocardial Infarction
Borzak S, Ridker PM (Henry Ford Hosp, Detroit; Harvard Med School, Boston)
Ann Intern Med 123:873–877, 1995   7–8

Introduction.—An ever-increasing number of clinical treatments are available, each supported by different types of clinical data. In the face of all this information, meta-analysis—a statistical technique to combine the results of different studies—has become useful in planning definitive trials. In some situations in which definitive trials are lacking, the results of meta-analysis have been used as a basis for decision making. The results of meta-analyses are often confirmed by subsequent studies; in other situations, however, the results of large-scale clinical trials have disagreed with those of preceding meta-analyses. Possible reasons for these disagreements were explored, using the examples of nitrate and magnesium therapy for acute myocardial infarction.

Nitrate and Magnesium Therapy.—In both examples, meta-analytic studies suggested that the treatments in question were efficacious for patients with acute myocardial infarction. This prompted large-scale clinical trials to test the hypotheses. Two trials of nitrate therapy found no significant reduction in mortality. One large trial of magnesium therapy did show a mortality benefit, but a subsequent trial did not. In the studies of nitrate therapy, difficulty in deciding which trials should be included in meta-analyses may have arisen from improving mortality rates and changing treatment strategies. Also, although meta-analyses may be considered "analytic" or "exploratory," they can in no way be considered experimental. In the instance of magnesium therapy, the issue is further complicated because the "fixed-effects" and "random-effects" models of meta-analysis found different estimates of the treatment effects. The difference in the results of the 2 clinical trials highlights the inability of meta-analytic techniques to resolve pathophysiologic issues.

Discussion.—The results of meta-analyses, even analyses of high statistical quality, can be misleading. Changes in medical practice, differences in study populations, and bias related to study selection can all contribute to conflicting results between meta-analyses or between meta-analyses and subsequent clinical trials. In using meta-analyses, the clinician should remember that these analyses can primarily generate—not test—hypotheses. If the meta-analysis is viewed as the prelude to a randomized clinical trial, then the differing results look less like discrepancies and more like the findings of an experiment whose results disagreed with its hypothesis.

▶ Meta-analysis needs both increased attention and increased critique. Such pooling of studies and continued analysis can lead to correct conclusions at times, and incorrect ones at other times.

L. Lasagna, M.D.

Translation of Clinical Trials Into Practice: A European Population-based Study of the Use of Thrombolysis for Acute Myocardial Infarction
European Secondary Prevention Study Group (Leicester Royal Infirmary, England)
Lancet 347:1203–1207, 1996   7–9

Introduction.—Thrombolytic treatment has been accepted as an important part of the standard management of acute myocardial infarction for the past 7 years. Controlled trials of 50,000 or more patients have resulted in precise estimates of treatment efficacy and risk. Nevertheless, only a minority of patients with acute myocardial infarction receive a thrombolytic drug on admittance to the hospital, with estimates ranging from 23% in the United States to 49% in the United Kingdom. To see how a shared knowledge base is interpreted in various health care systems, representative samples of patients admitted with acute myocardial infarction in 11 European regions were drawn.

Methods —A sample of 4,035 patients who were diagnosed with acute myocardial infarction and who were discharged from or died in the hospital was evaluated. A review of the medical records revealed the observed rate of thrombolytic use. A shortfall was defined as the proportion of patients who had no contraindication but did not receive a thrombolytic.

Results.—Thrombolytic treatment was used in a median of 36% of the patients, with a range of 13% to 52%. Three groups were identified among untreated patients: those causing diagnostic difficulty on admittance to the hospital or lacking ECG criteria for treatment; those with no apparent reason for withholding thrombolytic treatment, who were considered to comprise the shortfall and who accounted for 20%; and those whose symptom onset was more than 12 hours before admittance to the hospital. Older patients and women were less likely to receive thrombolytic treatment, according to logistic regression analysis in all patients without contraindications. In the clinical trials of thrombolytic therapy for acute myocardial infarction, older patients and women were underrepresented.

Conclusion.—A thrombolytic drug is given to only about one third of patients admitted to a European hospital with acute myocardial infarction. The maximum rate of thrombolysis is about 55%, allowing for delays to presentation and difficulty of early diagnosis. In the elderly, the lower use of thrombolytic treatment may result from their underrepresentation in the clinical trials. For women, however, the lower use of thrombolysis has no explanation. If the shortfall of 20% were abolished, up to 55% of patients admitted with acute myocardial infarction could receive thrombolytic treatment.

▶ This paper based on representative samples of patients from 11 European regions, reveals that a minority, about 36%, of patients actually received thrombolytic therapy. I have often wondered why clinical trials are not accepted readily by a population of doctors. In some cases, the problem may be that the patients in the study are not reflective of those seen by various physicians. However, that is probably not the case in these studies. A second reason may be that toxicity occurs in the general populations. Again, that does not seem to be the case here. The most important factor, which I think is operating here, is that some of the doctors are not up to date on the literature and are not aware of the trials. The physicians do not make a judgment to withhold thrombolytic therapy, they make an error.

The fact that women and elderly patients were underrepresented in this survey is very worrisome. The authors say that the small number of older patients may have been due to chance. However, the failure to include women is very indicative of what happens in many trials, and in many other settings where women are not treated in their proper proportion of the population. More women should be included in the trials. But, more important, we have to change the attitude of the physicians who are actually treating the patients and referring them to participate in clinical trials.

M. Weintraub, M.D.

Neutralising Antibodies After Streptokinase Treatment for Myocardial Infarction: A Persisting Puzzle
McGrath K, Hogan C, Hunt D, et al (Royal Melbourne Hosp, Parkville, Australia)
Br Heart J 74:122–123, 1995   7–10

Rationale.—Streptokinase (SK) is a bacterial protein that induces the formation of antibodies that can cause allergic changes. Neutralizing antibody may counter and even abolish thrombolytic activity. Patients who survive myocardial infarction may require ongoing thrombolytic therapy, and agents other than SK are relatively expensive.

Methods.—Antibody titers were monitored in 104 patients given a standard dose of 1.5×10^6 U of SK. No patient had previously received SK, and none of the patients received steroids. Fifty-three patients provided single serum samples 54 to 84 months after dosing, and 51 were tested at least once from 6 to 33 months after treatment. Twenty-seven patients from the coronary care unit who were not given SK served as a control group.

Results.—Sera from controls had a mean SK neutralizing capacity of 0.17×10^6 IU. Neutralizing antibody titers in SK-treated patients did not differ significantly from control values 2 years after treatment.

Implications.—Streptokinase might provide effective thrombolysis as early as 2 years after a single dose. More information on patency after standard doses of SK in patients with increased neutralizing antibody titers are needed before recommending retreatment.

▶ I do not know which physicians would be brave enough to attempt treatment with SK in a patient only on the basis of a laboratory result of a low neutralizing antibody. One could say that all a patient with a heart attack needs is a severe allergic reaction. Still, it is very interesting and very important to figure out whether a patient can receive SK a second time after a certain period has passed. Streptokinase continues to be much cheaper than tissue plasminogen activator, although the outcome may be not quite as good.

M. Weintraub, M.D

Comparisons of Characteristics and Outcomes Among Women and Men With Acute Myocardial Infarction Treated With Thrombolytic Therapy

Weaver WD, White HD, Wilcox RG, et al (Univ of Washington, Seattle; Green Lane Hosp, Auckland, New Zealand; Queen's Med Ctr, Nottingham, England; et al)

JAMA 275:777–782, 1996   7–11

Introduction.—Some studies comparing outcomes among women and men have found that women have higher rates of morbidity and mortality after acute myocardial infarction. A large, randomized, controlled trial compared baseline characteristics, complications, and outcomes in men and women treated with thrombolytic therapy after acute myocardial infarction.

Methods.—Participants were enrolled in the Global Utilization of Streptokinase and Tissue Plasminogen Activator for Occluded Coronary Arteries (GUSTO-I) trial. The patients, 30,653 men and 10,315 women, were drawn from 1,081 hospitals in 15 countries; 56.3% were from the United States. All had symptoms of acute infarction beginning 6 hours or less before randomization and the ECG finding of ST elevation. Each patient received 1 of 4 thrombolytic regimens: streptokinase with subcutaneous heparin; streptokinase with IV heparin; streptokinase plus alteplase, a tissue-type plasminogen activator, with IV heparin; or accelerated alteplase with IV heparin. The risk of death and stroke were compared after adjustments for baseline differences between men and women.

Results.—Compared with men, women were 7 years older, on average, and arrived at the hospital a median of 18 minutes later after symptom onset. Women also had higher age-adjusted incidences of diabetes and a history of hypertension and smoking. Overall, women had a significantly higher 30-day mortality than men (11.3% vs. 5.5%), and most of the excess mortality was attributed to older age. The age difference also contributed to an increased incidence of strokes among women (2.1% vs. 1.2% for men). Women continued to have a slight excess risk of mortality after adjustment for baseline characteristics. They also had a significantly higher incidence of certain nonfatal complications after treatment: shock, congestive heart failure, serious bleeding, and reinfarction. Alteplase was more beneficial in both men and women, decreasing mortality and nonfatal stroke. Differences in rates of angioplasty (35% for women; 32% for men) and bypass surgery (9% for men; 7% for women) were slight.

Conclusion.—In the GUSTO-I trial, in which previous treatment imbalances between men and women were corrected, women were at greater risk of both fatal and nonfatal complications after receiving thrombolytic therapy for acute myocardial infarction.

▶ The mortality rate of women with an acute myocardial infarct is higher than that of men, perhaps because this disease is manifested in women approximately 10 years later than in men.

This study involved female patients with baseline characteristics such as to render them representative of only 20% to 30% of all women hospitalized for acute heart attacks. Nevertheless, it is disturbing if women who receive thrombolytic therapy are really at greater risk of both fatal and nonfatal complications. Can we change this for the better in any way?

L. Lasagna, M.D.

Dietary Antioxidant Vitamins and Death From Coronary Heart Disease in Postmenopausal Women
Kushi LH, Folsom AR, Prineas RJ, et al (Univ of Minnesota, Minneapolis; Univ of Miami, Fla; Univ of Pittsburgh, Pa)
N Engl J Med 334:1156–1162, 1996   7–12

Background.—Because oxidative modification of low-density lipoprotein may promote atherosclerosis, the role of dietary antioxidant vitamins in the prevention of coronary heart disease (CHD) is of great interest. The relation between dietary antioxidant vitamins and death from CHD in postmenopausal women was investigated.

Methods.—A total of 34,486 postmenopausal women with no cardiovascular disease who completed a questionnaire early in 1986 were included. The questionnaire elicited information on the intake of vitamins A, E, and C from food sources and supplements. Two hundred and forty-two women died of CHD during the about 7 years of follow-up.

Findings.—Vitamin E intake appeared to be inversely related to the risk of death from CHD after adjustment for age and dietary energy intake. This relation was especially evident in a subgroup of 21,809 women who did not consume vitamin supplements. This inverse association persisted, with relative risks of 1.0, 0.70, 0.76, 0.32, and 0.38 from the lowest to the highest quintiles, respectively, after adjustment for possible confounders. Although there was little evidence that vitamin E intake from supplements was related to a reduced risk of death from CHD, the effects of high-dose supplementation and the duration of supplement use could not be addressed definitively. The risk of death from CHD apparently was unassociated with vitamin A or C intake.

Conclusions.—The intake of vitamin E from food appears to be inversely related to the risk of death from CHD in postmenopausal women. This risk may be reduced without using vitamin supplements. Vitamin A and C intake was uncorrelated with a lower risk of death from CHD.

▶ As I have already pointed out in this particular volume of the YEAR BOOK OF DRUG THERAPY, you do need to follow your grandmother's advice, especially if she told you to eat a diet that contained lots of vitamins from food. You do not have to be crazy to eat this diet, but just make sure you eat plenty of nuts, a concentrated source of vitamin E. Actually, it is a real interesting thing about eating food as opposed to taking vitamin supplements. It may be that the food contains something else besides the pure vitamin. Food may contain small amounts of very potent substances. Or, we may not absorb all the vitamine from food, and that might be a boon compared to supplements. Of course, your grandmother also should be listened to in terms of not smoking, wearing your seat belt, and even wearing a helmet when riding your bicycle.

M. Weintraub, M.D.

Effects of Antioxidant Vitamins C and E on Signal-averaged Electrocardiogram in Acute Myocardial Infarction
Chamiec T, Herbaczyńska-Cedro K, Ceremużyński L, et al (Grochowski Hosp, Warsaw, Poland)
Am J Cardiol 77:237–241, 1996   7–13

Background.—It has been suggested that oxygen-free radicals may induce injury that causes ventricular late potentials. Ventricular late potentials have been seen in patients after acute myocardial infarction (AMI) and during exercise-induced myocardial ischemia; they are a risk factor for ventricular tachycardia and sudden cardiac death. The hypothesis that supplementation with vitamins C and E could decrease the risk of late potentials by decreasing oxygen-free radical production was tested in a prospective, randomized trial.

Methods.—Sixty-one patients with AMI were randomly assigned to receive either conventional treatment alone or conventional treatment plus vitamins C and E. Signal-averaged electrocardiography (SAECG) was performed within 48 hours of the AMI and repeated between days 9 and 13. Leukocyte chemiluminescence, to assess oxygen-free radical production, was performed within 48 hours of the AMI and repeated between days 12 and 14.

Results.—In the control patients, repeated SAECG demonstrated significantly increased mean total QRS and low-amplitude signal durations and decreased root-mean-square voltage of the last 40 msec of the QRS. In contrast, these values were all relatively stable in the intervention group. The final SAECG revealed significant differences between the groups in these values and late potentials present in 8 patients in the intervention group, compared with 14 control patients. Late potentials at the final SAECG did not correlate with any clinical characteristics. The leukocyte chemiluminescence values decreased significantly between measurements in the intervention group but remained relatively unchanged in the control groups, reflecting a significant difference between the 2 groups at the final measurement.

Conclusions.—Supplementation with the antioxidant vitamins C and E decreased oxygen-free radical production in leukocytes and modified abnormal SAECG parameters. Supplementation with vitamins C and E may thus protect against myocardial injury caused by reactive oxygen metabolites in patients with acute myocardial ischemia and infarction. These findings require confirmation with a larger number of patients.

▶ This study was done because the investigators hypothesized that the antioxidant vitamins C and E could prevent ECG changes related to oxygen-free radicals in patients with AMI. It looks as though they were right. Should all patients who have heart attacks receive vitamins C and E prophylactically? Why not?

L. Lasagna, M.D.

Usefulness of Antioxidant Vitamins in Suspected Acute Myocardial Infarction (The Indian Experiment of Infarct Survival-3)
Singh RB, Niaz MA, Rastogi SS, et al (Med Hosp and Research Ctr, Moradabad, India)
Am J Cardiol 77:232–236, 1996   7–14

Background.—Previous studies have shown the protective effects of antioxidants against free radical production. Free radicals have been shown to be involved in reperfusion-induced damage and lipid peroxidation during acute myocardial infarction (AMI). Therefore, the effects of combined antioxidant vitamins on plasma levels, cardiac enzymes, oxidative stress, and complications were evaluated in patients with suspected AMI.

Methods.—A total of 125 patients with a clinical diagnosis of suspected AMI with onset within 24 hours were randomly assigned to receive either supplements of vitamins A, C, E, and β-carotene (63 patients) or placebo tablets (62 patients) orally for 28 days. The patients were monitored with 12-lead electrocardiography for 4–5 days. Laboratory data were analyzed during clinical follow-up and after 28 days. Clinical observations and complications were noted during the first 28 days.

Results.—Compared with the control group, the antioxidant group demonstrated greater decreases in serum glutamic oxaloacetic transaminase and lipid peroxides and a smaller increase in lactate dehydrogenase cardiac enzyme. As reflected by these changes in cardiac enzymes, the levels of gram-equivalent creatine phosphokinase and creatine phosphokinase-MB, and changes in the ECG findings, the antioxidant group demonstrated significant reductions in the infarct size, compared with the control group. The antioxidant group also had a significantly lower incidence of angina pectoris, poor left ventricular function, cardiac deaths, and re-infarction.

Conclusions.—Supplementation with vitamins A, C, E and β-carotene resulted in less cardiac necrosis, decreased infarct size, and a significant decrease in adverse cardiac events, suggesting than antioxidants provide myocardial protection by preventing cell death.

▶ Like the previous abstract, this one suggests that vitamin therapy can be useful in patients with AMI, but has the added merit of showing not just ECG changes but also important clinical benefit.

L. Lasagna, M.D.

A Randomised, Double-blind, Placebo-controlled Trial of L-Carnitine In Suspected Acute Myocardial Infarction

Singh RB, Niaz MA, Agarwal P, et al (Med Hosp and Research Centre, Moradabad, India; Univ of Tennessee, Knoxville)
Postgrad Med J 72:45–50, 1996   7–15

Background.—Normally, high concentrations of carnitine are found in cardiac muscle. However, carnitine deficiency occurs in the myocardium during acute myocardial infarction, particularly in the infarcted portion of the myocardium. Carnitine administration has been shown to have significant benefits in patients with recent myocardial infarction. The effect of L-carnitine administration on cardiac enzymes and lipid peroxides was studied in a randomized, double-blind, placebo-controlled trial.

Methods.—Patients with suspected acute myocardial infarction with symptom onset within 24 hours were randomly assigned to receive either L-carnitine 51 patients) or placebo (50 patients). Venous blood samples were obtained at baseline, every 4 hours for 24 hours, every 6 hours for 24 hours, and then daily for 8 days and analyzed for creatine kinase (CK) and its muscle-brain (MB) fraction, lactate dehydrogenase, aspartate transaminase, and lipid peroxides. Electrocardiographic assessment was performed at baseline and on days 3, 7, and 10 of treatment. Clinical data were also collected on cardiac events.

Results.—The myocardial infarct size was significantly reduced in the carnitine group, compared with the placebo group, as indicated by CK and CK-MB levels and QRS scores on the electrocardiograms. The cardiac enzymes and lipid peroxides were comparable in the 2 groups at baseline, but were significantly more reduced by carnitine treatment. Compared with the placebo group, the carnitine group had significantly fewer cases of angina pectoris, class III and IV left ventricular function, total arrhythmias, nonfatal infarction, and cardiac deaths.

Conclusions.—Carnitine supplementation significantly reduced the cardiac enzymes and lipid peroxides, indicating less cardiac necrosis and reduced infarct size. This effect was associated with fewer cardiac events and complications.

▶ This study was done in India and, therefore, may not apply to the United States. Carnitine deficiency is more common in poorer countries. Secondary carnitine deficiency may cause the accumulation of fatty acids, which can be toxic to the cardiac cell membranes. However, in this study, treatment with carnitine diminished angina pectoris related to left ventricular dysfunction, cardiac arrhythmias, and a variety of other causes. I think that physicians should give aspirin, a proven therapy, immediately after myocardial infarction, then they can worry about whether to add carnitine.

M. Weintraub, M.D.

Cost-effectiveness of Prescription Recommendations for Cholesterol-Lowering Drugs: A Survey of a Representative Sample of American Cardiologists
Gaspoz J-M, Kennedy JW, Orav EJ, et al (Univ Hosp, Geneva; Univ of Washington, Seattle; Brigham and Women's Hosp, Boston; et al)
J Am Coll Cardiol 27:1232–1237, 1996   7–16

Background.—Guidelines for the prescription of cholesterol-lowering drugs have been published, but little is known about the national prescription practices of physicians and how they compare with the recommendations of cost-effectiveness analyses. The cost-effectiveness of cardiologists' recommendations for the pharmacologic treatment of hypercholesterolemia was investigated.

Methods and Findings.—Three hundred forty-six cardiologists responded to a survey. The respondents were considered to be reasonably representative of the membership of the American College of Cardiology. Twelve hypothetical patients were described on the survey. The cardiologists recommended pharmacologic treatment more often for patients with conditions for which previously published studies estimated treatment to be more cost-effective. However, cardiologists tended to recommend such treatment for primary prevention even when its cost was estimated to exceed $100,000/year of life saved.

Conclusions.—Cardiologists' pharmacologic recommendations for lowering lipid concentrations appear to reflect published cost-effectiveness analyses. However, recommendations still vary markedly, with somewhat less aggressive therapy for secondary prevention and more aggressive therapy for primary prevention than is recommended by cost-effectiveness analyses.

▶ Consensus guidelines are not necessarily followed by practicing physicians, sometimes with good reason. Expert groups don't necessarily come to correct conclusions. This article indicates that some doctors seem to believe that, even though it costs more than $100,000, saving a year of life is justification for treatment. For patients in this situation, I suspect that their agreement or disagreement would be strongly affected by who pays for it.

L. Lasagna, M.D.

Cholesterol Lowering and the Use of Healthcare Resources: Results of the Scandinavian Simvastatin Survival Study

Pedersen TR, for the Scandinavian Simvastatin Survival Study Group (Aker Hosp, Oslo, Norway; Fredriksberg Hosp, Copenhagen; Hvidovre Hosp, Copenhagen; et al)
Circulation 93:1796–1802, 1996   7–17

Background.—Advances in the treatment of cardiovascular disease have unfortunately resulted in higher costs. The impact of treatment to lower cholesterol on healthcare resources was investigated.

Methods and Findings.—Data for the analysis were obtained from the Scandinavian Simvastatin Survival Study, which was a randomized, double-blind, placebo-controlled trial. In the trial, simvastatin decreased the risk of death by 30% during a mean 5.4 years in patients with previous myocardial infarction or stable angina pectoris as a result of a 42% decrease in the risk of coronary deaths. Nine hundred thirty-seven of 2,223 patients in the placebo group had 1,905 hospitalizations for acute cardiovascular events or coronary revascularization procedures. Seven hundred twenty of the 2,221 patients in the simvastatin group had 1,403 such hospitalizations. The corresponding numbers of hospital days in the 2 groups were 15,089 and 9,951, respectively. In the United States, these reductions would translate to a hospital cost savings of $3,872 per patient, which would decrease the cost of simvastatin by 88% to $0.28 per day.

Conclusions.—Simvastatin has been found to decrease mortality and morbidity in patients with coronary heart disease. In addition, this drug significantly decreases the use of hospital services, which offsets most of the drug's cost.

▶ Inhibitors of HMG coenzyme A are effective in reducing low-density lipoprotein cholesterol. Hence, if the cholesterol theory of atherosclerosis is correct, there should be fewer cardiovascular events in patients treated with one or another of these "statins." And indeed, that is what seems to be the case.

The drawback is the cost—the statins are not cheap. The analysis concludes that such treatment substantially reduces the cost of cardiovascular disease, to a degree that offsets a large part of the drug's cost. For a change, ethics, good medical care, and economics are in agreement.

L. Lasagna, M.D.

Design, Rationale, and Baseline Characteristics of the Prospective Pravastatin Pooling (PPP) Project—A Combined Analysis of Three Large-scale Randomized Trials: Long-term Intervention With Pravastatin in Ischemic Disease (LIPID), Cholesterol and Recurrent Events (CARE), and West of Scotland Coronary Prevention Study (WOSCOPS)

Furberg C, for the PPP Project Investigators (Bowman Gray School of Medicine, Winston-Salem, NC)

Am J Cardiol 76:899–905, 1995   7–18

Background.—The Prospective Pravastatin Pooling (PPP) project, begun in 1992, was designed to investigate the effects of pravastatin on all-cause and coronary mortality as well as total coronary events in special populations and to confirm long-term safety. The objectives of the PPP project, the studies included in it, the baseline characteristics of the study populations, outcome events definitions, and the power to test the study hypotheses were described.

The PPP Project.—The project includes data from 3 large, placebo-controlled, randomized trials—the Long-Term Intervention With Pravastatin in Ischemic Disease trial, the Cholesterol and Recurrent Events trial, and the West of Scotland Coronary Prevention Study. All have common design features, including drug, dose, and duration. Two thousand of the study participants, or 10%, are women. At study entry, 1,841 individuals were aged 70 years or older. More than 6,000 have a total cholesterol level of less than 5.5 mmol/L. The mean low-density lipoprotein cholesterol level among the study participants is 4.2 mmol/L, and the mean blood pressure is 134/81 mm Hg. Twenty percent of the participants are current smokers. Previous myocardial infarction is documented in half of the participants. More than 7% of the participants have a history of diabetes; 26% have a history of hypertension. Data on about 1,100 deaths from coronary artery disease (CAD), 500 non-CAD deaths, and more than 1,000 cancers will probably be available for analysis. With a pooled population of 19,768 patients and about 100,000 patient-years of follow-up, the PPP project should have enough power to determine the effects of treatment on total and CAD mortality and cancer incidence and to determine the effects of treatment on total CAD in the elderly, in women, in patients with diabetes, and in patients with lower serum cholesterol levels.

Conclusions.—The PPP is a prospective collaborative study involving 3 ongoing, long-term, large-scale, monotherapy trials of pravastatin. The large size of the study population provides the statistical power needed to test the study hypotheses about the effects of pravastatin on mortality from different causes and in important patient subgroups.

▶ There are many drawbacks to merging the Cholesterol and Recurrent Events and Long-Term Intervention With Pravastatin in Ischemic Disease studies with the West of Scotland Coronary Prevention Study because the patient characteristics are not the same at baseline. All of the patients in the Cholesterol and Recurrent Events study have had a myocardial infarction, as have most of the patients in the ischemic disease study. However, none of the patients in the Scottish study have had a myocardial infarction. In addition, as s common in Europe, their cholesterol level is much higher (a mean of 27? mg/dL), and these men from Scotland are much thinner than individuals i⁻ the other 2 studies.

Still, this very interesting paper lays out many important goals. The main benefit will ze the opportunity to test women, who make up about 10% of the participants; the elderly (those 70 years of age or older), who make up approximately 8% of the population, and lower cholesterol levels. I hope that there will be enough patient-years of study to tell us about cancer risk as well as the risk of accidents and violent death in the participants with lower cholesterol levels. Although some individuals might complain about the need for placebo groups in these studies, I believe that the questions under investigation are so important that a placebo group is necessary.

M. Weintraub, M.D.

Drug Therapy for Hypercholesterolemia in Patients With Cardiovascular Disease: Factors Limiting Achievement of Lipid Goals
Schectman G, Hiatt J (Milwaukee VA Med Ctr Med College of Wisconsin)
Am J Med 100:197–204, 1996   7–19

Background.—In the revised National Cholesterol Education Program (NCEP) guidelines, more aggressive diet and drug treatments are recommended for patients with cardiovascular disease. However, clinicians may be unable to help their patients achieve the target low-density lipoprotein (LDL) cholesterol levels recommended because cholesterol-lowering treatments have adverse effects that make compliance difficult. The ability of lipid-lowering drug therapy to achieve target LDL cholesterol levels in patients with cardiovascular disease followed up for 12 months or more was investigated.

Methods.—Two hundred forty-four consecutive patients with coronary artery disease or peripheral vascular disease were analyzed retrospectively. This cohort had been treated for hypercholesterolemia at a large veterans affairs medical center. Target LDL cholesterol levels were 130 mg/dL or less, and target triglyceride levels were 200 mg/dL or less.

Findings.—With lipid-lowering drug treatment, LDL cholesterol was reduced from 25% to 42% below baseline in patients with mild to severe hypercholesterolemia. This treatment enabled about 75% of patients with LDL cholesterol levels of 160 mg/dL or less to achieve their lipid goal. However, less than 50% of those with baseline LDL cholesterol values exceeding 160 mg/dL reached their target lipid values. In a multivariate analysis, variables that predicted the attainment of goal lipid levels were lower baseline LDL cholesterol and triglycerides, the use of drug combinations rather than monotherapy, and compliance with therapy.

Conclusions.—The effective use of current lipid-reducing drugs apparently still will not achieve the NCEP recommended lipid levels in many patients. To reach these goals, patients will often need combinations of cholesterol-reducing drugs, which will necessitate the frequent use of bile-acid sequestrants and niacin. New strategies for improving tolerance and compliance are greatly needed.

▶ These authors seem to have a low threshold for calling hypercholesterolemia "mild"; they define it as 130–160 mg/dL, which many people would consider trivially elevated.

Getting patients to take unpleasant drugs for a prolonged period of time to forestall or prevent far-off harm is always going to be difficult. The statins, although more expensive than niacin or bile-acid sequestrants, should be more tolerable.

L. Lasagna, M.D.

Cholesterol-lowering Therapy After Heart Transplantation: A 12-Month Randomized Trial
Pflugfelder PW, Huff M, Oskalns R, et al (Univ of Western Ontario, London, Canada)
J Heart Lung Transplant 14:613–622, 1995   7–20

Background.—Hypercholesterolemia is a common postoperative finding in heart transplant recipients. It may play an important role in the genesis and progression of allograft coronary artery disease. The efficacies of gemfibrozil, simvastatin, and cholestyramine for reducing cholesterol levels in heart transplant recipients were compared.

Methods.—Forty-eight patients with moderate hypercholesterolemia after heart transplantation were enrolled in a prospective, 1-year study. By random assignment, 17 patients received gemfibrozil, 600 mg twice a day; 13, simvastatin, 10 mg every day; and 18, cholestyramine, 4 g twice a day. Detailed analyses of lipoproteins were done at baseline and after 3, 6, and 12 months of therapy.

Findings.—After 3 months of simvastatin treatment, the total cholesterol level was decreased by 19% and the low-density lipoprotein (LDL) -cholesterol level by 29%. There was a sustained 25% reduction in total cholesterol level and a 39% reduction in LDL-cholesterol level at 1 year. Neither gemfibrozil nor cholestyramine lowered cholesterol levels. Apolipoprotein B levels were decreased by 29% at 1 year of simvastatin treatment and were unchanged by the other treatments. Gemfibrozil reduced serum triglyceride levels up to 36%, which was significant. The other treatments did not affect serum triglyceride levels. Patients treated with simvastatin and gemfibrozil had an initial increase in high-density lipoprotein cholesterol level. However, this effect was not maintained at 1 year. Simvastatin favorably affected the ratio of LDL to high-density lipoprotein, showing a 38% decrease by 1 year. The other treatments had no such effect. Fourteen patients dropped out of the study during the year—8 because of gastrointestinal intolerance. Four patients receiving gemfibrozil and 10 rece ʌing cholestyramine left the study early. All patients receiving simvastatin completed the study. None of the agents caused biochemical abnormaliti s, or significant changes in cyclosporine blood levels.

Conclusic 1s.—Of the 3 drugs studied, simvastatin most effectively reduced chole terol levels in patients after heart transplantation. The extent of total cho esterol, LDL-cholesterol, and apolipoprotein B reduction associated wi 1 simvastatin in these patients was comparable to that in patients wit hypercholesterolemia who did have a heart transplant. Simvastatin wa also the best tolerated of the 3 agents.

Effect of Pravastatin on Outcomes After Cardiac Transplantation
Kobashigawa JA, Katznelson S, Laks H, et al (Univ of California, Los Angeles; Brigham and Women's Hosp, Boston)
N Engl J Med 333:621–627, 1995   7–21

Background.—Hypercholesterolemia occurs frequently after patients have heart transplantation and is associated with the development of coronary va culopathy in these patients. Inhibitors of 3-hydroxy-3-methylglutaryl co-enzyme A reductase have been found to reduce blood cholesterol level and suppress natural killer cells, which may be involved in the developm nt of acute rejection and coronary vasculopathy. Pravastatin is a 3-hydro y-3-methylglutaryl co-enzyme A reductase inhibitor. Its effects on ser n cholesterol levels, cardiac rejection, survival, and the development c coronary vasculopathy were evaluated in a prospective, randomized, pen-label trial in patients with heart transplants.

Methods.—A total of 97 heart transplant recipients were randomly assigned to rece ve pravastatin or no pravastatin in addition to their immuno-

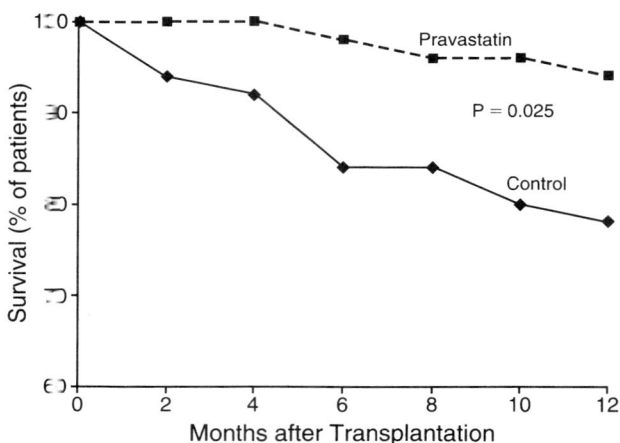

FIGURE 2.—Sur ival during the first year after cardiac transplantation in the study patients. (Courtesy of Kobashigawa J Katznelson S, Laks H, et al: Effect of pravastatin on outcomes after cardiac transplantation. *N Engl J Med* 333:621–627, 1995. Reprinted by permission of the New England Journal of Medicine. ©1995 Massachusetts Medical Society.)

suppressive regimen. The patients were monitored regularly for serum cholesterol levels and for signs of acute rejection. The presence of coronary vasculopathy was determined with coronary angiography and intracoronary ultrasonography performed at baseline and 1 year after transplantation. Peripheral blood natural killer cells were assayed in the last 20 patients randomized to assess immunosuppression in the 2 groups.

Results.—At 1 year after transplantation, the pravastatin group had a significantly lower mean cholesterol level than the control group. Although the 2 groups had a comparable average number of episodes of mild or moderate cardiac rejection, the pravastatin group had significantly fewer episodes of cardiac rejection accompanied by hemodynamic compromise. At l year, 94% of the pravastatin group and 78% of the control group survived (Fig 2). Three patients in the pravastatin group and 7 patients in the control group had angiographic evidence of coronary vasculopathy at 1 year after transplantation. An additional 3 patients from the control group were found to have coronary vasculopathy at autopsy. Intracoronary ultrasonography demonstrated less progression in maximal intimal thickness and the intimal index in the pravastatin group, compared with the control group. The pravastatin group had significantly lower natural killer cell cytotoxicity than the control group.

Conclusions.—Inclusion of pravastatin in the immunosuppression regimen after heart transplantation reduces cholesterol levels and the incidence of major rejection, improves 1-year survival, and limits the development of coronary vasculopathy. The reduction of natural killer cells also suggests that pravastatin increases the immunosuppressive effect of cyclosporine in patients with heart transplants.

▶ These 2 open but randomized studies (Abstracts 7–20 and 7–21) investigated therapy for hypercholesterolemia in patients with heart transplants. Perhaps because of the antirejection medications or other pretransplant factors, hypercholesterolemia is an unfortunate but common event. Previous studies have examined niacin (stopped secondary to hyperglycemia, lovastatin (concern over rhabdomyolysis and increased serum concentration of lovastatin), or probucol. A lack of effect, drug interactions, or adverse effects of the medications have prevented adequate therapy for patients with heart transplants. The first paper (Abstract 7–20) studied gemfibrozil, which lowered triglycerides significantly but did not lower cholesterol levels, and cholestyramine, which had more than 71% of patients dropping out secondary to gastrointestinal intolerance. In addition, simvastatin was tried. It was well tolerated and lowered cholesterol levels with a reasonable adverse-event profile. In contrast, the other paper (Abstract 7–21) studied patients who had just undergone a transplant, not patients 3 years posttransplant, and who had lower cholesterol levels. A larger group of patients was randomly assigned to receive either pravastatin or no therapy. In this group of patients, pravastatin was effective and, as shown in Figure 2, apparently improved survival. It looks as though simvastatin and pravastatin are well tolerated for up to a year with a good effect.

M. Weintraub, M.D.

Sheffield Risk and Treatment Table for Cholesterol Lowering for Primary Prevention of Coronary Heart Disease

Haq IU, Jackson PR, Yeo WW, et al (Royal Hallamshire Hosp, Sheffield, England)
Lancet 346: 467–1471, 1995   7–22

Background.—The use of a hydroxymethylglutaryl-co-enzyme-A reductase inhibitor as secondary prevention for coronary heart disease results in benefits that clearly exceed its risks in patients with a 1.5% or greater risk of coronary death. A logical extrapolation of this to primary prevention of coronary disease can be made, provided that treatment is targeted at patients with a similar or greater risk. A table that refines previously proposed methods of risk prediction was developed.

The Sheffield Risk and Treatment Table for Primary Prevention of Coronary Heart Disease.—In this table, research subjects with the specified degree of coronary risk are identified (Table). The table also shows the serum cholesterol level that confers that degree of risk in the individual and identifies research subjects without this risk, regardless of their cholesterol level. The table can be used easily in clinical practice. The predominant effect of age on coronary risk is highlighted. Some patients with serum cholesterol levels as low as 5.5 mmol/L are candidates for lipid-reducing drug therapy, whereas others with cholesterol levels as high as 9 mmol/L are not candidates.

Conclusions.—Although reducing cholesterol levels is an effective way to prevent coronary events in patients at high risk, cholesterol-level measurement by itself is not a good method for identifying patients at high coronary risk. This method is easily adapted to target a different level of coronary risk as new evidence on treatment risks and benefits becomes available.

▶ This paper is from the United Kingdom; therefore, a higher cholesterol level would be expected to trigger therapy. One has to remember a variety of other things in looking at the table. First, the conversion factor for cholesterol from mmol/L to mg/100 mL is approximately 0.26. Furthermore, the hypertension is defined in the European fashion; therefore, it is higher than on this side of the Atlantic (treatment goal for systolic pressure of 160 mm Hg and, if "not present," blood pressure equivalent to 139 mm Hg, which is the average blood pressure for British men).

Yet this material is really very interesting. It takes into effect the mortality rate of 1.5% per year, and it takes age into effect. It also considers hypertension, smoking, diabetes, and left ventricular hypertrophy. In other words, it tries to assess total cardiac risk. However, it takes a very strong-willed physician (at least, stronger than me) not to treat a smoker with diabetes and a cholesterol level of 9.2 who is younger than 64 years of age. You will really have to think about that one very carefully.

M. Weintraub, M.D.

TABLE—Sheffield Risk and Treatment Table for Primary Prevention of Coronary Heart Disease

Cholesterol concentration (mmol/L) in men

Hypertension	Yes	Yes	Yes	Yes	Yes	Yes	No	No	Yes	Yes	No	No
Smoking	Yes	Yes	Yes	No	Yes	No	Yes	Yes	No	No	No	No
Diabetes	Yes	No	Yes	Yes	No	No	Yes	No	Yes	No	Yes	No
LVH	Yes	Yes	No	Yes	No	Yes	No	No	No	No	No	No
Age (years)												
70	5·5	5·5	5·7	5·9	6·5	6·8	7·2	8·3	8·4			
69	5·5	5·5	5·9	6·1	6·8	7·0	7·5	8·6	8·8			
68	5·5	5·5	6·3	6·4	7·1	7·3	7·8	9·0	9·1			
67	5·5	5·5	6·4	6·7	7·3	7·6	8·1	9·3				
66	5·5	5·5	6·7	6·9	7·7	8·0	8·5					
65	5·5	5·6	7·0	7·2	8·0	8·3	8·8					
64	5·5	5·8	7·3	7·5	8·3	8·6	9·2					
63	5·5	6·1	7·6	7·9	8·7	9·0						
62	5·5	6·3	7·9	8·2	9·1							
61	5·8	6·6	8·3	8·6								
60	6·0	6·9	8·7	9·0								
59	6·3	7·3	9·1									
58	6·6	7·6										
57	7·0	8·0										
56	7·3	8·4										
55	7·7	8·8										
54	8·1	9·3										
53	8·5											
52	9·0											
<52												

Cholesterol concentration (mmol/L) in women

Hypertension	Yes	Yes	Yes	No	Yes	Yes	No	Yes	Yes	No	Yes	No
Smoking	Yes	Yes	No	Yes	No	Yes	No	Yes	No	Yes	No	No
Diabetes	Yes	Yes	Yes	Yes	Yes	No	Yes	No	No	No	No	No
LVH	Yes	No	Yes	No	No	Yes	No	No	Yes	No	No	No
Age (years)												
70	5·5	7·1	7·4	9·0								
69	5·5	7·4	7·7	9·4								
68	5·5	7·7	8·0	9·8								
67	5·6	8·0	8·3									
66	5·8	8·4	8·7									
65	6·1	8·7	9·1									
64	6·4	9·1	9·4									
63	6·6	9·5	9·9									
62	6·9	9·9										
61	7·2											
60	7·6											
59	7·9											
58	8·3											
57	8·7											
56	9·2											
55	9·6											
54	10·1											
<54												

Note: A patient whose value falls in the *unshaded area* has an estimated risk of coronary death of less than 1.5%.
Abbreviation: LVH, left ventricular hypertrophy.
(Courtesy of Haq IU, Jackson PR, Yeo WW, et al: Sheffield risk and treatment table for cholesterol lowering for primary prevention of coronary heart disease. *Lancet* 346:1467–1471, 1995. Copyright by The Lancet Ltd., 1995.)

Usefulness of Beta-blocker Therapy in Patients With Non–Insulin-dependent Diabetes Mellitus and Coronary Artery Disease

Reicher-Reiss H, for the Bezafibrate Infarction Prevention (BIP) Study Group
(Sheba Med Ctr, Tel Hashomer, Israel)
Am J Cardiol 77:1273–1277, 1996   7–23

Background.—Although long-term β-blocker treatment has been shown to reduce mortality, few studies have examined its use in patients with diabetes melitus (DM) and coronary artery disease (CAD). In this high-risk group, β-blockers could have undesirable effects in masking or prolonging hypoglycemia, altering glucose tolerance, increasing lipid blood levels, or worsening congestive heart failure. The long-term effects of β-blocker treatment in diabetic patients with CAD were evaluated.

Methods.—The study used data from the Bezafibrate Infarction Prevention study, an Israeli secondary prevention trail. Of 14,417 patients with CAD who were screened for participation in the trial, 2,723 had non–insulin-dependent DM. One third of this group, or 911 patients, received β-blocker therapy; the remainder of patients did not. These 2 groups were compared for their baseline characteristics and 3-year mortality rates.

Results.—The 3-year overall mortality rate was 8% in the DM patients with CAD who were treated with β-blockers vs. 14% in those who were not, for a 4×% mortality reduction. Similarly, β-blocker use was associated with a =2% reduction in the cardiac mortality rate (Table 2). The 3-year survival curves showed an increasingly divergent difference in mortality (Fig 1). β-Blocker therapy was significantly and independently associated with improved survival on multivariate analysis (relative risk, 0.58). Older patients with DM derived the greatest benefit from β-blocker treatment, along with patients with a history of myocardial infarction, those with limited functional capacity, and lower-risk patients.

TABLE 2—Mortality in Diabetic Patients According to β-Blocker Therapy

	Diabetics	
Mortality	Beta Blockers (n = 911)	No Beta Blockers (n = 1,812)
Total	7.8%*	14.0%
Cardiac	4.9%*	8.4%
Cerebrovascular accident	0.7%	0.8%
Neoplasm	0.5%	0.9%
Other	1.3%	2.4%
Unknown	0.3%	1.3%

*P < 0.05 vs. those not receiving β-blocker therapy.

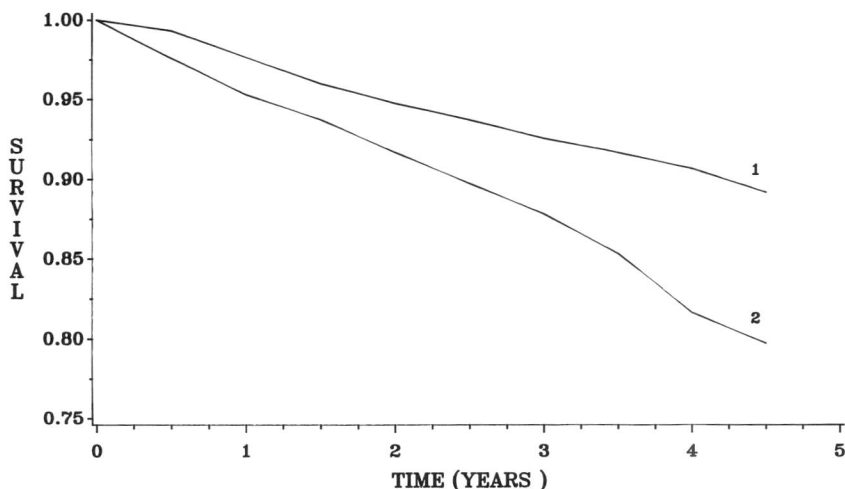

FIGURE 1.—Survival curves for diabetic patients treated with (*1*) or without (*2*) β-blockers. *P* log rank = 0.0001. (Reprinted by permission of the publisher, courtesy of Reicher-Reiss H, for the Bezafibrate Infarction Prevention (BIP) Study Group: Usefulness of beta-blocker therapy in patients with non–insulin-dependent diabetes mellitus and coronary artery disease. *Am J Cardiol* 77:1273–1277. Copyright 1996 by Excepta Medica, Inc.)

Conclusion.—β-Blocker therapy appears to improve long-term survival for patients with non–insulin-dependent DM and CAD. This benefit is especially important because of the poorer long-term survival of this high-risk patient group. Only a randomized, prospective, placebo-controlled trial can settle the controversial issue of whether patients with combined DM and CAD should receive β-blocker therapy.

▶ β-blockers have been shown to be effective in reducing mortality after myocardial infarction, but there has been controversy regarding their use in diabetic patients with coronary artery disease because of the possibility that these drugs may produce undesirable effects, namely, masking or prolonging hypoglycemia, affecting glucose tolerance, increasing blood lipids, or exacerbating congestive heart failure.

Accordingly, this study is a welcome contribution to the debate. It is *not* a randomized trial, but the data are so encouraging that one might question the ethicality of a new controlled trial.

L. Lasagna, M.D.

Pet Ownership, Social Support, and One-year Survival After Acute Myocardial Infarction in the Cardiac Arrhythmia Suppression Trial (CAST)

Friedmann E Thomas SA (Brooklyn College of City Univ of New York; New Life Directions, Ellicott City, Md)

Am J Cardic 76:1213–1217, 1995   7–24

Objective and Methods.—Both social support and owning a pet—an alternative form of social support—reportedly enhance the survival of patients with coronary artery disease. The independent effects of pet ownership, social support, and other psychosocial factors on 1-year survival were examined in patients enrolled in the Cardiac Arrhythmia Suppression Trial. Questionnaires were used to assess social support in 369 participants who had a history of acute myocardial infarction, 30% of whom owned pets.

Findings.—Twenty patients (5.4%) died within 1 year. Logistic regression analysis indicated that both a high level of social support and owning a pet independently predicted survival after controlling for functional status, demographic status, and other psychosocial factors. Only 1 dog owner died, compared with 9 of 282 participants who did not own dogs. Owning a cat also contributed to survival but not as obviously.

Conclusion.—Patients who have had an acute myocardial infarction are likelier to do well if they receive a relatively high level of social support and also if they own a pet, particularly a dog.

▶ I love this article! Before reading it I had no idea of the abundant literature suggesting that having animal pets (a term not liked by animal lovers; I think they prefer "companion animals") helped patients with coronary disease to survive longer This seems especially true for dogs, as opposed to other pets. Why this is so is another story.

I must, however, confess that I have not hurried to buy a dog.

L. Lasagna, M.D.

Triiodothyronine Therapy Lowers the Incidence of Atrial Fibrillation After Cardiac Operations

Klemperer JD. Klein IL, Ojamaa K, et al (New York Hosp-Cornell Univ, New York; North Shore Univ Hosp, Manhasset, NY)

Ann Thorac Surg 61:1323–1329, 1996   7–25

Background.—Atrial fibrillation occurs commonly after cardiac operations. Cardiopulmonary bypass results in the euthyroid sick state. Therefore, the effect of perioperative triiodothyronine (T3) on the incidence of atrial fibrillation was prospectively investigated in patients undergoing coronary artery bypass grafting (CABG) in a randomized, double-blind, placebo-controlled clinical trial.

Methods.—Patients aged 40–85 years with depressed ejection fractions and no evidence of thyroid disease, who underwent CABG, were randomly assigned to receive either placebo (5% dextrose solution) or T3 infused at the time of aortic cross-clamp removal and continued for 9 hours, with a 3-hour taper infusion. Continuous monitoring of cardiac rhythm was used to detect arrhythmias and fibrillation.

Results.—There were no differences between the 2 groups in the incidence of supraventricular or ventricular arrhythmias during the first 24 postoperative hours. However, the prevalence of atrial fibrillation was significantly greater in the placebo group during the next 96 hours, with 29 episodes in 16 patients in the T3 group compared with 69 episodes in 30 patients in the placebo group. Most episodes of atrial fibrillation occurred between the second and fourth postoperative days. The T3-treated patients also required fewer treatment interventions, including procainamide therapy, anticoagulation, or cardioversion.

Conclusions.—Perioperative treatment with T3 decreased the incidence of atrial fibrillation after CABG. Additional clinical trials are needed to confirm these findings.

▶ Patients undergoing cardiovascular bypass frequently have atrial fibrillation develop, which is associated with strokes and malignant ventricular arrhythmias. Because a low T3 state often is present as a result of such bypasses, giving T3 perioperatively is logical. The results described above demonstrate that the theoretical notion is correct, and has important therapeutic implications.

L. Lasagna, M.D.

Interaction of Ischaemia and Encainide/Flecainide Treatment: A Proposed Mechanism for the Increased Mortality in CAST I

Greenberg HM, Dwyer EM Jr, Hochman JS, et al (St Luke's/Roosevelt Hosp, New York; Columbia Univ, NY; New Jersey Med School, Newark; et al)
Br Heart J 74:631–635, 1995   7–26

Background.—The Cardiac Arrhythmia Suppression Trial (CAST I) was a randomized, double-blind, placebo-controlled study in which patients with a recent myocardial infarction received drugs (encainide/flecainide) to suppress premature ventricular contractions and ventricular tachycardia. In this study, the active drug groups had a higher cardiac and sudden death mortality rate than the placebo group. The CAST I database was analyzed to determine which occurred first—cardiac death or arrest, angina pectoris or nonfatal recurrent infarction—to examine whether the relation between intercurrent ischemia and encainide or flecainide could explain the increased mortality observed in the treatment groups in this study.

Results.—Although there were the same number of nonfatal infarctions and angina pectoris incidents in the treatment and placebo groups in the CAST I study, the treatment groups had a significantly higher fatality rate than the placebo group. When nonischemic end points, congestive heart failure and syncope, were analyzed, fatality was more common in the placebo group.

Conclusions.—In the CAST I study population, the mortality from ischemia-related events was higher in the treatment groups, whereas the mortality from nonischemic events was higher in the placebo group. This suggests that an interaction between encainide or flecainide and active ischemia may have been responsible for the unexpected increased mortality in the treatment group in this study. Future antiarrhythmic drug screening should include ischemic models.

▶ The CAST I study created quite a furor some years ago. Now, of course, in addition to scientific articles, there has even been an important "muckraking" book written on the subject. The authors of this study believe that the problem was an interaction between the antiarrhythmic drugs and ischemia in the patients. Their analysis and their suggestion for the development of further antiarrhythmic drugs should be studied. This clinical trial is an example of several in which the placebo group did better than the treatment groups. Some of them have not been as famous as this one, because the outcome here of therapy was supposed to be, and was thought to be, lifesaving. However, there are several other clinical trials in which the plaintive plea of the patient, "Doc, only if I can be in the active treatment group," was an ill-advised request. Too often, we believe that we know the outcome of a trial and that the treatment groups that receive the active therapy will do better than the comparable placebo group. At the same time, we all know that the active moiety may not be effective for this or any therapy. That is just one reason for using randomization and for doing clinical trials.

M. Weintraub, M.D.

Influence of *Metoprolol* on Heart Rate Variability in Survivors of Remote Myocardial Infarction
Keeley EC, Page RL, Lange RA, et al (Univ of Texas, Dallas; Parkland Mem Hosp, Dallas)
Am J Cardiol 77:557–560, 1996   7–27

Purpose.—Long-term β-blocker therapy reduces mortality in survivors of myocardial infarction, perhaps by decreasing heart rate variability (HRV). Diminished HRV is a powerful predictor of mortality in this group of patients. The effects of metoprolol treatment on HRV in survivors of myocardial infarction were assessed.

Methods.—The study included 43 patients who had had myocardial infarction 12 to 18 months previously. There were 26 men and 17 women, aged 38 to 69 years. All patients had 2 24-hour ambulatory ECG recordings made 2 weeks apart. Twenty-eight of the patients, comprising group A, had taken metoprolol for the previous year but discontinued it for 2 weeks before the first ECG was made. Then, 2 weeks after they restarted metoprolol treatment, the second ECG was made. The other 15 patients, comprising group B, were not taking metoprolol for either of the 2 recordings.

Results.—For patients in group A, metoprolol treatment increased the time domain variables suggesting increased vagal tone (i.e., root-mean-square successive difference in normal RR [NN] intervals and proportion of NN that differed by more than 50 msec). Frequency domain variables—the logarithms of the 24-hour very–low-frequency and the 24-hour high-frequency power, reflecting parasympathetic activity—also were increased with metoprolol.

Conclusions.—As evaluated by the time and frequency domain measures of HRV, parasympathetic cardiac activity in survivors of myocardial infarction is increased by metoprolol. This antiarrhythmic effect may account for the ability of β-blockers to reduce life-threatening arrhythmias and sudden death in survivors of myocardial infarction.

▶ When the theory first was presented that by diminishing HRV, one increased the chances for adverse effects, and, in fact, increased the chances for sudden cardiac death, it was counterintuitive. However, as one thinks about the setting of heart failure, in which there is increased sympathetic tone and decreased HRV, it also seems likely that increased parasympathetic tone would be beneficial.

M. Weintraub, M.D.

Digoxin or Flecainide for Prophylaxis of Supraventricular Tachycardia in Infants?
O'Sullivan JJ, Gardiner HM, Wren C (Freeman Hosp, Newcastle Upon Tyne, England)
J Am Coll Cardiol 26:991–994, 1995   7–28

Purpose.—Infants with supraventricular tachycardia are at high risk of spontaneous recurrence of tachycardia. Digoxin is usually recommended for prophylaxis. However, there have been no controlled clinical trials testing its efficacy, nor is there agreement about which drug should be used when digoxin fails. Digoxin and flecainide were compared for safety and efficacy in the prophylaxis of supraventricular tachycardia in infants.

Patients.—The retrospective study included 39 infants with supraventricular tachycardia caused by atrioventricular re-entry. The infants (median age, 12 days) were treated during an 8-year period. Six patients required IV flecainide to gain immediate control of the tachycardia, after which they received oral flecainide. The remaining 33 patients received oral digoxin.

Findings.—Forty-two percent of the patients receiving digoxin were free from recurrent tachycardia. The remaining 58% had multiple recurrences of tachycardia and required replacement of digoxin with oral flecainide.

All 19 of these patients had full control of their tachycardia, as did 5 of the 6 patients receiving IV followed by oral flecainide. The overall effectiveness rate of flecainide was therefore 96%, with a 95% confidence interval of 80% to 100%.

Conclusions.—Digoxin, the conventional drug of first choice for prevention of recurrent supraventricular tachycardia in infants, seems less effective than oral flecainide. This small study suggests that flecainide is highly effective and has no apparent adverse effects. The authors now use flecainide as the preferred drug for prophylaxis of supraventricular tachycardia in infants.

▶ Supraventricular tachycardia in infants can be readily restored to sinus rhythm, but because recurrences are common prophylactic treatment is generally recommended. Digoxin is generally regarded as the drug of choice, but this study challenges the traditional wisdom and puts in a plug for oral flecainide.

L. Lasagna, M.D.

Effects of *Bisoprolol* on Heart Rate Variability in Heart Failure
Pousset F, Copie X, Lechat P, et al (Hôpital Broussais, Paris)
Am J Cardiol 77:612–617, 1996   7–29

Background.—Heart rate variability (HRV) is associated with low vagal activity and poor outcome in patients with heart failure. Heart rate variability may provide a noninvasive test of autonomic nervous system activity. Although data have indicated that β-blockers are beneficial for patients with heart failure, their effect on HRV is not known. Twenty-four–hour HRV was analyzed in a group of patients with congestive heart failure to determine whether the long-term benefit of β-blockers is related to the restoration of a better sympathetic-parasympathetic balance.

Methods.—Fifty-four patients from the randomized, double-blind, placebo-controlled Cardiac Insufficiency Bisoprolol Study comprised the study group. Heart rate variability was analyzed before randomization and after 2 months of treatment.

Results.—After 2 months, the patients in the bisoprolol treatment group had a significantly reduced average heart rate compared to the patients in the placebo group. Bisoprolol increased 24-hour root-mean-square successive differences in heart rate, 24-hour percentage of adjacent RR differences greater than 50 msec, daytime standard deviation of RR intervals, and daytime high-frequency (0.16 to 0.40 Hz) power.

Conclusions.—The treatment of patients with heart failure using the β-blocker, bisoprolol, was associated both with RR interval changes and with partial restoration of HRV. This suggests that part of the beneficial effects of β-blockers may result from increased vagal activity. The link between β-blockers, increased HRV, and beneficial prognosis requires further confirmation.

▶ It is actually quite refreshing to realize that HRV can be a good thing. At least it correlates well with outcome in the treatment of congestive heart failure. Changing the heart rate with medications may be somewhat backwards in our understanding of what we are trying to treat, however, if the outcome really is variability change. In other words, the drugs we give could, in fact, change the heart rate without changing the effect on mortality. In some cases, the pathology that causes the regularization, usually at a high heart rate, will not be altered by our treatment and the patients will still suffer the consequences of the underlying congestive heart failure. That is why the current study, part of a multicenter, placebo-controlled, randomized study, were so encouraging.

M. Weintraub, M.D.

Pulmonary Embolism:—The Role of Thrombolytic Therapy in Its Management
More RS, Chauhan A (St Mary's Hosp, London; Papworth Hosp, Cambridge, England)
Postgrad Med J 72:157–161, 1996   7–30

Background.—Pulmonary embolism (Fig) can cause pulmonary hypertension and an acute increase in right ventricular afterload, which can lead to right ventricular failure and increases in right atrial pressure, resulting in clinical shock. The mortality rate associated with pulmonary embolism is approximately 14%. Its treatment is discussed.

Anticoagulation or Thrombolysis.—Historically, patients were treated with anticoagulation, which prevented further thromboembolic events during the natural lysing process by the fibrinolytic system. However, recent studies have shown that patients can benefit from the use of thrombolytic therapy, which actively dissolves the embolus. The benefits of thrombolytic therapy include quicker anatomic and hemodynamic improvement and better prevention of recurrent emboli. However, thrombolytic therapy may increase bleeding complications.

Management Options.—Studies have not demonstrated the superiority of any 1 thrombolytic agent. The agents can be administered either centrally, with catheters placed within either the right ventricle or the pulmonary circulation, or peripherally, with apparently equal efficacy. Short administration regimens are as effective as the longer regimens and can be administered more simply.

Conclusions.—Patients in all age groups and postoperative patients have benefitted from thrombolytic therapy. Given its efficacy, thrombolytic therapy should always be considered in the absence of contraindications for patients with massive pulmonary embolism associated with acute pulmonary hypertension, right ventricular dysfunction, or systemic hypotension.

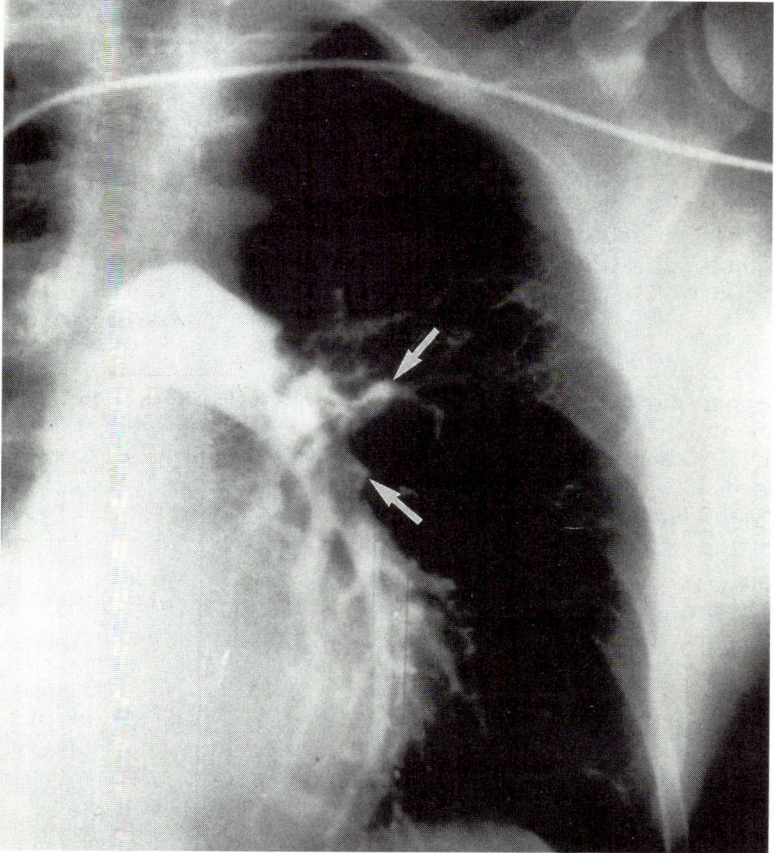

FIGURE.—Pulmonary angiogram obtained using a pulmonary artery catheter. Multiple intraluminal clots are present (*arrows*) in the left upper and lower lobe pulmonary arteries. (Courtesy of More RS, Chauhan A: Pulmonary embolism: The role of thrombolytic therapy in its management. *Postgrad Med J* 72:157–161, 1996.)

► Because thromboembolism is often undiagnosed, the estimate of 50,000 U.S. deaths annually from this condition is probably too low. The classic presentation shouldn't be missed—acute pleuritic pain, shortness of breath, hemoptysis, tachypnea, tachycardia with or without hypoxia, hypotension, and right heart strain changes in EKG.

Thrombolytic therapy for massive embolism makes very good sense.

L. Lasagna, M.D.

Hemorrhagic Complications of Thrombolytic Therapy

Lauer JE, Heger JJ, Mirro MJ (Fort Wayne Ctr for Med Education, Ind; Fort Wayne Cardiology Inc, Ind)
Chest 108:1520–1523, 1995   7–31

Background.—The administration of thrombolytic drugs, early in myocardial infarction, has been demonstrated to salvage ischemic myocardium and improve outcome. The most dangerous adverse effects of this therapy are hemorrhagic complications, especially cerebral hemorrhage. The incidence of hemorrhagic complications was evaluated and the risk factors identified in a retrospective study of patients who underwent thrombolytic therapy after myocardial infarction.

Methods.—Three hundred and fifty patients were obtained from a chart review at 1 hospital of all patients receiving IV thrombolytic therapy for acute myocardial infarction from July 1987 to May 1992.

Results.—Of the 350 patients, 20 had a bleeding complication, including 4 with cerebral hemorrhage. The risk factors associated with hemorrhage were age greater than 65 years and female gender. The risk factors associated with cerebral hemorrhage were age greater than 65 years and a history of hypertension.

Conclusions.—The overall incidence of hemorrhage was 5.7% and the incidence of cerebral hemorrhage was 1.1%. Age, hypertension, and female gender were associated with an increased risk of hemorrhagic complications. Caution should be exercised in using thrombolytic therapy in patients with these risk factors.

▶ It is really a shame that this group of investigators did not weigh their patients and add the data to the Thrombolytic Therapy for Acute Myocardial Infarction-7 (TAMI-7) study. In that study, weight-adjusted doses were used. In any case, perhaps a lesser dose, adjusted for weight, would be useful in decreasing the toxicity of thrombolytic therapy and anticoagulation in elderly women.

M. Weintraub, M.D.

A Comparison of Continuous Intravenous Epoprostenol (Prostacyclin) With Conventional Therapy for Primary Pulmonary Hypertension

Barst RJ, for the Primary Pulmonary Hypertension Study Group (Columbia Univ, New York; Univ of Maryland, Baltimore; Univ of North Carolina, Chapel Hill; et al)
N Engl J Med 334:296–301, 1996   7–32

Background.—To date, no treatment studied in prospective, randomized trials has improved survival among patients with primary pulmonary hypertension. The efficacy of continuous epoprostenol infusion was investigated in a 12-week, open-label, prospective, randomized, multicenter study of patients with severe primary pulmonary hypertension who remained in New York Heart Association (NYHA) functional class III or IV despite conventional treatment.

Methods —Eighty-one patients were included. Continuous IV infusion of epoprostenol plus conventional treatment was given to 41 patients, and conventional treatment alone was given to 40. Epoprostenol treatment improved exercise capacity. In the patients given conventional treatment alone, exercise capacity declined. Quality-of-life indices and hemodynamics also improved only in the epoprostenol-treated group. The changes in mean pulmonary artery pressure for patients given epoprostenol were −8%, compared with +3% for the patients receiving conventional therapy alone. Mean changes in pulmonary vascular resistance were −21% and +9%, respectively. Eight patients died, all of whom received only conventional therapy. Four episodes of catheter-associated sepsis and 1 thrombotic event occurred.

Conclusions.—Compared with conventional therapy alone, continuous IV epoprostenol infusion plus conventional treatment improves hemodynamics, exercise endurance, quality of life, and survival in patients with primary pulmonary hypertension. Epoprostenol used as a bridge to transplantation may enable hemodynamic stabilization, which may lower perioperative rates of morbidity and mortality.

▶ Primary pulmonary hypertension is a mysterious disease that we don't really understand. (Why does calling a disease "primary" or "idiopathic" or "essential" make some people think we understand the cause? In fact, these words mean just the opposite.)

Giving epoprostenol (formerly called prostacyclin) seems helpful in all sorts of ways, even if only used as a bridge to transplantation.

L. Lasagna, M.D.

Immunosuppressive Therapy Prevents Recurrent Pericarditis
Marcolongo R, Russo R, Laveder F, et al (Padua Univ, Italy)
J Am Coll Cardiol 26:1276–1279, 1995   7–33

Background.—Repeated relapses of acute pericarditis can occur despite anti-inflammatory therapy. Steroid treatment for recurrent pericarditis is controversial. Clinical outcomes in 1 group of patients with recurrent pericarditis before and after immunosuppressive treatment were reported.

Methods.—Twelve patients, aged 15–65 years, were included. Recurrent pericarditis in this group was unrelated to any systemic disease. In all patients, short-term low-dose steroid treatment had been ineffective previously. A total of 39 relapses had occurred during a 14.2-month follow-up. Prednisone therapy was initiated at 1–1.5 mg/kg body weight per day for 4 weeks, then gradually withdrawn, for a total course of 3 months. When prednisone doses were reduced, the patients began a 5-month course of aspirin therapy, starting at 1.6 g/day until steroid suspension, then decreased to 0.8 g/day. The mean follow-up was 41.6 months.

Findings.—High-dose prednisone induced a stable remission in all but 1 patient, who had 1 relapse. Adding azathioprine to the prednisone treatment in this patient resulted in continued remission. Severe steroid-related adverse effects developed during treatment in 3 patients. Prednisone had to be replaced with azathioprine in 1 patient and cyclophosphamide in another patient. This variation did not negatively affect clinical outcomes.

Conclusions.—Preventing recurrent pericarditis depends on an adequate dose and duration of steroid therapy. These should be evaluated before alternative treatments are begun. For patients who do not respond to anti-inflammatory treatment, high-dose prednisone plus aspirin may be indicated. Only patients who do not respond to high-dose prednisone or in whom serious complications result from steroid treatment should receive cyclophosphamide or azathioprine.

▶ Primary pericarditis is an unpleasant condition even when acute and limited; it is disabling in that minority of patients who have recurrent painful bouts with or without pericardial effusion. Because an immunologic basis has been postulated, it's not surprising that immunosuppressive therapy is sometimes invoked.

The authors of this study have come up with a proposed long-term therapeutic agenda on the basis of their clinical experience with 12 patients with a recurring syndrome seemingly unrelated to any systemic disease. The data are not those of a controlled trial, but deserve attention.

L. Lasagna, M.D.

Economic Outcomes of Withdrawal of Digoxin Therapy in Adult Patients With Stable Congestive Heart Failure

Ward RE, Gheorghiade M, Young JB, et al (Henry Ford Health System, Detroit; Northwestern Univ, Chicago; Baylor College of Medicine, Houston; et al)
J Am Coll Cardiol 26:93–101, 1995   7–34

Background.—Two large digoxin-withdrawal studies have used identical design variables and have researched data on patients with congestive heart failure who either are or are not receiving angiotensin-converting enzyme inhibitors. They have shown that continued digoxin therapy decreases the risk of treatment failures requiring changes in congestive heart failure treatment or resulting in congestive heart failure–related emergency visits and hospitalization in such patients. In the current clinical policy analysis, the benefits, risks, and costs of continuing digoxin treatment were determined, and the national economic implications of digoxin withdrawal were assessed.

Methods.—A decision-analytic model was used to test the alternative strategies of continuing and withdrawing digoxin. The patients had congestive heart failure with normal sinus rhythm, New York Heart Association functional class II or III, and left ventricular ejection fraction of 35%

or less. The analysis was based on expert opinion and epidemiologic assumptions in published reports.

Findings.—Continuing digoxin treatment would prevent about 185,000 clinic visits, 27,000 emergency visits, and 137,000 hospitalizations for congestive heart failure on a national level. With an estimated 12,500 cases of digoxin toxicity, the net annual savings would be about $406 million. In a 1 way sensitivity analysis assuming an annual incidence of toxicity of 33% or less, digoxin treatment was found to be cost-saving.

Conclusions.—Clinicians should consider continuing digoxin treatment in patients with stable congestive heart failure. This strategy will probably lower costs and increase health benefits.

▶ After more than 2 centuries of use, digitalis remains controversial. This study applies a decision-analytic model to quantify the benefits of continuing digoxin treatment in patients with congestive heart failure and normal heart rhythm. (The benefits of digitalis glycosides in patients with atrial fibrillation are generally accepted.)

The authors' analysis suggests substantial cost and health benefits from the continuation of digoxin therapy in patients with stable congestive heart failure. Thank you, Dr. Withering.[1]

L. Lasagna, M.D.

Reference

1. Withering W: An account of the foxglove and some of its medical uses with practical remarks on dropsy and other diseases, in Willins FA, Keyes TE (eds): *Classics of Cardiology.* New York, Henry Schuman, 1941, pp 231–252.

8 Ear, Nose, Throat, and Eye Disorders

Increasing Incidence of Penicillin- and Ampicillin-Resistant Middle Ear Pathogens
Rodriguez WJ, Schwartz RH, Thorne MM (Children's Natl Med Ctr, Washington, DC; Vienna Pediatric Assocs, Va)
Pediatr Infect Dis J 14:1075–1078, 1995   8–1

Purpose.—Acute otitis media (AOM) is very common among babies and young children. Its management is complicated by the emergence of antibiotic-resistant organisms. Clinical trial data on the results of cultures of middle-ear exudates were used to document an increasing incidence of drug-resistant pathogens among children with AOM.

Methods.—Specimens of middle-ear exudate were collected from 151 children participating in comparative trials of antibiotics for AOM. A total of 159 samples were obtained and cultured, almost all by tympanocentesis. All children (mean age, 35 months) were enrolled at 1 U.S. pediatric practice. The study used specified diagnostic criteria for AOM: outward bulging of the eardrum, opacification of the eardrum regardless of color, and impaired mobility to positive and negative pressure through the pneumatic otoscope.

Results.—In all but 5% of patients, a bacterial pathogen was isolated. The isolated organisms included *Streptococcus pneumoniae*, 27%; *Moraxella catarrhalis*, 25%; group A streptococcus, 4%; and *Staphylococcus aureus*, 2%. Mixed bacterial culture results were obtained in 6 patients, 3 of whom had 1 or more ampicillin-resistant bacteria. Of 8 patients with persistent AOM, 3 had different organisms on follow-up culture and 5 had ampicillin- or penicillin-resistant cultures. Penicillin resistance was noted in 21% of recovered strains of *S. pneumoniae*; ampicillin resistance was found in 62% of *Haemophilus influenzae* isolates and 98% of *M. catarrhalis* isolates.

Conclusions.—The incidence of penicillin and ampicillin resistance in the pathogens causing AOM appears to be increasing. The empiric use of amoxicillin for AOM needs to be re-evaluated, at least in the authors' community. Drug-resistant pathogens here seem most likely to be found in infants with AOM and high fever or irritability; in older children who are in significant pain; and children in day care with pain; and children in day care with moderate pain, fever, and AOM.

▶ The pneumococcus continues to develop resistance to penicillin, but other bugs also show decreased sensitivity to antibiotics over time. Hence the need for eternal vigilance to guide therapy appropriately to the local conditions.

L. Lasagna, M.D.

Results of an Epidemiological Study on Drug-Treated Intraocular Hypertension in Belgium

Walckiers D, Sartor F (Inst of Hygiene and Epidemiology, Brussels, Belgium)
J Clin Epidemiol 49:489–493, 1996   8–2

Background.—Because age is an important risk factor for glaucoma, the frequency of this disease is likely to increase as the populations of Western countries continue to age. Epidemiologic aspects of this public health problem in Belgium were assessed.

Findings.—In 1992, 1,513 patients attending a sample of 209 pharmacies (4% of all pharmacies open to the public in Belgium) for the purchase of eye drops or ointments for the treatment of intraocular hypertension completed questionnaires (58% response rate). Mean participant age was 67 years; after adjustment for age, the prevalence of diabetes mellitus among the participants was 1.7 times greater than that among the general Belgian population. Ninety-six percent of the participants purchased beta-blocker eye drops for use either alone or in combination. The frequency of prescription of parasympathomimetics increased with patient age. Twenty-eight percent of participants had a family history of glaucoma or blindness. A quarter of the patients who had been treated with drugs for less than 1 year had seen an ophthalmologist more than 4 times a year. However, of those treated for at least 5 years, only 11% saw an ophthalmologist that often. Both eyes were treated by 86% of patients. Per-person annual consumption of eye drops containing parasympathomimetics was 12.4 bottles; of eye drops containing beta-blockers, 13.6 bottles; and of those containing epinephrine or dipivefrine, 12.3 bottles. Per-person annual consumption of parasympathomimetic-containing ointments was 9.9 tubes. The prevalence of drug-treated intraocular hypertension in Belgium was estimated at 77 per 10,000 inhabitants based on these data and sales figures.

Conclusions.—The mean age of patients in the sample was much greater than the mean age of the Belgian population (67 years vs. 39 years), supporting age as a risk factor for increasing mean intraocular pressure. The prevalence calculation is in agreement with that reported in Scandinavian countries.

▶ In this study, many of the patients were treated with beta-blockers, parasympathomimetics, and epinephrine. More recently, in the United States, drugs that inhibit prostaglandin synthesis and that are alpha-blockers have become available. The old stand-by, systemically administered carbonic anhydrase inhibitors, are used to treat some patients. All these therapies, including the new ones, are attempts to control the disease so that laser trabeculoplasty or filtering surgeries may be avoided. Ophthalmologists really do have more arrows in their quiver now than compared to even 5 years ago.

M. Weintraub, M.D.

A Six-Month, Randomized, Double-Masked Study Comparing Latanoprost With Timolol in Open-angle Glaucoma and Ocular Hypertension
Watson P, for the Latanoprost Study Group (Addenbrooke's Hosp, Cambridge, England; Pharmacia AB, Uppsala, Sweden)
Ophthalmology 103:126–137, 1996   8–3

Introduction.—The prostaglandin analogue latanoprost, formerly known as PhXA41, was developed for use in lowering intraocular pressure (IOP) in patients with glaucoma. Latanoprost, like prostaglandin $F_{2\alpha}$, works by increasing uveoscleral outflow rather than influencing aqueous humor production. Latanoprost was compared with timolol for its IOP-lowering effects and its systemic and ocular side effects.

Methods.—The study included 294 patients with open-angle glaucoma or ocular hypertension. The patients were randomized to receive 6 months of treatment with 0.005% latanoprost, administered once daily in the evening, or 0.5% timolol, administered twice daily. The IOP-reducing effect and side effects of the 2 treatments were compared.

Results.—After 6 months of treatment, diurnal IOP was reduced by about 33%—from 25 to 17 mm Hg—in both the latanoprost and timolol groups. Neither treatment was associated with upward drift in IOP, and both treatments were well tolerated. Conjunctival hyperemia was significantly more frequent with latanoprost, but this complication was very mild. Corneal punctate epithelial erosions were also more common with latanoprost. Latanoprost did cause increased iris pigmentation in 10% of patients, but systemic side effects were more common with timolol.

Conclusions.—For patients with open-angle glaucoma or ocular hypertension, once-daily dosing with 0.005% latanoprost is as effective as twice-daily dosing with 0.5% timolol in lowering IOP. Systemic and ocular tolerance of latanoprost treatment is good. Its main side effect, noted especially in patients with green-brown or blue-brown eyes, is increased iris pigmentation.

▶ In this particular study, 15 patients (10.1%) had the typical change in iris pigmentation seen with latanoprost. However, before you go out and become a spy or assume another identity, remember that the increased pigmentation is generally seen with people who have blue-brown or green-brown eye color. In addition, it doesn't occur until later in the treatment; it usually takes at least a couple of months and possibly as long as 6 months to develop. Nonetheless, latanoprost administered in a very low concentration (0.005% daily) is a remarkably potent and effective medication for glaucoma.

M. Weintraub, M.D.

9 Endocrine and Metabolic Disorders

The Economic Cost of Obesity: The French Situation
Lévy E, Lévy P, Le Pen C, et al (Université Paris-Dauphine; Hôtel Dieu, Paris)
Int J Obes 19:788–792, 1995   9–1

Background.—Obesity is associated with an increased risk of many major diseases, societal burden in terms of increased health care costs and lost productivity, and individual burden in terms of reduced quality of life, increased morbidity, and premature mortality. The burden of obesity in France in terms of direct and indirect costs and in terms of overmortality was estimated.

Methods.—A prevalence-based approach was used to identify the costs incurred in a given year (1992) by obese residents (body mass index greater than or equal to 27). All costs for obese patients were considered, irrespective of grade of obesity or stage of associated disease. Direct costs measured included personal health and hospital care, physician's services, drugs, and other resources that could find other use if obesity were not present. Production losses were estimated as indirect costs. The economic benefit of obesity, a reduced incidence of hip fractures, also was considered.

Results.—The direct costs of obesity in France (about 12 billion French francs) were equivalent to 2% of all the expenses of the French health care system. Costs associated with hypertension amounted to more than one third of the total direct costs of obesity. Indirect costs were estimated at 0.6 billion French francs. Because of the methods of data collection used, these figures are considered conservative estimates.

Conclusions.—The monetary burden of obesity in France is substantial. Indirect costs and loss of lifetime earnings were likely to be underreported by these study methods; however, the figures estimated are similar to those of previous reports from Western countries.

▶ If it is true that obesity accounts for somewhere between 2% and 5% of all health care expenditures, using a conservative estimate, the introduction of new therapies for obesity can really make an impact on patients' pocketbooks as well as their pannus. We usually do not think of the Europeans, such as the French people, as having much obesity. And, in fact, they have less than Americans. However, the incidence of obesity is increasing in Europe, as it is in the United States. In all the Western countries, although people are living longer, they also are getting more obese. Among the reasons for this are the facts that food is relatively inexpensive, deliciously prepared, and varied, and that intake, even with a recent change in fat content, is too large. Exercise, although it is increasing for some people in our society has not really increased as a general rule throughout the population. Thus with higher intake and less caloric expenditure, obesity has increased. Physicians are facing the conundrum of people who are living longer but are both heavier and demanding medications to help them lose weight.

M. Weintraub, M.D.

Resting Metabolic Rate and Postabsorptive Substrate Oxidation in Morbidly Obese Subjects Before and After Massive Weight Loss
Buscemi S, Caimi G, Verga S (Univ of Palermo, Italy)
Int J Obes 20:41–46, 1996   9–2

Background.—Previous studies suggest that obese people may have an energy-sparing metabolism. Because of the high incidence of weight relapse, it is difficult to perform long-term studies of changes in energy expenditure on obese people who have lost a lot of weight. Changes in resting metabolic rate (RMR) and in postabsorptive substrate oxidation were studied in morbidly obese patients who lost massive amounts of weight after surgical biliopancreatic bypass.

Methods.—The study included 10 morbidly obese patients (mean body mass index [BMI] 54 kg/m²) who underwent biliopancreatic bypass. This procedure permits massive, stable weight loss over a prolonged period. The patients were studied before surgery, during massive weight loss, and 36 to 42 months after weight loss. Measurements made at each point included RMR, postabsorptive oxidation of carbohydrates (CHO), lipids, and proteins; body composition; and plasma concentrations of glucose, free fatty acids, insulin, and thyroid hormones. A group of control subjects, mean BMI 21 kg/m², also was studied.

Results.—The patients' mean BMI at the final evaluation was stable at 33 kg/m². Their RMR fell progressively during the weight loss period, both in absolute terms and normalized for fat-free mass. At the final evaluation, the normalized RMR of the patients was even lower than that of the control subjects. Oxidation of CHO increased over the long term, whereas oxidation of lipids decreased. There was no significant change in oxidation of proteins.

Conclusions.—Subjects with previous morbid obesity appear to have an energy-sparing metabolism that, coupled with high energy intake, could favor high body weight. Their pattern of substrate oxidation normalizes when they lose weight, probably reducing their risk of abnormal glucose tolerance. Whether it is possible for these subjects to maintain long-term weight loss without a surgical procedure remains open to debate.

▶ Many people believe that obesity is the result of energy sparing, and perhaps it is in some cases. We certainly know it is not all due to markedly excessive intake. Certainly, intake could be excessive in terms of the RMR. These postoperative patients give us a fair amount to think about in terms of the treatment of obesity.

M. Weintraub, M.D.

Body Fatness and Waist Circumference Are Independent Predictors of the Age-Associated Increase in Fasting Insulin Levels in Healthy Men and Women
Colman E, Toth MJ, Katzel LI, et al (Univ of Maryland, Baltimore; Baltimore Veterans Affairs Med Ctr, Md)
Int J Obes 19:798–803, 1995   9–3

Background.—Elevated levels of fasting insulin increase risk of coronary artery disease and have been associated with advancing age. Factors that might independently affect this age-associated increase in healthy men and women were examined in a cross-sectional analysis.

Methods.—Participants included healthy men (427) and women (293) ranging in age from 18 to 90 years. Fasting plasma glucose and insulin levels were measured. Factors considered were age, total body fatness (via underwater weighing), abdominal fat distribution (waist circumference), peak VO_2 (treadmill test to exhaustion), leisure time physical activity (structured interview), and dietary intake (3-day food diary). Stepwise multiple regression analysis was used to determine independent predictive values.

Results.—As expected, fasting insulin concentrations increased with age in participants of both sexes. Waist circumference and percent body fat were major independent predictors of fasting insulin concentrations in men. Smaller independent contributions were found for age, glucose concentration, and peak VO_2. Among women, fasting insulin levels correlated independently with waist circumference and fasting glucose concentration. After adjustment for waist circumference, the rate of increase in insulin levels with increasing age was not significant in women.

Conclusions.—In healthy men and women, total adiposity and central body fat distribution are the primary determinants of increasing fasting insulin levels. Less important contributors include age, dietary intake, and fitness and activity levels. Age-associated increases in insulin levels may be attenuated by maintenance of an appropriate level and distribution of body fat.

▶ The degree of central obesity seems to be very much related to hypertension, at least in obese patients. Some believe that the level of serum insulin is related to this phenomenon and really is the cause of a syndrome that involves coronary artery disease, hypertension, hyperlipoproteinemia and adult-onset diabetes mellitus. We know that the "apple-shaped" person is more prone to hypertension than is the "pear-shaped" person. Well, as I survey my increasing "beer belly," I know that I'll have to go on a caloric-restricted regimen and increase my own exercise. Do any other readers of the YEAR BOOK OF DRUG THERAPY have to do the same?

M. Weintraub, M.D.

Dexfenfluramine Treatment of Obesity: A Double Blind Trial With Post Trial Follow Up
O'Connor HT, Richman RM, Steinbeck KS, et al (Royal Prince Alfred Hosp, Camperdown, Australia)
Int J Obes 19:181–189, 1995   9–4

Background.—Successful weight management necessitates a long-term approach. Thus, a better understanding of weight changes during and after dexfenfluramine treatment is essential to determine the efficacy of this drug in clinical practice.

Methods.—Sixty obese patients were enrolled in a randomized, placebo-controlled, 6-month trial. Twenty-seven patients receiving dexfenfluramine and 24 receiving placebo completed the study.

Findings.—After a 1-month run-in phase and the 6 months of treatment, weight loss in the patients given dexfenfluramine was 9.7 kg, compared with 4.9 kg in the placebo group. This difference was significant. The active treatment and placebo groups had differing body fat reductions (5 kg vs. 1 kg) and waist circumference reductions (10.5 cm vs. 5.7 cm). These differences were also significant. Patients receiving dexfenfluramine had a significantly greater incidence of nausea, dry mouth, and dizziness, which tended to decrease as treatment continued. None of the patients dropped out of the study because of side effects. The dexfenfluramine group had an improved cardiovascular risk profile, with reduced serum triglyceride levels, increased high-density lipoprotein cholesterol levels, and decreased fasting insulin levels. Even though the patients receiving placebo lost a significant amount of weight, these risk factor measurements worsened in them. When dexfenfluramine treatment was discontinued, the patients regained significantly more weight than those receiving placebo, indicating the loss of a treatment effect. Five months after the discontinuation of treatment, the benefits of dexfenfluramine over placebo were negated. At that time, the amount of weight lost in the dexfenfluramine group was 5 kg, compared with a 6.2-kg loss in the placebo group.

Conclusions.—When dexfenfluramine treatment is combined with diet and lifestyle modification, additional benefits occur. The greater weight loss in patients receiving dexfenfluramine is apparently associated with improvement in serum lipid profile and reduction of insulinemia. The long-term use of dexfenfluramine in patients with chronic obesity is supported.

▶ This study shows, as so many have, that weight loss with dexfenfluramine is possible and beneficial, at least in the short run. This study had 1 thing that very few weight-control studies have: a run-in period in which lifestyle alterations (behavior modification, caloric restriction, and, in some cases, exercise) are instituted. These programs have to last for a significant period of time so that the patients can learn how to help control their weight without using a medication. At the end of this study, the participants regained almost all the weight they had lost, but more in the dexfenfluramine group than in the placebo group. Of course, the main reason is that the patients who had received dexfenfluramine had more to regain because they had lost more weight. This factor was not mentioned by the authors of the study.

Nonetheless, this study is helpful because it explains some material about dexfenfluramine and compares it with other medications. Many physicians have become interested in medications for obesity. Physicians are attempting to reevaluate the usefulness of such medications. Some are already jumping on the bandwagon and using medications, perhaps in patients who do not really need them, as a way to make money. Why is treating obesity not the same as treating hypertension?

M. Weintraub, M.D.

Effect of Dexfenfluramine on Body Weight, Blood Pressure, Insulin Resistance and Serum Cholesterol in Obese Individuals
Holdaway IM, Wallace E, Westbrooke L, et al (Auckland Hosp, New Zealand)
Int J Obes 19:749–751, 1995   9–5

Background.—The serotonergic agent dexfenfluramine can effectively reduce weight in obese individuals. In addition, it may have direct pharmacologic effects on various cardiovascular risk factors. The metabolic effects of dexfenfluramine in obese patients were studied in an attempt to differentiate between the direct pharmacologic effects and the effects of weight loss.

Methods.—The randomized, double-blind, placebo-controlled trial included 50 obese adults with body mass indices ranging from 30 to 44 kg/m^2. All but 5 individuals were women. The patients were assigned to take either placebo or dexfenfluramine, 15 mg twice daily. The effects of dexfenfluramine on weight loss, blood pressure, insulin sensitivity, and serum lipid levels were examined during a 3-month period.

Results.—The mean weight loss was 3.8 kg with dexfenfluramine vs. 1.1 kg with placebo. Dexfenfluramine was also associated with a greater reduction in diastolic blood pressure, 5.0 vs. 1.5 mm Hg, and in cholesterol level, 0.38 vs. 0.06 mmol/L. Insulin sensitivity improved by 11% with dexfenfluramine vs. 4% with placebo. The blood pressure and insulin sensitivity changes began within 1 week after the start of dexfenfluramine, before weight loss had occurred.

Conclusions.—For obese patients, dexfenfluramine treatment reduces body weight and improves certain cardiovascular risk factors associated with obesity. The changes in risk factors appear to represent a direct effect of dexfenfluramine, independent of weight loss. More research is needed into pharmacologic approaches to the management of obesity.

▶ Dexfenfluramine, one of the isomers in fenfluramine, received FDA approval in 1996. It has been sold for years in many other countries and clearly can lead to weight loss and to concomitant improvement in blood pressure, cholesterol levels, and insulin sensitivity. Ordinarily, these latter changes are attributed to the weight loss, but this study suggests that a direct effect, independent of weight loss, may exist. Fascinating.

L. Lasagna, M.D.

Insulin Resistance in Systemic Hypertension: Pharmacotherapeutic Implications
Mediratta S Fozailoff A, Frishman WH (Albert Einstein College of Medicine/ Montefiore Med Ctr, Bronx, NY; Lenox Hill Hosp, New York; Mt Sinai Med Ctr, New York)
J Clin Pharmacol 35:943–956, 1995   9–6

Background.—The pathophysiology of essential hypertension has been associated with subtle abnormalities in glucose metabolism, including hyperinsulinemia and insulin resistance (Fig 1). Insulin resistance in the pharmacotherapy of hypertension was discussed.

Pharmacotherapeutic Implications of Insulin Resistance in Systemic Hypertension.—Hyperinsulinemia and insulin resistance may produce systemic hypertension through many mechanisms. Insulin has a salt-retaining effect on the kidney and augments catecholamine release, increases vascular sensitivity to vasoconstrictor substances, and reduces vascular sensitivity to vasodilator substances. Insulin can also increase tissue growth factor production and help retain sodium and calcium in cells. Treatment for insulin resistance includes regular aerobic exercise, weight reduction, and a high-fiber diet. Hypoglycemic drugs, weight-reducing agents, and certain antihypertensive drugs with possible favorable effects on blood pressure and insulin resistance are pharmacologic approaches to treatment.

Conclusion.—The best treatment for correcting insulin resistance in hypertensive patients is unknown. Treatment should at least not aggravate insulin resistance or other metabolic or genetic abnormalities. Antihypertensive therapy must be individualized based on the mechanisms of hypertension, which include insulin resistance, to best reduce the risk of cardiovascular morbidity and mortality.

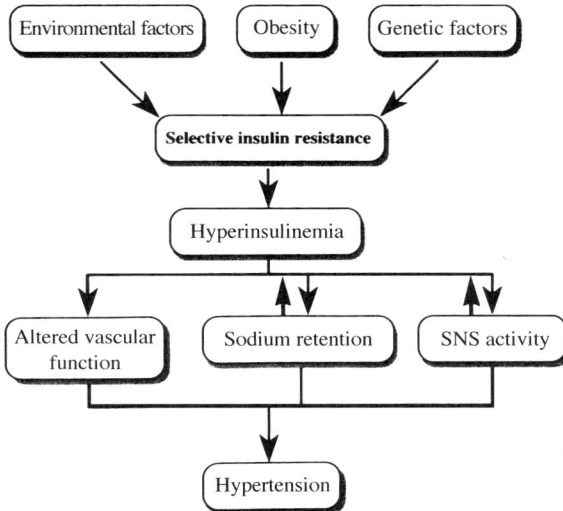

FIGURE 1.—Insulin resistance, hyperinsulinemia, and mechanisms for hypertension. *Abbreviation:* *SNS*, sympathetic nervous system. (Courtesy of Mediratta S, Fozailoff A, Frishman WH: Insulin resistance in systemic hypertension: Pharmacotherapeutic implications. *J Clin Pharmacol* 35:943–956, 1995.)

▶ This article provides the theoretical underpinning for the observation that many people with diabetes, hyperlipoproteinemia, and central obesity can be linked through the insulin concentration as shown on the figure reproduced here. It is really very therapeutically important because there are a lot of drugs that one can use to attack the various components of this syndrome. I think that the weight-reducing agents should be tried because obesity is central to the entire syndrome. Fenfluramine lowers blood sugar by 2 mechanisms: weight loss and a non–insulin-dependent one.

M. Weintraub, M.D.

Review of Limited Systemic Absorption of Orlistat, a Lipase Inhibitor, in Healthy Human Volunteers

Zhi J, Melia AT, Eggers H, et al (Hoffmann-La Roche Inc, Nutley, NJ; F Hoffmann-La Roche Ltd, Basel, Switzerland)

J Clin Pharmacol 35:1103–1108, 1995   9–7

Background.—Orlistat is a lipase inhibitor and represents a new concept in obesity treatment. Although systemic absorption is not required for efficacy, information about absorption is necessary for safe use of this drug. The pharmacokinetics of orlistat were investigated in healthy human volunteers.

Methods.—Pharmacokinetic screening data were collected from 23 phase 1 clinical studies performed over a 7-year period in 50 normal and obese healthy men and women who ingested a hypocaloric, well-balanced diet with 20% to 30% of the calories derived from fat. Plasma samples were monitored for orlistat. Two single-dose studies using radiolabeled orlistat were performed in 14 healthy male volunteers. Samples of blood, urine, and fecal material were collected before and at intervals of up to 9 days until no radioactivity was present in any of these specimens.

Results.—Very little systemic absorption of orlistat was detected in the pharmacokinetic screening studies. After labeled orlistat was ingested, almost the entire dose was recovered exclusively from the fecal samples.

Conclusions.—The systemic absorption of orlistat appears to be negligible, with almost the entire dose excreted fecally. At therapeutic doses, orlistat is likely to be safe, without any inhibition of systemic lipases.

▶ Orlistat is another step in the important and exciting cascade of therapy for non-insulin–dependent diabetes mellitus. The reason that it is so exciting to be working in this field is the onset of new therapeutic interventions. You can use acarbose, which is already on the market. You may be able to use orlistat, if it gets to the market. Neither of these drugs would cause hypoglycemia. You can use metiformin, and you can use some of the newer modalities of weight control. In a short time, you may be able to use drugs that are sensitizers to insulin—very exciting!

M. Weintraub, M.D.

Multicentre Trial of a Programmable Implantable Insulin Pump in Type I Diabetes
Selam J-L, for the Point Study II Group (Strasbourg, France; Vienna; Milano, Italy; et al)
Int J Artif Organs 18:322–325, 1995   9–8

Background.—Near-normoglycemic control through intensive subcutaneous insulin therapy may decrease microvascular diabetic complications. The main adverse effect of intensive subcutaneous insulin therapy is severe hypoglycemia. Continuous intraperitoneal infusion with a programmable implantable pump reduces the incidence of this complication. However, the use of this new technique has not become routine. System-related complications such as flow reduction from insulin precipitation and catheter obstructions limit its use. An improved version of the Siemens implantable system was evaluated in a multicenter trial in Europe.

Methods and Findings.—Thirty-one patients with type I diabetes were treated at 6 European centers for 10 to 30 months. No proven pump malfunctions were documented, in contrast to other pump models. In addition, there was only 1 no-flow reduction, which was unrelated to catheter obstruction. The no-flow reduction resulted in 12 surgical catheter replacements. Two incidents of programmer malfunctions occurred per patient-year. These incidents were easily managed by reconfiguration or replacement. Insulin remained clear and active in the pump reservoir. Glycemic control stayed in the near-normoglycemic range (Fig 1).

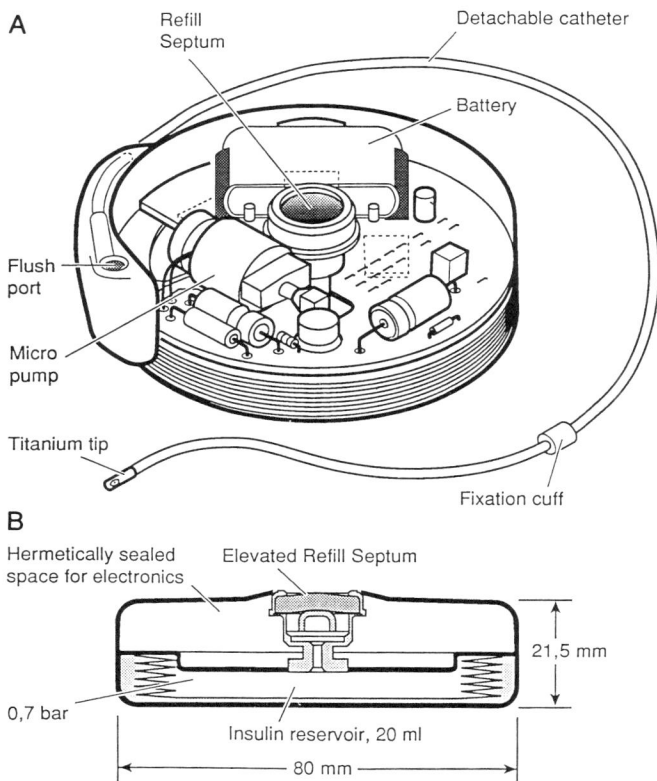

FIGURE 1.—Schematic opened (**A**) and sectioned (**B**) views of the Promedos 3 insulin pump. (Courtesy of Selam J-L, for the Point Study II Group: Multicentre trial of a programmable implantable insulin pump in type I diabetes. *Int J Artif Organs* 18:322–325, 1995.)

Conclusions.—If the current findings can be replicated in longer-term studies and the pump programmers improved, insulin therapy with implantable pumps may become the treatment of choice for patients with diabetes who are unresponsive to more traditional methods of intensive insulin therapy. If this goal is to be achieved, clinicians, medical engineers, and insulin manufacturers must work together more closely and intensively.

▶ The idea of an implantable insulin pump that will mimic the lovely biofeedback seen in nondiabetics is very attractive, but its realization in routine use eludes us, despite a doubling of implantations internationally over the last 3 years.

L. Lasagna, M.D.

A Double-blind Placebo-controlled Trial Evaluating the Safety and Efficacy of Acarbose for the Treatment of Patients With Insulin-requiring Type II Diabetes

Coniff RF, Hoogwerf BJ, Shapiro JA, et al (Miles Pharmaceutical, West Haven, Conn; Cleveland Clinic Found, Ohio; Lions Gate Hosp, North Vancouver, BC, Canada)
Diabetes Care 18:928–932, 1995   9–9

Background.—Administered orally, the complex oligosaccharide acarbose delays hydrolysis and absorption of carbohydates, thus reducing postprandial increments in blood glucose and insulin. There are insufficient data regarding the safety and effectiveness of acarbose in treating patients w th type II diabetes who require insulin injections to achieve adequate metabolic control. The ability of forced titration of acarbose—along with diet and insulin therapy—to improve glycemic control and reduce insulin requirements in this group of patients was studied.

Methods.—Two hundred nineteen patients with insulin-requiring type II diabetes were randomly assigned to receive acarbose or insulin. After a 6-week run-in period, patients in the treatment group received forced titration of acarbose, from 50 to 300 mg 3 times daily, over 24 weeks, and then had a 6-week follow-up period. The main outcome variables in the double-blind trial were the mean change in Hb A1c levels and the mean percentage change in total daily insulin dose.

Results.—A positive clinical response, according to specified criteria, was noted in 45% of patients receiving acarbose vs. 14% of those receiving placebo. Patients in the acarbose group had a 0.40% reduction in Hb A1c level and an 8.3% reduction in total daily insulin dose. Plasma glucose variables declined as well: fasting glucose decreased by 0.9 mmol/L, glucose C_{max} by 2.6 mmol/L, and glucose area under the curve by 270 mmol/min^{-1}/L^{-1}. Adverse events, especially flatulence and diarrhea, were more frequent in the acarbose group.

Conclusions.—In conjunction with insulin and diet therapy, acarbose treatment can produce a significant improvement in overall glycemic control for patients with insulin-requiring type II diabetes. Despite some relatively mild gastrointestinal disturbances, the treatment is well tolerated.

▶ The treatment of type II diabetes has undergone a number of important changes in the recent past. One change was the availability of metformin in the United States. This treatment, common elsewhere in the world, was not available to physicians here until recently because of its relation to phenformin and its lactic acidosis induction. Apparently, this is less common in metformin treatment except in the presence of renal dysfunction. More recently, acarbose has become available. It delays the hydrolysis and absorption of carbohydrates, decreasing the meal-related increases in insulin and blood glucose. Neither of these drugs causes serious hypoglycemia. Some patients also are receiving benefit from a drug called fenfluramine, which acts primarily by decreasing body weight and secondarily by lowering glucose through a non–insulin-mediated mechanism that is poorly understood. This new attack on the various causes of type II diabetes will help many patients whose disease is unresponsive to diet and sulfonylureas.

M. Weintraub, M.D.

Improvement of Insulin Sensitivity by Metformin Treatment Does Not Lower Blood Pressure of Nonobese Insulin-resistant Hypertensive Patients With Normal Glucose Tolerance

Dorella M, Giusto M, Da Tos V, et al (Univ of Padova, Italy)
J Clin Endocrinol Metab 81:1568–1574, 1996   9–10

Objective.—In normal-weight, hypertensive, insulin-resistant patients, drugs that lower insulin resistance, such as metformin, have yielded mixed results with respect to lowering blood pressure. A randomized, placebo-controlled, cross-over study examined the mechanism of action of metformin in normal-weight, hypertensive, normal glucose-tolerant patients; the relationship, if any, of changes in insulin regulation to changes in blood pressure; and other features of blood pressure regulation and its effect on renal and red cell cation handling.

Methods.—After a 4-week washout period, 9 normal-weight, hypertensive, normal glucose-tolerant patients (4 women), 29–67 years of age, were given either metformin (850 mg) twice daily or placebo for 4 weeks. Patients had a least 1 postchallenge insulin level greater than 360 pmol/L. Treatments were switched for the next 4 weeks. After each arm of the study, insulin sensitivity, urinary cation excretion, hormone and substrate concentrations, red cell cation heteroexchange, and blood pressures were determined. Euglycemic-hyperinsulinemia clamp studies were conducted.

Results.—Metformin significantly lowered insulin concentrations by increasing elimination and raised high-density lipoprotein cholesterol levels. Metformin significantly increased glucose oxidation, and reduced glycogen deposition. During the clamp study, metformin increased whole body glucose disposal and glucose oxidation and significantly increased glycogen deposition. Metformin increased blood lactate levels significantly at baseline and during the clamp study. No significant changes in blood pressure, panel-reactive antibodies, or plasma and urinary aldosterone, and plasma epinephrine and norepinephrine were observed for either metformin or placebo groups. Metformin increased the excretion of plasma cations but did not affect Na^+/Li^+ countertransport.

Conclusion.—Although treatment with metformin for 4 weeks lowered plasma insulin concentration, improved glucose disposal, and increased high-density lipoprotein cholesterol, it did not lower arterial blood pressure in normal weight, hypertensive, insulin-resistant patients with normal glucose tolerance.

▶ Idiopathic hypertension often develops in this patient group. The theory is that they have certain degree of insulin resistance and if this could be reverted back to normal, the patient's blood pressure would be reduced as well. It is unfortunate that in this small group of patients, although the treatment with metformin was quite effective in changing the biochemistry, it did not lower arterial blood pressure. Of course, the number of patients (9) and the short-term therapy (1 month) are problematic in a cross-over study. There seem to be newer insulin sensitizers coming down the road. Perhaps they'll be more effective. Or the theory, so beautiful and interconnected, will prove to be unfounded.

M. Weintraub, M.D.

Metformin Treatment in NIDDM Patients With Mild Renal Impairment
Connolly V Kesson CM (Victoria Infirmary NHS Trust, Glasgow, Scotland)
Postgrad Med J 72:352–354, 1996   9–11

Background.—The biguanides have been shown to provide substantial benefits in the treatment of non–insulin dependent diabetes mellitus (NIDDM). Although phenformin was withdrawn after it was associated with lactic acidosis, metformin has remained available. The effects of mildly elevated serum creatinine levels on the plasma lactic acid levels of patients treated with metformin were evaluated.

Methods.—Venous blood samples were obtained from patients with modestly elevated serum creatinine values, from age-matched patients with normal serum creatinine levels, and from age-matched healthy nondiabetic controls. The patients in the 2 case groups had NIDDM and had been treated with metformin for at least 6 months. Plasma lactate was measured in each sample.

Results.—Both groups of patients received a similar mean dose of metformin, but the patients with elevated serum creatinine levels had a longer duration of diabetes and metformin use. The plasma lactate levels were significantly higher in both patient groups than in the control group, but there was no significant correlation between the plasma lactate levels and the serum creatinine levels. There were no significant differences in serum B12 values. None of the patients had a history of illnesses associated with acidosis.

Conclusion.—Although the patients with elevated serum creatinine values had a longer duration of diabetes and metformin treatment, they did not have higher lactate levels than the diabetic patients with normal serum creatinine levels. Therefore, metformin treatment does not appear to be contraindicated in patients with mild renal impairment.

▶ Because of the risk of lactic acidosis, we really have to know what is meant by "mild renal impairment" in this study of optimal use of metformin. The authors report the serum creatinine level as 132.2 ± 9.5 mmol/L. Unfortunately, although they only had 17 patients in this group, they do not report the specific creatinine levels. Fortunately, metformin has a relatively short half-life, which is enhanced by tubular secretion. More important, metabolism to active agents does not occur. What this means, of course, is that spreading out the doses will be effective in decreasing the potential danger of lactic acidosis, even in patients with mild renal impairment.

M. Weintraub, M.D.

Efficacy of Metformin in Patients With Non-Insulin-Dependent Diabetes Mellitus

DeFronzo RA, Goodman AM, and the Multicenter Metformin Study Group (Univ of Texas, San Antonio; Lipha Pharmaceuticals, New York)
N Engl J Med 333:541–549, 1995   9–12

Purpose.—Until recently, sulfonylurea drugs were the only available oral therapy for patients with non–insulin-dependent diabetes mellitus (NIDDM) in the United States. Metformin has now been approved for use in the treatment of NIDDM. The efficacy of metformin treatment in moderately obese patients with NIDDM whose disease was poorly controlled with diet alone or diet plus a sulfonylurea drug was assessed in 2 randomized, placebo-controlled studies.

Methods.—Both studies evaluated the effects of 29 weeks of metformin treatment. In protocol 1, 289 patients whose diabetes was poorly controlled by diet alone were assigned to either metformin or placebo. In protocol 2, 632 patients whose diabetes was poorly controlled by diet plus glyburide were assigned to metformin, glyburide, or both. Efficacy was assessed by measurement of plasma glucose (while the patients were fasting and after oral glucose administration), lactate, lipids, insulin, and glycosylated hemoglobin.

Results.—In protocol 1, the mean fasting plasma glucose concentration at the end of the study was 189 mg/dL in the metformin group vs. 244 mg/dL in the placebo group. Glycosylated hemoglobin values were 7.1% vs. 8.6%, respectively. In protocol 2, the mean fasting plasma glucose concentration was 187 mg/dL in the metformin-plus-glyburide group, compared with 261 mg/dL in the glyburide-only group. Glycosylated hemoglobin values were 7.1% vs. 8.7%, respectively. The metformin-only group had values similar to those of the glyburide-only group. Symptoms consistent with hypoglycemia occurred in 18% of patients receiving metformin and glyuride, compared with 3% of those in the glyburide-only group and 2% of those in the metformin-only group.

Patients in both protocols who received metformin showed significant decreases in plasma total and low-density-lipoprotein cholesterol and triglyceride concentrations. These values were unchanged in the control groups. None of the treatments was associated with a significant change in fasting plasma lactate concentration.

Conclusions.—For patients with NIDDM whose disease is poorly controlled with diet or sulfonylurea therapy, metformin can be helpful. Metformin, given alone or combined with sulfonylurea, is well tolerated and can improve glycemic control as well as lipid concentrations. The main benefit of metformin appears to be mediated through inhibition of hepatic glucose production.

▶ Diet and exercise are the first things to try in patients with NIDDM, but they often fail to achieve optimal carbohydrate control. Sulfonylurea therapy is then usually tried, but its effects are also often disappointing.

Metformin as monotherapy or in combination with a sulfonylurea seems to improve both glycemic control and serum lipid concentrations in patients not otherwise well controlled. This makes sense, because sulfonylureas primarily act by enhancing insulin secretion, whereas metformin inhibits hepatic glucose production and increases the sensitivity of peripheral tissues to insulin.

Metformin has only 1 serious potential drawback—the production of lactic acidosis, which can be fatal and led to the removal from the market of its predecessor, phenformin. Quantitation of this risk is not easy, but the incidence of metformin-related acidosis is said to be one tenth to one twentieth of that reported with phenformin, for reasons that are not clear. The drug does, however, cause nausea and diarrhea, which are usually mild and transient but if not, will subside after a reduction in dose.

L. Lasagna, M.D.

Effect of Intensive Therapy on the Development and Progression of Diabetic Nephropathy in the Diabetes Control and Complications Trial
The Diabetes Control and Complications Trial (DCCT) Research Group
Kidney Int 47:1703–1720, 1995   9–13

Background.—The Diabetes Control and Complications Trial (DCCT), a multicenter, randomized clinical trial, compared the efficacy of intensive diabetes treatment, which sought to keep glucose levels as consistently close to normal as possible, with conventional diabetes treatment in regards to the development and progression of long-term complications in patients with insulin-dependent diabetes mellitus (IDDM). Previous reports have documented the superior efficacy of intensive diabetes therapy in delaying the onset or progression of retinopathy, microalbuminuria, and overt nephropathy. Changes in renal function were also studied in relation to the 2 treatment protocols in primary prevention and secondary intervention cohorts.

Methods.—At baseline, the 726 patients in the primary-prevention cohort had IDDM for 1–5 years, a stimulated serum C-peptide level less than 0.5 pmol/mL, no retinopathy, and a urinary albumin excretion rate (AER) less than 28 μg/min. The 715 patients in the secondary-intervention cohort had IDDM for 1–15 years, stimulated C-peptide levels less than 0.2 pmol/L in those with IDDM for at least 5 years, minimal or moderate retinopathy, and urinary AER levels less than 139 μg/min. Serum creatinine levels were measured after breakfast and the morning dose of insulin. Four-hour urine collections were analyzed for urine albumin and creatinine. The glomerular filtration rate was measured after 3 years and at the end of the study. Associations were examined between treatment assignment and albuminuria, renal insufficiency, and hypertension.

Results.—The incidence of microalbuminuria (≥ 28 µg/min) was 16% after 9 years of intensive therapy and 27% after 9 years of conventional therapy in the primary-prevention cohort. Intensive treatment resulted in a 34% reduction in risk of microalbuminuria developing. In the secondary-intervention cohort, the 9-year incidence of microalbuminuria (≥ 28 µg/min) was 26% in the intensive-therapy group and 42% in the conventional-therapy group. Intensive therapy resulted in a 43% reduction in risk in this cohort. In the primary prevention cohort, the 9-year incidence of a more advanced level of microalbuminuria (≥ 70 µg/min) was 3.3% with intensive treatment and 7% with conventional treatment, whereas the 9-year incidence was 10% with intensive treatment and 20.2% with conventional treatment in the secondary-intervention cohort. The 9-year incidence of clinical albuminuria (≥ 208 µg/min) was 2.6% with intensive therapy and 2.3% in the conventional-therapy group in the primary-prevention cohort, and 5.3% with intensive therapy and 11.3% with conventional therapy in the secondary-intervention cohort. Intensive therapy reduced the risk of sustained elevations of AER developing by 51% to 67%. Treatment assignment did not affect creatinine clearance or the development of hypertension. The glomerular filtration rate was nonsignificantly lower with intensive therapy.

Conclusions.—Intensive therapy was associated with a 39% reduction in the risk of microalbuminuria developing and a 54% reduction in the risk of clinical albuminuria developing. In the secondary intervention, AER levels increased 6.5% per year with conventional therapy and stayed consistent with intensive therapy. The use of intensive therapy is therefore recommended for most patients with IDDM.

▶ At least a third of insulin-dependent patients have in the past eventually had end-stage renal disease. This study describes in detail the benefits obtained by such patients when given intensive diabetes treatment. The data are very encouraging—at the very least, such therapy delays the progression of nephropathy and may indeed even prevent or delay the development of advanced renal disease.

L. Lasagna, M.D.

Prediction of the Human Pharmacokinetics of Troglitazone, a New and Extensively Metabolized Antidiabetic Agent, After Oral Administration, With an Animal Scale-Up Approach

Izumi T, Enomoto S, Hosiyama K, et al (Sankyo Co Ltd, Tokyo; Kyoto Univ, Japan; Univ of Tokyo)
J Pharmacol Exp Ther 277:1630–1641, 1996   9–14

Purpose.—Prediction of a drug's pharmacokinetics in humans often is attempted by evaluation of its pharmacokinetics in animals, but the drug usually is administered to the animals intravenously. Data derived after oral drug administration to animals were used to predict the human pharmacokinetics of troglitazone, an antidiabetic agent with a high metabolic clearance that is metabolized primarily in the liver. Data were obtained after intravenous and oral administration of troglitazone to mice, rats, monkeys, and dogs.

Procedure.—First, allometric equations involving the oral plasma clearance of total or unbound drug or the hepatic intrinsic clearance of unbound drug and animal body weight were used to predict the area under the plasma concentration–time curve and bioavailability (F) in humans after oral administration. Predictability did not differ markedly among the 3 methods. A series of steps then were followed to predict the range of plasma profiles after oral administration to humans. (1) Based on animal data, the exponent and coefficients in the allometric relation between body weight and factors such as total body plasma clearance and various distribution volumes were calculated. (2) The absorption rate constant was estimated from allometric relation to body weight and the F value from the predicted area under the plasma concentration–time curve. (3) Plasma concentration–time profiles after oral administration were described with an equation involving the allometric exponents and coefficients, the absorption rate constant, F, and body weight.

Outcome —Observed plasma profiles were similar to the simulated profiles. Predicted values for area under the plasma concentration–time curve were 60% to 120% of those observed. The technique described may be valuable for using animal data to predict a range of plasma profiles for humans receiving an orally administered drug.

▶ The development of troglitazone for treating type II diabetes may place it among the other new approaches, metformin and acarbose. Another treatment of type II diabetes may be the reduction of obesity using some of the new medications, of which there are many coming down the pike and some already on the market. All these will, of course, be added to the standard oral antidiabetic agents, making type II diabetes easier to treat. Of course, one can say this is necessary because Americans are getting fatter and the development of obesity leads to type II diabetes in susceptible people.

M. Weintraub, M.D.

Treatment of Symptomatic Diabetic Peripheral Neuropathy With the Anti-oxidant α-Lipoic Acid: A 3-Week Multicentre Randomized Controlled Trial (ALADIN Study)

Ziegler D, and the ALADIN Study Group (Heinrich-Heine-Universität, Düsseldorf, Germany)
Diabetologia 38:1425–1433, 1995   9–15

Background.—Antioxidant treatment prevents nerve dysfunction in experimental models of diabetes mellitus. The potential value of such treatment for diabetic patients was investigated.

Methods and Findings.—Three hundred twenty-eight patients with non-insulin-dependent diabetes with symptomatic peripheral neuropathy were assigned randomly to IV infusion of α-lipoic acid (ALA) at 1,200, 600, or 100 mg or placebo. The total symptom score in the feet declined by a mean of 4.5 points from baseline to day 19 in patients receiving 1,200 mg of ALA, by 5 points in those receiving 600 mg of ALA, and by 3.3 points in those receiving 100 mg of ALA. In the placebo group, the mean decline in symptom score was 2.6 points. After 19 days, response rates were 70.8% in the 1,200 mg-group, 82.5% in the 600-mg group, 65.2% in the 100-mg group, and 57.6% in the placebo group. After 19 days, there was a significant decrease in the total scale of the Pain Adjective List in patients receiving 1,200 and 600 mg of ALA, compared with those receiving

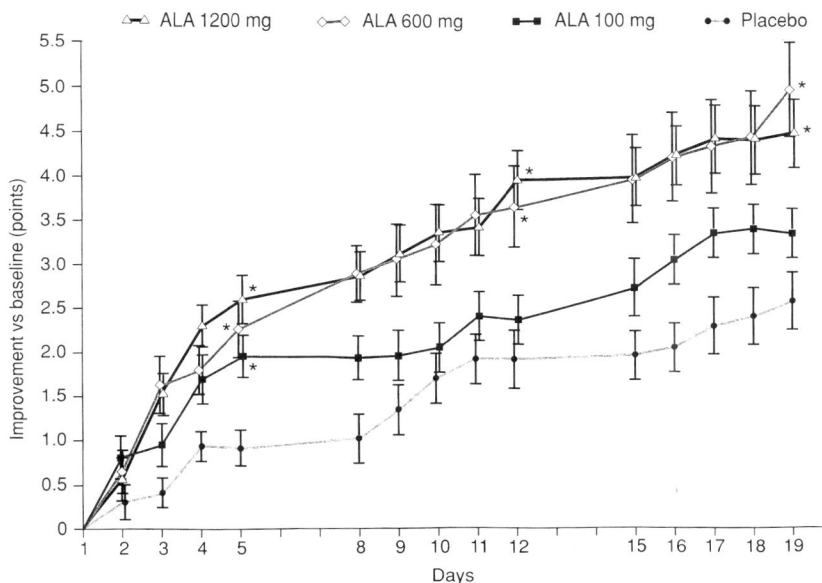

FIGURE 1.—Changes (improvement) in the total symptom scores from baseline on a daily basis in the four groups studied (mean ± SEM). * p < 0.05 vs. changes in placebo for statistical testing after 5, 12, and 18 days. (Courtesy of Ziegler D and the ALADIN Study Group: Treatment of Symptomatic Diabetic Peripheral Neuropathy With the Anti-Oxidant α-Lipoic Acid: A 3-Week Multicentre Randomized Controlled Trial (ALADIN Study). *Diabetologia* 38:1425–1433, 1995.)

placebo. Adverse events occurred in 32.6% of the patients receiving 12 mg, 18.2% of those receiving 600 mg, 13.6% of those receiving 100 mg, and 20.7% of those receiving placebo (Fig 1).

Conclusion.—Intravenous ALA in a dose of 600 mg/day over 3 weeks is superior to placebo in reducing the symptoms of diabetic peripheral neuropathy. Furthermore, this treatment is not associated with significant adverse reactions.

▶ This study was really too short for something like diabetic peripheral neuropathy which has a long history. However, ALA appears to be worthy of further study. All of the treatments showed improvement, even with the chronic, long-lasting nature of neuropathic pain which prevents improvement with placebo. Nonetheless, it is common for placebo-treated patients to improve in clinical trials. This is one of the causes for a drug to do somewhat better in actual clinical practice than it does in clinical trials. The improvement can be seen in the accompanying figure.

M. Weintraub, M.D.

Effect on Lipoprotein Profile of Replacing Butter With Margarine in a Low Fat Diet: Randomised Crossover Study With Hypercholesterolaemic Subjects
Chisholm A Mann J, Sutherland W, et al (Univ of Otago, Dunedin, New Zealand; Lincoln Univ, Canterbury, New Zealand)
BMJ 312:93 –934, 1996   9–16

Introduction.—An appreciable reduction in saturated fatty acids is necessary to decrease the risk of coronary heart disease in most Western countries. There is an association between total and low-density lipoprotein cholesterol and saturated fatty acids. As replacement fats for butter, which is relatively high in saturated fatty acids, margarines rich in unsaturated fatty acids often are recommended. It has been suggested that the use of margarine may be inappropriate in diets aimed at reducing the lipoprotein-mediated risk of coronary heart disease because most margarines contain at least some trans unsaturated fatty acids. A comparison of butter and margarine high in monounsaturates used as a source of "hard" fat in an overall reduced-fat diet was conducted to assess the effects on lipid and lipoprotein concentrations.

Methods.—Forty-nine volunteers who had polygenic hyperlipidemia and baseline total cholesterol concentrations in the range of 5.5–7.0 mmol/L participated in the 21-week protocol. For 4 weeks, they had their usual diet and completed a 4-day food record. They completed questionnaires about their past, present, and family medical history. They were randomly assigned to 2 groups who followed the margarine diet or the butter diet for 6 weeks. They had a 5-week washout period and were crossed over into the opposite group for another 6 weeks. Lipid and lipoprotein concentrations were measured, as were triglyceride fatty acids.

Results.—Throughout the study, body weight and blood pressure did not change. In the margarine group, concentrations of low-density lipoprotein cholesterol and apolipoprotein B were about 10% lower than in the butter group. With the 2 diets, Lp(a) lipoprotein and high-density lipoprotein cholesterol concentration were similar. All other measurements also were similar. An average of 17 g of butter or margarine was used each day for cooking and spreading.

Conclusion.—The use of unsaturated margarine rather than butter by patients with hypercholesterolemia is associated with a lipoprotein profile that could reduce cardiovascular risk. This is the result despite concerns about the adverse effects on lipoproteins of trans fatty acids in margarines. The conclusion is strengthened that margarine is an appropriate replacement fat for butter for those with raised cholesterol concentrations.

▶ More trees and computer disks were sacrificed to margarine's effect on cholesterol than to many other theories. Fortunately, results such as these put to rest the idea that margarine's concentration of "trans unsaturated fatty acids" would be inappropriate, or in fact harmful, in patients with hyperlipoproteinemia or hypercholesterolemia. Margarine still seems to be the best fat choice in hypercholesterolemic diets. Now all we have to do is wait until the next study comes along and throws cold water on that hypothesis.

M. Weintraub, M.D.

Apparent Discontinuation Rates in Patients Prescribed Lipid-lowering Drugs
Simons LA, Levis G, Simons J (Univ of New South Wales, Australia; St Vincent's Hosp, Sydney, New South Wales, Australia)
Med J Aust 164:208–211, 1996   9–17

Background.—Lipid-lowering drugs are commonly prescribed to patients with hyperlipidemia for long-term treatment so that the risk of coronary heart disease is reduced and survival is improved. Discontinuation rates were studied prospectively over a 1-year period in several community pharmacies to examine compliance with long-term treatment with lipid-lowering drugs.

Methods.—Data were obtained from 138 pharmacies on 610 patients who filled a first prescription for simvastatin, pravastatin, or gemfibrozil and who had not been treated with a lipid-lowering drug in the preceding 3 months. Patients who were at least 4 weeks late in filling repeat prescriptions were identified. These patients were questioned by the pharmacist at the next opportunity regarding reasons for discontinuation. Factors predicting discontinuation were analyzed using demographic and other prescription data from the pharmacy records.

Results.—After 1 year, 60% of the patients had discontinued treatment, half discontinued within 3 months, and a quarter discontinued within 1 month of treatment initiation. The dominant reasons for discontinuation were being unconvinced about needing treatment (32%), poor efficacy (32%), and adverse events (7%). Although the treatment was considered ineffective by the physicians of 32% of the patients, only half of these patients were prescribed another drug. A lower risk of discontinuation was significantly and independently predicted by an age of at least 65 years, concurrent treatment with other cardiovascular drugs, and using analgesic drugs. The risk of discontinuation was higher among patients treated with antidepressant drugs and among patients treated with gemfibrozil compared with those treated with simvastatin.

Conclusions.—A large proportion of patients in whom lipid-lowering drug therapy was initiated discontinued the drug within 1 year, which resulted in a high cost of wasted treatment and a substantial loss of opportunity to prevent heart disease. Many of the early discontinuations were patient initiated, for reasons that may be counteracted with informational intervention.

Treating Elevated Cholesterol Levels: The Great Satan in Perspective
Gibaldi M, Kradjan W (Univ of Washington, Seattle)
J Clin Pharmacol 36:189–197, 1996   9–18

Introduction.—Serum cholesterol is inextricably linked to coronary heart disease, and the results of primary prevention trials have led to the recommendation that people with moderately to severely elevated cholesterol levels should be identified and treated, by drugs if necessary. However, there is ongoing debate over the relative value of cholesterol-lowering drugs for primary and secondary prevention. Issues related to the optimal use of lipid-lowering drugs for the treatment of high cholesterol levels were reviewed.

Discussion.—The debate centers on whether lipid-lowering drugs should be used to treat all patients with elevated cholesterol levels—even those with no clinical signs of coronary disease—or limited to patients with previous angina, coronary angioplasty, coronary artery bypass surgery, or myocardial infarction. Recommendations based on the results of primary prevention trials have included blood cholesterol measurement in all young adult patients and even in children older than 2 years with a family history suggesting an increased risk of coronary disease. Such approaches would be extremely expensive and may do more harm than good. Furthermore, the results of primary prevention trials do not show that reducing cholesterol prolongs overall survival. It is even possible that low cholesterol levels may lead to increased noncardiovascular morbidity, either directly or indirectly.

In contrast, a growing body of evidence suggests that interventions to reduce serum cholesterol can reduce morbidity and mortality in patients with known coronary disease. These effects become apparent after about 1 year of therapy, and become still greater thereafter. One study suggested that treating 100 patients with coronary heart disease would save the lives of 4 of 9 patients who would otherwise die, prevent nonfatal myocardial infarction in 7 of 21 patients, and avoid revascularization procedures in 6 of 19 patients.

Summary.—The available evidence is not strong enough to support the screening of large populations for high cholesterol or the use of primary preventive therapy in patients with known high cholesterol. However, aggressive cholesterol-reducing therapy appears to be highly effective in patients with known coronary heart disease. Further research is needed to determine whether there are any risk factors that can identify patients who would benefit from primary prevention.

▶ Although the study on discontinuation rates was centered in Australia, the figures are unlikely to be different here in the United States. In fact, the causes are unlikely to be different. The very easy to take "statin" drugs seem to be no problem at all. In most cases, you only have to prescribe 1 a day, they rarely cause side effects at that dosage, and if they do, the patient can be transferred to another drug. They are incredibly effective. More importantly, the 4S Study and the West of Scotland Study, discussed elsewhere in this edition of the YEAR BOOK, indicated a primary preventive effect of the lipid-lowering agents.

On the other hand, the great "Satan" is really the cholesterol molecule, which is being beaten back from the walls of our city, no matter how high or how low it is in a particular individual. We do need more data, however, to determine whether there exists a group of patients with risk factors who would benefit from primary prevention.

M. Weintraub, M.D.

Excessive Thyroid Hormone Replacement Therapy
Nuovo J, Ellsworth A, Christensen DB, et al (Univ of California, Davis; Univ of Washington, Seattle)
J Am Board Fam Pract 8:435–439, 1995   9–19

Background.—Accelerated osteoporosis and other long-term metabolic complications are possible in patients receiving excessive thyroid hormone replacement therapy. The chances of iatrogenic hyperthyroxinemia have increased with the increased bioavailability of newer commercial products. Laboratory assays for thyrotropin (TSH) have improved as well, making detection of hyperthyroxinemia more likely. To determine how often excessive prescribing occurs, thyroid replacement therapy at 1 clinic was audited. The contribution of changes in replacement thyroid hormone preparations and thyroid function tests on the incidence of the problem was evaluated as well.

Methods.—The audit included 78 patients receiving thyroid hormone for hypothyroidism at a family medicine residency training program. In-formation on the specific thyroid medication used and the thyroid laboratory test results was gathered from each patient's chart. One-way analysis of variance was used to compare data from the years 1975 to 1981 and 1982 to 1989.

Results.—The mean serum thyroxine level in the earlier period (about 8 µg/dL) was similar to that of the later period (about 9 µg/dL). This was so even though the mean TSH level decreased from 25 to 7 mIU/mL and the mean daily levothyroxine dose declined from 184 to 145 µg/day. Thirty-three percent of the patients had supersuppressed TSH levels from 1982 to 1990, compared with 10% from 1975 to 1981. After controlling for study period, age was not significantly related to either TSH or thyroxine.

Conclusions.—Patients with hypothyroidism are at risk of receiving excessive thyroid hormone replacement therapy, with resultant iatrogenic hyperthyroxinemia. Clinicians should bear in mind that the currently used levothyroxine preparations are more potent than those used in the past. Accurate dose titration can be achieved using the sensitive TSH assay. All patients receiving thyroid hormone replacement therapy need long-term monitoring as part of their health care maintenance regimen.

▶ Patients on thyroid hormone need TSH monitoring. Levothyroxine is a popular drug in the United States, although I have long been certain that everyone receiving it cannot possibly have hypothyroidism. The reformulation of thyroid products has led at times to increased bioavailability, so that changes in supplier (or changes in the same product over time) can lead to trouble. Current levothyroxine formulations are more potent than the older ones.

L. Lasagna, M.D.

Genetic and Clinical Features of 42 Kindreds With Resistance to Thyroid Hormone: The National Institutes of Health Prospective Study
Brucker-Davis F, Skarulis MC, Grace MB, et al (Natl Inst of Diabetes, Digestive, and Kidney Diseases, Bethesda, Md; Natl Cancer Inst, Bethesda, Md)
Ann Intern Med 123:572–583, 1995   9–20

Background.—Patients with resistance to thyroid hormone exhibit decreased pituitary and tissue responsiveness to thyroid hormone. The condition is usually transmitted in autosomal dominant fashion; its prevalence is low but uncertain. Resistance to thyroid hormone may be defined as generalized resistance and pituitary resistance, and its manifestations range from subclinical to highly symptomatic. The genetic and clinical findings of 42 kindreds with resistance to thyroid hormone are reported.

Methods.—The study included 104 patients from 42 unrelated kindreds with resistance to thyroid hormone, all studied prospectively at a single institution. Also studied as controls were 114 unaffected relatives of similar environmental and genetic backgrounds to those of the patients. The initial evaluation included thyroid, cardiovascular, psychometric, hearing, speech, and growth testing. Thyroid tests were performed at baseline and again after stimulation with thyroid-stimulating hormone-releasing hormone. The research subjects also underwent DNA analysis to detect mutations of the thyroid hormone receptor β gene on exons 9 and 10 and evaluation of tissue-specific compensation for resistance.

Results.—Twenty-two kindreds demonstrated autosomal dominant inheritance, 14 had sporadic inheritance, and 6 had unknown transmission. Sixty-four patients in 25 kindreds showed genetic mutations: 16 of them in exon 9 and 9 in exon 10 of the TRβ gene.

Nineteen percent of the patients had undergone thyroidectomy. Sixty-five percent of the patients with resistance to thyroid hormone had goiter, 60% had attention-deficit hyperactivity disorder, 38% had intelligence quotients less than 85, 35% had speech impediments, and 18% had short stature. A number of previously unreported clinical features were noted as well: 56% had frequent ear, nose, and throat infections; 32% were children with low weight for height; 21% had hearing loss; and 18% had cardiac abnormalities. The phenotype varied with genotype, age, presence of resistance to thyroid hormone in the mother, and sex. Tissue resistance also differed between families. Pituitary resistance was the most common, followed by brain, bone, liver, and heart resistance (Fig 1).

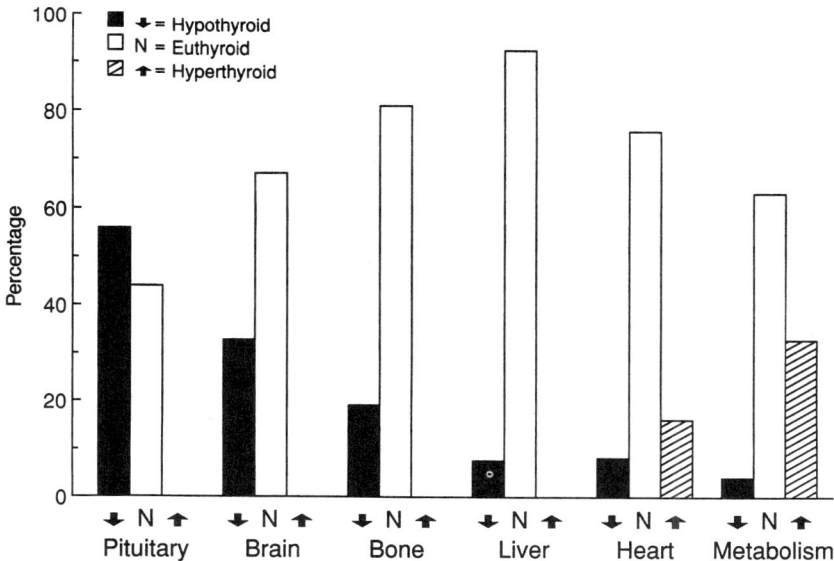

FIGURE 1.—Degree of resistance to thyroid hormone in various organs in patients with resistance to thyroid hormone. The variables studied were basal and TSH-releasing hormone-stimulated TSH levels for the pituitary gland; full-scale IQ for the brain; percentile of the height and bone age for the bone; cholesterol, testosterone-binding globulin, and ferritin levels for the liver; resting pulse for the heart; and basal metabolic rate for the metabolism. For the pituitary gland, the liver, the heart, and the metabolism, the results were from patients with no history of thyroidectomy who were not receiving thyroid medication. Patients receiving cardiac medication were excluded for the evaluation of the heart. *Abbreviations:* *TSH*, thyroid-stimulating hormone; *IQ*, intelligence quotient. (Courtesy of Brucker-Davis F, Skarulis MC, Grace MB, et al: Genetic and clinical features of 42 kindreds with resistance to thyroid hormone: The National Institutes of Health prospective study. *Ann Intern Med* 123:572–583, 1995.)

Conclusions.—This large study highlights the variability of resistance to thyroid hormone. The incidences of the classic clinical features of this condition are reported, along with some previously unreported clinical characteristics. Resistance to thyroid hormone is often viewed as a relatively benign problem. However, some affected families have cardiac disorders, and the associated behavioral disorders may have important personal, familial, and social consequences. Newborns from families with known resistance should be screened and possibly started on early thyroid hormone replacement therapy, although this treatment approach needs further study.

▶ Resistance to thyroid hormone was first described by Refetoff et al.[1] The phenotype is heterogeneous, but there are classic clinical features: attention-deficit hyperactivity disorder, growth delay, and tachycardia. During the last 20 years 104 such patients and 114 unaffected relatives have been studied at the National Institutes of Health.

Resistance to thyroid hormone is commonly mistaken for Graves' disease, but the hormonal profile is usually unambiguous provided the patient has not undergone thyroidectomy. The diagnosis should not be missed if a proper family history is taken and is supplemented by measurement of free thyroxine and thyroid-stimulating hormone, and an MRI scan of the pituitary.

This article supports earlier studies in some respects but reports a number of new clinical features, such as frequent ear, nose, and throat infections, hearing loss, low weight, and cardiac problems.

L. Lasagna, M.D.

Reference

1. Refetoff S, DeWind LT, DeGroot LJ: Familial syndrome combining deaf-mutism, stuppoed epiphyses, goiter and abnormally high PBI: Possible target organ refractorines to thyroid hormone. *J Clin Endocrinol Metab* 27:279–294, 1967.

Silent Myocardial Ischemia in Hypothyroidism
Bernstein R, Müller C, Midtbø K, et al (Oslo City Univ, Norway; Ullevaal Hosp, Oslo, Norway; Aker Hosp, Oslo, Norway)
Thyroid 5:443–447, 1995   9–21

Background.—In some patients with severe hypothyroidism, thyroxine treatment can improve, aggravate, or precipitate angina pectoris. Myocardial infarction and sudden death are not uncommon among those whose angina is worsened with thyroxine replacement therapy. A recent study using radionuclide ventriculography suggests that the effect of thyroxine is related to the presence of reversible coronary dysfunction rather than to asymmetric septal hypertrophy. Six patients were followed up to confirm these findings.

Methods.—All patients had severe, untreated primary hypothyroidism without evidence of coexisting coronary artery disease. Blood pressure was

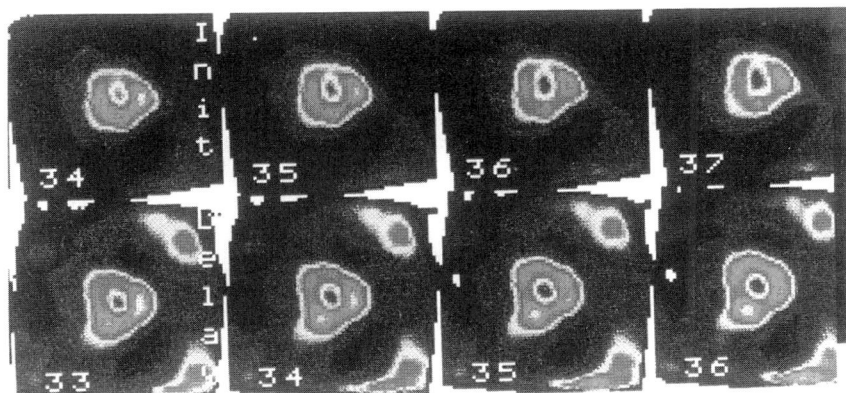

FIGURE 1.—Short-axis [201] Tl tomograms obtained immediately after exercise (**top strip**) and after 3 hours of rest (**bottom strip**) in a woman, 34, with severe hypothyroidism (height, 1,740 mm; weight, 67 kg) before thyroxine replacement therapy. Tomographic sections oriented from apex (**left**) to base (**right**) display anterior myocardial perfusion defects immediately after stress, which normalize completely after 3 hours. (Courtesy of Bernstein R, Müller C, Midtbø K, et al: Silent myocardial ischemia in hypothyroidism. *Thyroid* 5:443–447, 1995.)

normal in 5, and none were receiving any medication. Echocardiography and redistribution tomographic myocardial thallium-201 imaging (single photon emission CT [SPECT]) were performed before thyroxine replacement therapy; SPECT was repeated at 10 days and after 2 months of therapy. Thyroxine was started at 0.025 mg daily for 3 days, increased to 0.05 mg daily for 1 month, then continued at 0.1 mg daily.

Results.—Two patients achieved only 81% of the target heart rate during exercise ECG stress testing limited by fatigue and 4 achieved heart rates from 85% to 97% of age-predicted maximal heart rate. Tomograms in 4 patients showed substantial regional perfusion defects after exercise that were normalized at rest before thyroxine therapy (Fig 1); in 1 case, normalization also occurred after 10 days on thyroxine. Exercise and redistribution SPECT were normal in each patient with restoration of euthyroidism. Statistical evaluation of SPECT results suggests that the proportional incidence of myocardial perfusion defects in hypothyroidism will be at least 22% with 95% probability.

Conclusion.—Although the sensitivity of [201] Tl stress imaging by SPECT is approximately 90% in detection of coronary artery disease, specificity is relatively low. Despite this low specificity, it does appear that impaired myocardial perfusion as assessed by SPECT is the result of reversible coronary dysfunction characteristic of the hypothyroid state.

▶ A small but not trivial percentage of patients with severe hypothyroidism have angina pectoris before or after treatment. Hence, angiography has been recommended for many such patients. The availability of a new kind of myocardial imaging has provided these authors with a way to evaluate whether patients with hypothyroidism have impaired cardiac perfusion as a result of reversible coronary dysfunction. This situation seems to be not uncommon.

L. Lasagna, M.D.

Monitoring of Growth Hormone Replacement Therapy in Adults, Based on Measurement of Serum Markers
de Boer H, Blok GJ, Popp-Snijders C, et al (Free Univ, Amsterdam, The Netherlands. Royal North Shore Hosp, St Leonards, NSW, Australia)
J Clin Endocrinol Metab 81:1371–1377, 1996   9–22

Background.—Adult growth hormone deficiency (GHD) is associated with clinically relevant abnormalities that are at least partially reversed by growth hormone (GH) replacement therapy. The optimal dosage and the most appropriate method of monitoring treatment remain controversial. The usefulness of insulin-like growth factor (IGF-I), IGF-binding protein-3, and the acid-labile subunit as markers for monitoring GH replacement therapy in adults was investigated.

Methods.—Forty-six men with GHD participated in a 1-year, double-blind, placebo-controlled, dose-response study of GH replacement therapy. The dosages of recombinant human GH ranged from 0.33 to 3.0 IU/m² day.

Results.—Significant, dose-dependent increases in all 3 markers were observed with the lowest GH dosages. Insulin-like growth factor required lower dosages than the other 2 markers for normalization of serum levels and was more likely to rise to abnormally high concentrations than were the other 2 markers at higher GH dosages.

Conclusions.—Serum levels of IGF-I appeared to be the most sensitive marker for the detection of excessive GH replacement therapy in growth-hormone–deficient adults. Using this standard, the predicted optimal GH dosage for men 20 to 40 years of age with GHD was 1.4 IU/m² day.

▶ The use of serum markers to determine a drug effect, in this case GH, is plagued with the same problems as other surrogate markers for drug effect. One has to know, or establish, whether the marker relates to the effect of the drug or hormone in a meaningful way. Having to stick to certain numbers as the end point for the treatment is rarely a beneficial course of action. However, in this case, the IGF-I does bear some relation to outcome and would be a reasonable first cut at a goal. Of course, as we have learned from previous examples, with the changes and improvements in scientific methodology, IGF-I will soon yield to IGF-Ia, b, c, d, and e, and only 1 of those will be seen to change with GH.

M. Weintraub, M.D.

Treatment of Children With Congenital Heart Disease and Growth Retardation With Recombinant Human Growth Hormone

Sasaki H, Baba K, Nishida Y, et al (Kurashiki Central Hosp, Okayama, Japan; Kyoto Univ, Japan; Shimane Med Univ, Japan)
Acta Paediatr 85:251–253, 1996   9–23

Background.—Growth retardation is a significant problem associated with severe congenital heart disease in children. The value of growth hormone (GH) treatment in such patients has not been well documented. The outcomes of recombinant human GH treatment in 7 prepubertal children with congenital heart disease who had had corrective cardiac surgery were reported.

Methods.—The children were 6 boys and 1 girl, aged 5.3–12.7 years. Their height, standardized in years, ranged from 3.2 to 9 at the beginning of the study. The surgical correction of heart disease had been completed at least 2 years before GH therapy was initiated. Growth hormone was given in 6 or 7 divided doses of 0.5 international units kg^{-1} $week^{-1}$ for 2 years or longer.

Findings.—The mean growth rate increased from 4.3 cm $year^{-1}$ before treatment to 7.8 cm $year^{-1}$ in the first year of treatment and to 6.3 cm $year^{-1}$ in the second year of treatment. After 2 years, mean standardized height increased from -3.31 to -2.54. With treatment, mean height age difference minus bone age difference was positive.

Conclusions.—Although the precise mechanism of increased growth was not clearly defined, this study shows that recombinant GH improves growth rate in children with growth retardation associated with congenital heart disease after surgical correction. The ultimate benefit of GH treatment for such patients cannot be determined until a final assessment of height is made.

▶ Growth hormone used to be administered only to people with GH deficiency in the days when cadaver pituitaries were the source of GH. Now, with recombinant GH readily available (and free of Creutzfeld-Jakob disease risk), the hormone is being studied in other clinical situations. It looks as if it helps correct growth retardation as a result of congenital heart disease. One nice aspect of this approach was the failure to increase the rate of skeletal maturation in the face of increased linear growth velocity, which should lead to improved adult height.

L. Lasagna, M.D.

Long Term Sequelae of Sex Steroid Treatment in the Management of Constitutionally Tall Stature

de Waal WJ, Torn M, de Muinck Keizer-Schrama SMPF, et al (Erasmus Univ Rotterdam, The Netherlands)
Arch Dis Child 73:311–315, 1995   9–24

Background.—Many constitutionally tall adolescent patients receive high doses of sex steroids to reduce their final height. Most of the reported side effects of this practice have occurred only during or shortly after the end of treatment, and in any case have been mild and reversible. The potential long-term side effects of sex steroid treatment during adolescence were studied, emphasizing the possible effects on hypothalamic-gonadal function.

Methods.—Sixty-four men and 180 women who had received supraphysiologic doses of sex hormones during puberty for constitutionally tall stature were studied a mean of 10 years after the end of treatment, when they underwent a standardized interview. For both sexes, the interview included questions about satisfaction, possible side effects of hormone treatment, and reproductive issues. Also studied were 61 tall men and 94 tall women who elected not to undergo hormone treatment after evaluation.

Results.—Ninety-three percent of the women and eighty-six percent of the men expressed satisfaction with their decision to undergo sex steroid treatment. One or more side effects occurred during treatment in 77% of the women and 78% of the men. The side effects were generally mild, however; they led to treatment cessation in 3% of the women and none of the men. Women reported more frequent side effects during high-dose estrogen treatment than during oral contraceptive treatment. Five percent of the women had amenorrhea lasting more than 6 months after the end of hormone therapy. The patients and controls were not significantly different in their menstrual cycle characteristics. No cases of malignancy were reported. The data collected on pregnancies—127 total—showed no notable differences in details and outcomes between the patients and the controls.

Conclusions.—Through 10 years after the end of treatment, sex steroid treatment for constitutionally tall adolescents appears to have no long-term effects on reproductive function or cancer risk. Longer follow-up is needed, however. The increased incidence of side effects in female patients receiving high-dose estrogen therapy suggests a possible dose-dependent relationship.

▶ Short people often wish they were taller, and tall boys and especially girls (except for basketball players!) often wish they weren't quite so different from the average.

This study suggests that long-term side effects from sex steroid treatment in the teenage years are probably not a problem.

L. Lasagna, M.D.

Aspirin and NSAID Use in Older Women: Effect on Bone Mineral Density and Fracture Risk

Bauer DC, for the Study of Osteoporotic Fractures Research Group (Univ of California, San Francisco; Kaiser Permanente Ctr for Health Research, Portland, Ore; Oregon Health Sciences Univ, Portland; et al)
J Bone Miner Res 11:29–35, 1996   9–25

Background.—The relation between prostaglandins and bone metabolism is not clear. In vitro and animal studies suggest that prostaglandin inhibition by aspirin or nonsteroidal anti-inflammatory drugs (NSAIDs) may inhibit bone loss and preserve bone mineral density (BMD). However, the effect of these agents on BMD and fracture risk in postmenopausal women is not known.

Methods.—The risk factors for osteoporosis and aspirin and NSAID use were studied in 7,786 white women older than 65 years. Axial BMD also was measured. Fractures were documented prospectively during the subsequent 4 years of follow-up.

Findings.—In an age-adjusted analysis, daily aspirin or NSAID use was associated with a 2.3% to 5.8% increase in BMD of the hip and spine, which persisted after adjustment for weight, medications, self-reported arthritis, and radiographic findings of osteoarthritis. However, the multiply adjusted increase in BMD was only 1% to 3.1%. Daily users of aspirin and NSAIDs had a fracture risk comparable to that of nonusers. The relative risk of hip fracture was 1.1 among daily aspirin users after adjustment for potential confounders. Among daily NSAID users, this risk was 0.9. When all nonspine fractures were considered together, the risk was 1.0 among both aspirin users and NSAID users.

Conclusions.—In elderly women, regular aspirin or NSAID use may have a modestly beneficial effect, which persists after adjustment for obesity and osteoarthritis. However, there is no clinically significant protective effect on the risk of fractures associated with regular aspirin or NSAID use.

▶ This paper is very interesting in that it reminds us that people who have osteoarthritis can have an increase of bone mass by a mechanism that is, as yet, unknown. Higher aspirin and NSAID use in this population was greater in women who had osteoarthritis by self-report. The fact that the study showed no difference in fracture rate, although there was a difference in BMD, probably could be related to the 2-year follow-up period. Perhaps the registry of older women, totaling more than 5,000 people at this point, will be looked at again 4 and 6 years after they first entered the study.

M. Weintraub, M.D.

Individualised Low-dose Alglucerase Therapy for Type 1 Gaucher's Disease

Hollak CEM, Aerts JMFG, Goudsmit R, et al (Academic Med Centre, Amsterdam)

Lancet 345: 1474–1478, 1995   9–26

Introduction.—For patients with type 1 Gaucher's disease, a common lysosomal storage disorder, enzyme supplementation is effective at doses of 30–130 U of alglucerase per kilogram per month. Individualized dosing would appear to be the best approach, especially given the high cost and unknown side effects of alglucerase. Individualized, very low doses of alglucerase were studied to investigate their effects.

Methods.—The study included 25 patients with symptomatic type 1 Gaucher's disease, 13 of whom had undergone splenectomy. They began treatment at a dose of 1.15 U of alglucerase per kilogram 3 times weekly, or 15 U/kg/month. The patients' responses to treatment were monitored on the basis of hematologic variables and liver and spleen volume, and the alglucerase dose was halved, maintained, or doubled accordingly.

Results.—Seventy-two percent of the patients had a response after 6 months of alglucerase treatment. There were 17 moderate responses and 1 good response in this group. At 12 to 18 months, all evaluable patients had sustained improvement. Hematologic response was slower to occur in patients with severe splenomegaly.

Conclusions.—In patients with type 1 Gaucher's disease, very low initial doses of alglucerase can produce good results at lower cost than higher doses. The results appear similar to those reported with higher doses of alglucerase and better than those reported for a low-dose regimen of 10 U/kg every 2 weeks. The clinical response to alglucerase varies greatly, and the only way to find out which patients can benefit from a low dose is to use very low doses initially.

▶ Here is another great surprise. Being a clinician and adjusting the dose to the outcome allows you to arrive at an apparently good response. Physicians can do better than either being restricted to the low-dose 10 U of alglucerase per kilogram every 2 weeks or prescribing a fixed higher dose. The dose adjustment saves enormous amounts of money for this very expensive but effective treatment. The dose in this study was individualized using 3 criteria: the hemoglobin level, the platelet count, and the organ-volume response. Actually, it took a good clinician to assess these 3 variables. Nonetheless, the criteria used were quite clear and are outlined in the paper.

M. Weintraub, M.D.

10 Gastrointestinal Disorders

A Cost Analysis of Alternative Treatments for Duodenal Ulcer

Imperiale TF, Speroff T, Cebul RD, et al (Case Western Reserve Univ, Cleveland, Ohio)

Ann Intern Med 123:665–672, 1995   10–1

Background.—Duodenal ulcer disease, a very common disorder, is associated with substantial morbidity. The costs of alternative strategies for the treatment of this condition were compared.

Methods.—Using a decision model, the costs per cure of 3 initial treatment strategies for an endoscopically proved duodenal ulcer were compared. These strategies were H_2-receptor antagonist therapy given for 8 weeks, antibiotic treatment for *Helicobacter pylori* infection plus H_2-receptor antagonist treatment, and urease test–based treatment. Secondary treatments for symptomatic recurrences included empirical therapy based on a second endoscopy-guided urease test or biopsy. Subsequent cure was assumed. Patients at low risk for malignant ulcer comprised the cohort in this analysis.

Findings.—For all secondary strategies, initial treatment with antibiotics for *H. pylori* infection plus an H_2-receptor antagonist was associated with the lowest mean cost per symptomatic cure when the prevalence or likelihood of *H. pylori* infection exceeded 66% to 76%. Initial therapy with an H_2-receptor antagonist was the most expensive. These findings were not sensitive to the rates of duodenal ulcer recurrence after either treatment, to the cost of either treatment, or to the prevalence of *H. pylori*.

Conclusions.—Initial treatment with antibiotics for *H. pylori* infection plus an H_2-receptor antagonist has the lowest cost per symptomatic cure, regardless of the secondary treatment used for ulcer recurrence. Eradicating *H. pylori* should be part of the initial treatment strategy for patients with duodenal ulcer.

▶ Duodenal ulcer disease racks up 500,000 new cases annually in the United States, plus 4 million recurrences per year. Usually not a fatal disease, the disease is nevertheless responsible for a lot of medical care cost, morbidity, and absence from work. These total costs are estimated to be between $3 and $4 billion annually.

Now that we know that duodenal ulcer usually has an infectious origin, cure is possible. (The exceptions to this generality include such causes as nonsteroidal anti-inflammatory drugs and Zollinger-Ellison syndrome.)

Absent these noninfectious causes, physicians should promptly treat with antimicrobial and antisecretory drugs. The savings in both monetary and quality-of-life terms will be very, very large.

L. Lasagna, M.D.

Double-blind Trial of Omeprazole and Amoxicillin to Cure *Helicobacter pylori* Infection in Patients With Duodenal Ulcers
Bayerdörffer E, Miehlke S, Mannes GA, et al (Univ of Munich; Krankenhaus der Barmherzigen Brüder, Munich; Private Practice, Cologne, Germany; et al)
Gastroenterology 108:1412–1417, 1995   10–2

Purpose.—"Triple therapy" with bismuth salts and 2 antibiotics is an effective treatment for *Helicobacter pylori*-related duodenal ulcer disease. Researchers are seeking new regimens that will reduce the associated problems of side effects and antibiotic resistance. The combination of omeprazole and amoxicillin was investigated for its capability to cure *H. pylori* infection in patients with duodenal ulcers.

Methods.—The double-blind, randomized trial included 270 patients with *H. pylori*-related duodenal ulcer from 10 German centers. One group of patients received omeprazole, 40 mg 3 times a day, and amoxicillin, 750 mg 3 times a day, for the first 14 days, followed by omeprazole alone, 20 mg once a day until day 42. The other group received omeprazole plus amoxicillin placebo, 750 mg 3 times a day, for 42 days. Cure rates of *H. pylori* infection were assessed by performing endoscopic biopsies.

Results.—The *H. pylori* infection was cured in 91% of patients receiving omeprazole plus amoxicillin as compared with none of those receiving omeprazole plus placebo. On intention-to-treat analysis, infection cure rates were 89% for the omeprazole plus amoxicillin group and 0% for the control group. Just 58% of patients who were pretreated with omeprazole in the 4 weeks before the study were cured of *H. pylori* infection compared with 95% of those who were not pretreated. By the end of 1 year, relapses occurred in 11% of patients receiving omeprazole plus amoxicillin compared with 44% in those treated with omeprazole plus placebo. Relapse rates were 2% in patients negative for *H. pylori* compared with 49% in patients positive for *H. pylori*.

Conclusions.—The combination of omeprazole and amoxicillin used in this study is an effective treatment for *H. pylori* infection and duodenal ulcer. The treatment is well tolerated, and all strains of *H. pylori* are sensitive to amoxicillin.

▶ Recently, the FDA approved clarithromycin to be used with omeprazole for this indication. Amoxicillin is quite a bit cheaper and may be as effective.

Certainly, it is very well tolerated. One only very rarely sees outcome criteria such as the investigators found in this particular study. An 89% outcome rate in the omeprazole plus amoxicillin group vs. 0 in the omeprazole plus placebo group is really remarkable. Most often, many drugs require fancy statistics and only show an outcome rate that is 15% or 20% better than the placebo (not that that outcome rate is bad; it just occurs more commonly).

M. Weintraub, M.D.

Bismuth-based Combination Therapy for *Helicobacter pylori*–Associated Peptic Ulcer Disease (Metronidazole for Eradication, Ranitidine for Pain)
Tefera S, Berstad A, Bang CJ, et al (Haukeland Univ, Bergen, Norway; Stord Hosp, Norway)
Am J Gastroenterol 91:935–941, 1996   10–3

Background.—The eradication of *Helicobacter pylori* infection in patients with peptic ulcers is effective but difficult to achieve. Triple therapy, including bismuth salt and 2 antibiotics, appears to be the most successful treatment. The roles of ranitidine and metronidazole in this treatment were investigated.

Methods.—One hundred eighty patients with peptic ulcer disease and positive results for *H. pylori* were assigned randomly to 1 of 4 regimens. Regimen 1 included bismuth subnitrate suspension, 150 mg 4 times daily; oxytetracycline, 500 mg 4 times daily; metronidazole, 400 mg 3 times daily for 10 days; or ranitidine, 300 mg twice daily for 4 weeks. Regimens 2, 3, and 4 were the same as regimen 1, except that regimen 2 was without ranitidine, regimen 3 was without metronidazole, and regimen 4 was without metronidazole and ranitidine. Gastroscopy and ^{14}C-urea breath tests were done 4 weeks after treatment was stopped. Breath tests alone were done 6 months after treatment was stopped.

Findings.—In an intention-to-treat analysis, *H. pylori* was eradicated in 96% of patients on regimen 1, 91% on regimen 2, 20% on regimen 3, and 9% on regimen 4. When regimens 1 and 2 were compared with 3 and 4, eradication rates were 93% and 14% with and without metronidazole, respectively. The occurrence of diarrhea and abdominal pain was increased with metronidazole. When regimens 1 and 3 were compared with 2 and 4, it was found that ranitidine did not significantly affect *H. pylori* eradication or ulcer healing, but reduced the occurrence of pain. Three patients who were *H. pylori* negative at 4 weeks became positive again by 6 months after treatment cessation. All had received placebo instead of metronidazole. The remaining 85 patients continued to be *H. pylori* negative.

Conclusions.—In this type of bismuth-based treatment, *H. pylori* eradication depends critically on metronidazole. The inclusion of ranitidine in such treatment decreases the occurrence of abdominal pain.

▶ Successful treatment of *H. pylori* infection not only makes patients with peptic ulcer feel better, but saves money for the health care budget.

This study certainly found metronidazole a necessary addition if one wants success from a bismuth-oxytetracycline regimen. It is unfortunate that metronidazole resistance is not uncommon and that many find the drug unpleasant to take.

L. Lasagna, M.D.

Mucosal Erosions in Longterm Non-steroidal Anti-inflammatory Drug Users: Predisposition to Ulceration and Relation to *Helicobacter pylori*

Taha AS, Sturrock RD, Russell RI (Royal Infirmary, Glasgow, Scotland)
Gut 36:334–336, 1995   10–4

Introduction.—Gastroduodenal erosions are a common finding on endoscopy in patients taking short courses of nonsteroidal anti-inflammatory drugs (NSAIDs). The significance of these erosions in long-term NSAID users and their link to *Helicobacter pylori* have not been established. The presence or absence of erosions was evaluated in a group of long-term NSAID users, including associations between erosions, peptic ulcer development, and *H. pylori* infection.

Methods.—The study included 50 patients with arthritis who had been taking NSAIDs for at least 4 weeks. They continued treatment throughout the study, which included endoscopic examinations performed at baseline and at 4, 12, and 24 weeks. Patients in whom the initial examination revealed ulcers were excluded from the study. Patients with and without erosions and with and without *H. pylori* infection were compared for the development of peptic ulcers.

Results.—Twenty-three of the patients had erosions and 27 did not. Peptic ulcers developed in 39% of the patients with erosions as compared with 22% of those without. *H. pylori* infection was present in 30 patients. Sixty percent of patients with *H. pylori* infection had erosions compared with 25% of noninfected patients. Forty percent of infected patients as compared with 15% of noninfected patients had ulcers; the proportion of patients with ulcers complicating previous erosions was 27% for infected patients as compared with 5% for noninfected patients. Peptic ulcer development was unrelated to the initial number of erosions but was strongly related to the presence of *H. pylori*-positive erosions.

Conclusions.—In patients with long-term NSAID exposure, peptic ulcers are associated with the presence of mucosal erosions, even though the erosions may be transient or recurrent. Ulcers are also associated with the presence of *H. pylori* infection, especially when duodenal erosions are present as well.

▶ It used to be said that people who had gastroduodenal erosions from taking NSAIDs would not necessarily get ulcers. This study proves the error of that statement. Of course, the patients who had ulcers in this population were more likely to be positive for *H. pylori*. Another interesting point about this study is the underrepresentation of men in the study population by a factor of approximately 4½. I'm sure one could come up with some explanation for this based on the patients' diagnoses, particularly rheumatoid arthritis. Still, it's a little bit of a wonder in these generally older patients that the preponderance of women was so great. It always makes me think that elderly women are not only more numerous but also may be overdosed on a milligram per kilogram basis.

M. Weintraub, M.D.

Symptom Improvement from Prokinetic Therapy Corresponds to Improved Quality of Life in Patients With Severe Dyspepsia
Cutts TF, Abell TL, Karas JG, et al (Univ of Tennessee, Memphis)
Dig Dis Sci 41:1369–1378, 1996   10–5

Background.—Cisapride and domperidone, both prokinetic agents, have been shown to improve symptoms related to gastrointestinal motility disorders and severe dyspepsia. The effects on quality of life and psychological parameters of long-term treatment with prokinetic agents were investigated.

Methods.—Twenty-seven patients with severe dyspepsia for at least 6 months duration were treated with either cisapride (22 patients) or domperidone (5 patients) at a daily dose of 60–80 mg/day for 1 year. The patients were assessed before and after treatment for symptomatic improvement, psychological traits (using the Minnesota Multiphasic Personality Inventory), psychological state (using the Million Behavioral Health Inventory), and quality of life (using the Sickness Impact Profile).

Results.—All patients had some symptomatic improvement. The patients were stratified into quartiles of symptomatic response. Change in symptom scores correlated with all 25 parameters, with significant group differences in 12 of the 25 psychological and quality-of-life parameters.

Conclusion.—The symptomatic improvement achieved with prokinetic therapy is correlated with improvements in psychological and quality-of-life parameters in patients with dyspepsia. Greater symptomatic improvement corresponds with greater quality-of-life improvements. The findings support the theory that psychological distress is a result, rather than a cause, of physiologic distress in these patients.

▶ Gastrointestinal motility disorders really can upset the quality of life. In these days of getting drugs on formularies or available in managed care organizations, the drug companies are going to gather lots of quality-of-life data before drug approval. This will provide them with a shot at getting the drug on the formulary or displacing a drug that is on the formulary already. This particular analysis of quality of life was not done double-blind, however. I think that quality-of-life studies will have to be done as part of a randomized, controlled, double-blind study, however, if done before approval.

M. Weintraub, M.D.

A Randomised Trial Comparing Mesalazine and Prednisolone Foam Enemas in Patients With Acute Distal Ulcerative Colitis

Lee FI, Jewell DP, Mani V, et al (Victoria Hosp, Blackpool, England; John Radcliffe Hosp, Oxford, England; Leigh Infirmary, Manchester, England; et al)
Gut 38:229–233, 1996   10–6

Background.—Oral and/or rectal mesalazine can be used in the treatment of distal ulcerative colitis. The efficacy and safety of a foam enema preparation of mesalazine were compared with those of prednisolone foam enemas in patients with acute distal ulcerative colitis.

Methods.—Adults with distal ulcerative colitis relapse were assigned randomly to foam enema or prednisolone foam enema for 4 weeks. At the end of treatment, 149 patients in the first group and 146 in the second group were evaluable.

Findings.—Fifty-two percent of patients receiving mesalazine and 31% receiving prednisolone achieved clinical remission. There was a trend toward more patients in the mesalazine group achieving sigmoidoscopic remission. Histologic remission occurred in 27% of the mesalazine group and in 21% of the prednisolone group. Both groups had improvement in their symptoms. Sixty-seven percent of patients receiving mesalazine had no blood in their stools after 4 weeks, compared with 40% receiving prednisolone. Patients given prednisolone had significantly fewer days with liquid stools than patients given mesalazine, the median being 0 and 1 day, respectively, by the fourth week.

Conclusion.—Mesalazine foam enema appears to be better than prednisolone foam enema in achieving clinical remission. Favorable trends in sigmoidoscopic and histologic remission rates supported this. Both mesalazine and prednisolone were well tolerated.

▶ The history of the use of mesalazine or 5-aminosalicylic acid (5-ASA) represents an attempt to bring the active medication to the place of inflammation in the large bowel. Unfortunately, stomach acid, various bacteria, etc., have all worked to diminish the amount of 5-ASA that gets to the large colon intact. That is why the combination with a sulfapyridine carrier in the sulfasalazine formation has been used for many, many years. More recently, the 5-ASA has been put in a enteric coating or a slow release formulation, an enema, or a suppository. Because many of the adverse effects came from the sulfonamide portion of the molecule, the removal of it, as in 5-ASA, has been adopted by many physicians, to the benefit of many patients.

M. Weintraub, M.D.

An Oral Preparation of Mesalamine as Long-term Maintenance Therapy for Ulcerative Colitis: A Randomized, Placebo-controlled Trial

Hanauer SB, for the Mesalamine Study Group (Univ of Chicago)
Ann Intern Med 124:204–211, 1996   10–7

Objective.—Sulfasalazine is the drug of choice for the treatment of mild to moderate ulcerative colitis and to maintain remission, but it has a substantial incidence of side effects and idiosyncratic reactions mainly as a result of the sulfapyridine carrier molecule. Other methods of delivering the active molecule mesalamine have been studied and include coating the drug to prevent the adverse effects of stomach acid. The safety and efficacy of a pH-sensitive, polymer-coated oral formulation of mesalamine for the maintenance of remission in patients with ulcerative colitis was studied in a multi-center, double-blind, placebo-controlled, randomized clinical trial.

Methods.—A total of 264 ulcerative colitis patients (146 males), 18–75 years of age, received either 0.8 g/d, 1.6 g/d, or placebo, administered as 4 tablets a day. Tablets were coated with a pH sensitive resin that breaks down only at a pH of 7 or higher. Patients received endoscopic examinations at baseline, and 1, 3, and 6 months. Findings were graded on a 0–3 scale in which 0 represented normal or mild granularity and other mild symptoms, 2 represented marked erythema or granularity, and 3 represented spontaneous bleeding and ulcerations. Efficacy was measured as treatment outcome. Safety was evaluated at each visit, and adverse events were documented.

Results.—Failure to meet study criteria and protocol violations resulted in the exclusion of 75 patients. The percentage of treatment successes in the low dose ($n = 68$) and high dose ($n = 58$) groups were 58.8% and 65.5%, significantly more than in the placebo group ($n = 63$) with 37%. Similarly, in the intent-to-treat group, significantly more low and high dose patients, 63.3% and 70.1%, were considered treatment successes than in the placebo group 48.3%. Age, sex, and race did not affect the analyses. In the intent-to-treat analysis, the high dose group, but not the low dose group, had a significantly longer time to relapse when compared with the placebo group. Adverse events were reported 81 times by placebo-treated patients, 72 times by patients in the low dose group, and 106 times in the high dose group. Most adverse events were mild to moderate and included headache, flu syndrome, diarrhea, rhinitis, and abdominal pain.

Conclusion.—Coated mesalamine at daily doses of 0.8 g and 1.6 g was well tolerated and was significantly more effective than placebo for the maintenance of remission in patients with ulcerative colitis.

▶ The relapse rate in this study ranged from just over 30% in the treatment groups to over 50% in the placebo group after 180 days of treatment. Unfortunately, this relatively high level is substantiated by other investigators, but it is still too high for ulcerative colitis. Nevertheless, the data are quite clear and compelling.

M. Weintraub, M.D.

Oral Budesonide as Maintenance Treatment for Crohn's Disease: A Placebo-controlled, Dose-ranging Study

Greenberg GR, and The Canadian Inflammatory Bowel Disease Study Group (Univ of Toronto)
Gastroenterology 110:45–51, 1996

10–8

Background.—Because of its rapid hepatic metabolism, the corticosteroid budesonide has high topical anti-inflammatory activity and low systemic activity. The safety and efficacy of an oral controlled-release preparation of this agent for maintaining remission in patients with ileal or ileocecal Crohn's disease were investigated.

Methods.—One hundred five patients were enrolled in the double-blind, multicenter trial. Placebo or budesonide, 3 to 6 mg daily for 1 year, was prescribed. The main outcome measure was relapse as defined by a Crohn's Disease Activity Index score of more than 150 and a minimum increase of ≤0 points.

Findings.—The median time to relapse or treatment cessation was 178 days in patients given 6 mg of budesonide. Corresponding medians were 124 days in those given 3 mg of budesonide and 39 days in those given placebo. At 1 year, the relapse rate in the group receiving 6 mg of budesonide was comparable to that in the 3-mg and placebo groups. The 3 groups were comparable in basal plasma cortisol levels and incidence of corticosteroid-associated effects (Fig 1).

Conclusion.—Oral budesonide at a daily dose of 6 mg can lengthen time to relapse in patients with recently treated, quiescent Crohn's disease. However, this effect is not sustained at 1 year. Further clinical studies are

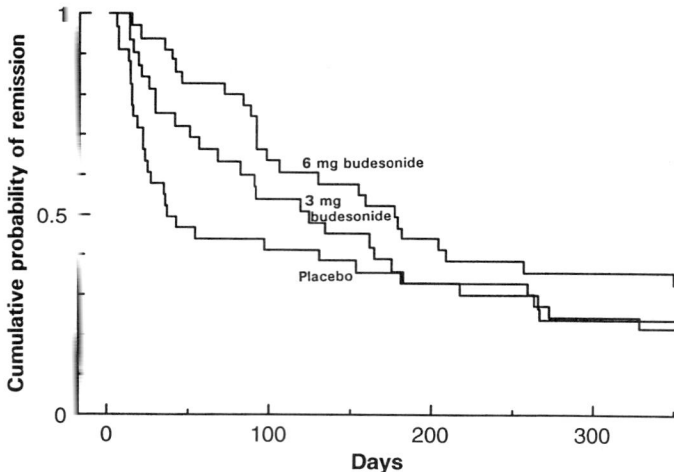

FIGURE 1.—Life table analysis based on time to relapse or discontinuation for all patients treated. (Courtesy of Greenberg GR, and The Canadian Inflammatory Bowel Disease Study Group: Oral budesonide as maintenance treatment for Crohn's disease: A placebo-controlled, dose-ranging study. *Gastroenterology* 110:45–51, 1996.)

needed to determine the effects of higher doses of budesonide or more flexible dosing schedules on the long-term outcomes of patients with this disease.

▶ This study was very well done and seems to use a correct experimental design. The figure shows that the effect of the 3-mg dose of budesonide did not have any more value after about 100 days and that the 6-mg dose probably did not have much effect after 200 days. We should ask, with the relatively low incidence of serious side effects, should not patients try the drugs and have a different kind of intervention at 3 or 6 months, perhaps mesalamine? It would be a shame to say that this study showed that budesonide was totally ineffective in preventing a recurrence of a flair of Crohn's disease. However, the authors of this particular paper say that the efficacy of mesalamine may not have been established in this patient population. Somebody needs to do a clinical trial.

M. Weintraub, M.D.

Prophylactic Mesalamine Treatment Decreases Postoperative Recurrence of Crohn's Disease
McLeod RS, Wolff BG, Steinhart AH, et al (Univ of Toronto; Toronto Hosp; Mayo Clinic, Rochester, Minn; et al)
Gastroenterology 109:404–413, 1995   10–9

Background.—About 80% of patients with Crohn's disease eventually need surgery. Unfortunately, the disease often recurs after such treatment. The value of mesalamine in reducing the risk of recurrent Crohn's disease after surgical resection was investigated.

Methods.—One hundred sixty-three patients with no evidence of residual disease after surgical resection were enrolled in the study. By random assignment, patients received 1.5 g of mesalamine twice a day or placebo within 8 weeks of surgery. Maximum follow-up was 72 months.

Findings.—Symptomatic recurrence was documented in 31% of the patients in the active treatment group, compared with 41% of those in the control group. The relative risk of recurrence in the treatment group was 0.63 using an intention-to-treat analysis and 0.53 using an efficacy analysis (Fig 2). In addition, the endoscopic and radiologic rate of recurrence was significantly reduced, with relative risks of 0.65 and 0.64 in the 2 respective analyses. One serious side effect—pancreatitis—was documented in the mesalamine group.

Conclusions.—Mesalamine effectively reduces the symptomatic, endoscopic, and radiologic rate of recurrence after surgery for Crohn's disease. Additional research is needed to determine the best pharmacologic agents and dosage for prophylaxis and whether prophylaxis is of value in patients with residual disease after surgery.

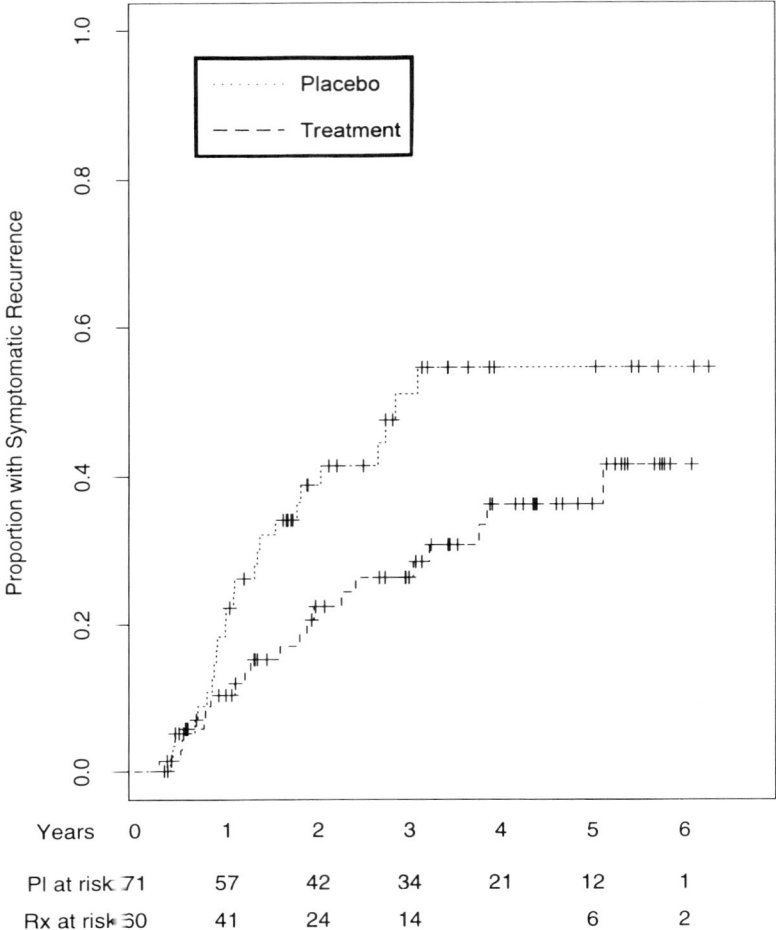

FIGURE 2.—Symptomatic recurrence rate in treatment and control groups (efficacy analysis). *Dotted line* is the placebo group, and *solid line* is the treatment group. (Courtesy of McLeod RS, Wolff BG, Steinhart AH, et al: Prophylactic mesalamine treatment decreases postoperative recurrence of Crohn's disease. *Gastroenterology* 109:404-413, 1995.)

▶ The treatment of Crohn's disease has undergone important changes since the introduction of mesalamine and newer medical therapies. Although the investigators used the "intention-to-treat" analysis, they did a more important series of analyses, including the efficacy analysis shown in Figure 2. Whereas some believe that the intention-to-treat analysis is the most clear-cut and the least likely to contain any bias, it is only 1 of a number of ways of looking at the data, many of which should be included in papers on clinical trials.

M. Weintraub, M.D.

Long-term Follow-up of Patients With Crohn's Disease Treated With Azathioprine or 6-Mercaptopurine

Bouhnik Y, Lémann M, Mary J-Y, et al (Hôpital Saint-Lazare, Paris; Hôpital Saint-Louis, Paris; Université Paris)
Lancet 347:215–219, 1996   10–10

Objective.—Various medical and surgical approaches are available for the management of Crohn's disease, with the selection depending on the severity of illness. One efficient maintenance therapy for patients with Crohn's disease is the immunosuppressant drug azathioprine (AZA), or its metabolite 6-mercaptopurine (6-MP). However, this treatment carries potential risks of bone marrow suppression, liver damage, malignancy, and other adverse effects. The duration of treatment has not been established. The long-term results of treatment with AZA/6-MP for Crohn's disease were reported, including identification of the risk factors for relapse.

Methods.—The analysis included 157 patients with Crohn's disease who took AZA or 6-MP for more than 6 months and remained in clinical remission for longer than 6 months without steroid treatment. Time to relapse was evaluated as a function of time in this group of patients, in 42 patients who ceased AZA/6-MP treatment for reasons other than a relapse, and in the entire sample of patients with Crohn's disease, regardless of whether they could be treated with AZA/6-MP. The Cox proportional hazard model was used to assess the influence of other factors on relapse rate, both during and after immunosuppressive therapy.

Results.—The cumulative probability of relapse in patients who continued taking AZA/6-MP therapy was 11% at 1 year and 32% at 5 years. Relapse was more likely to occur in female patients, younger patients, and those who took more than 6 months to go into remission. The probability of relapse for patients who stopped taking AZA/6-MP was 38% at 1 year and 5% at 5 years. Factors associated with an increased risk of relapse were male sex, younger age, and remission lasting fewer than 4 years. Beyond 4 years, the risk of relapse was about the same whether therapy was continued or stopped.

Conclusions.—Maintenance therapy with AZA or 6-MP has long-term benefits for patients with Crohn's disease. This treatment is probably best withdrawn once the patient has been in remission for 4 years, because the risk of relapse appears to be the same whether treatment is continued or stopped. A placebo-controlled withdrawal trial is being performed to confirm this recommendation.

▶ If a patient with Crohn's disease can't be cured by surgical resection or bypass and has chronic active lesions, AZA and its active metabolite 6-MP are extremely helpful in controlling symptoms and allowing reduction or discontinuation of corticosteroids.

This study suggests that a prudent approach might be to stop these drugs in patients who have been in remission for 4 years. Because the drugs do carry risks (even if they don't lead to lymphoma, a controversial point), the advice seems sensible.

L. Lasagna, M.D.

Randomized, Double-Blind Phase II Trial of Lexipafant, a Platelet-activating Factor Antagonist, in Human Acute Pancreatitis
Kingsnorth AN, Galloway SW, Formela LJ (Univ of Liverpool, England)
Br J Surg 82:1414–1420, 1995   10–11

Background.—The role of platelet-activating factor (PAF) in acute experimental pancreatitis has been studied by observing the effects of therapy with pharmacologic PAF antagonists. Lexipafant, a potent PAF antagonist structurally different from other PAF antagonists, has been shown to reduce morphologic damage in acute experimental pancreatitis when given shortly after disease induction. It has also been found to alleviate acute lung injury by decreasing pulmonary capillary permeability. A phase II trial of Lexipafant in human acute pancreatitis was reported.

Methods.—Eighty-three patients were enrolled in the double-blind, placebo-controlled study. Forty-two received IV Lexipafant, 60 mg for 3 days, and 41 received placebo. The 2 groups were matched initially for age, sex, cause of pancreatitis, Acute Physiology and Chronic Health Evaluation (APACHE II) score, and organ failure score (OFS). Twenty-nine patients had severe disease, as evidenced by an APACHE II score of 8 or greater.

Findings.—After 72 hours of Lexipafant, the incidence of organ failure and total OFS were significantly reduced. Seven of 12 patients with severe acute pancreatitis receiving Lexipafant recovered from organ failure during treatment compared with only 2 of 11 placebo recipients. New organ failure developed in another 2 patients receiving placebo. Lexipafant significantly decreased serum interleukin (IL)-8. A decline in IL-6 was documented on day 1. Plasma polymorphonuclear elastase-α_1-antitrypsin complexes peaked on day 1, then, in placebo recipients only, declined gradually to baseline levels during the next 5 days. Lexipafant treatment did not affect C-reactive protein.

Conclusions.—Platelet-activating factor antagonism is a logical treatment for limiting damage in patients with acute pancreatitis. Lexipafant is a potent PAF antagonist that minimizes organ dysfunction and suppresses some aspects of the inflammatory response in such patients, Further research on this agent is warranted.

▶ Lexipafant s an imidazolyl derivative of a heterocyclic nitrogen compound. This is a very fascinating drug because the imidazole class contains within it many compounds that help all kinds of diseases. They cure fungal infections, lower blood pressure, treat cancer, are vitamins, and so on. And, I don't mean just drugs in theory but those in actual clinical use today. If we only knew why this particular nucleus was so important to so many drugs that do so many things, we'd be way ahead of the game. We'd also be ahead of our understanding of pancreatitis if we could figure out why and how damage occurred. In this case we have the 2 mysteries merged together. We have to hope that they will be untangled sometime soon.

M. Weintraub, M.D.

Prospective Randomised Study of Effect of Octreotide on Rebleeding From Oesophageal Varices After Endoscopic Ligation
Sung JJY, Chung SCS, Yung MY, et al (Chinese Univ, Shatin, Hong Kong)
Lancet 346:1666–1669, 1995   10–12

Purpose.—Endoscopic variceal ligation is safer than injection sclerotherapy for the treatment of esophageal varices, but it is associated with early rebleeding rates of 20% to 40%. Octreotide, a synthetic analogue of somatostatin, has been used to treat variceal hemorrhage when endoscopic expertise is not available. The use of octreotide infusion as an adjunct to endoscopic variceal ligation to lower the risk of early rebleeding was studied.

Patients.—The study population consisted of 94 patients with endoscopically confirmed esophageal variceal bleeding, of whom 47 with a mean age of 56 years were randomly allocated to endoscopic variceal ligation alone and 47 with a mean age of 58 years to octreotide infusion plus endoscopic variceal ligation. All patients underwent a second variceal ligation 5 days after the first treatment.

Results.—Bleeding was controlled in 44 patients treated with variceal ligation alone and in 45 patients who received the combination treatment. None of the patients treated with octreotide experienced drug-related side

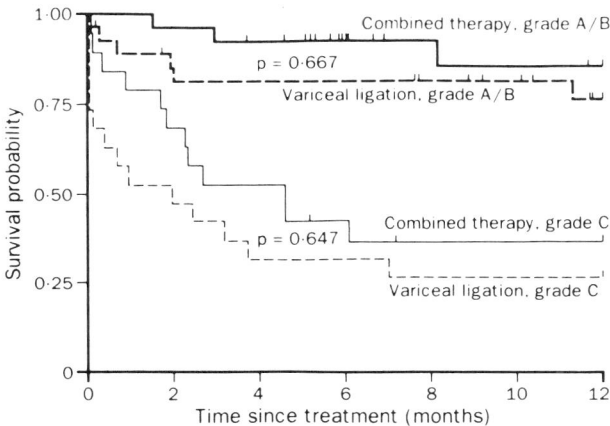

FIGURE.—Kaplan Meier survival plots at 1 year for patients who received variceal ligation alone or combined octreotide and variceal ligation according to severity of liver dysfunction. (Courtesy of Sung JJY, Chung SCS, Yung MY, et al: Prospective randomised study of effect of octreotide on rebleeding from oesophageal varices after endoscopic ligation. *Lancet* 346:1666–1669. Copyright by The Lancet, Ltd., 1995.)

effects that required discontinuation of the infusion. Early rebleeding occurred in 18 patients (38%) treated with ligation alone and in 4 patients (9%) who had the combination treatment. The difference was statistically significant. Ten patients in the ligation alone group and 1 patient in the combination treatment group required balloon tamponade for massive hematemesis and hemodynamic instability. Nine patients (19%) in the ligation alone group and 4 (9%) in the combination treatment died in the hospital, but this difference did not reach statistical significance. The 30-day mortality rates were 23% in the ligation alone group and 11% in the combination treatment group. The cumulative survival at 1 year was significantly better in both groups for patients of Child-Pugh A or B grades than for those with grade C ($P = 0.0004$ and $P = 0.0007$, respectively) (Figure).

Conclusions.—Octreotide infusion, when used as an adjunct to endoscopic variceal ligation in the management of variceal hemorrhage, significantly lowers early rebleeding rates and reduces the need for balloon tamponade

▶ Even though the treatment of esophageal varices has changed dramatically since my own training—from tamponade to sclerotherapy to endoscopic variceal ligation with and without various adjunctive therapies—the mortality in the hospital remains near 25%. In addition, bleeding after treatment recurs in about 20% to 40% of patients. The investigators of this study tried variceal ligation in addition to the drug octreotide, a synthetically made analogue of the hormone somatostatin. There was some benefit, and that benefit appears to have been significant. Although I hate to be labeled one of those we-need-more-data types, in this case, we do.

M. Weintraub, M.D.

11 Genitourinary Tract Disorders

Aspirin, A Silent Risk Factor in Urology: Review Article
Zhu J-P, Davidsen MB, Meyhoff HH (Hillerød Hosp, Denmark)
Scand J Urol Nephrol 29:369–374, 1995   11–1

Background.—An increasing number of operative hemorrhagic complications in patients taking aspirin daily have been reported. Such adverse effects have been described in patients undergoing cardiothoracic surgery, hip surgery, tonsillectomy, cholecystectomy, head injuries, and, more recently, prostatectomy. The normal hemostatic mechanism, the main pharmacologic effects of aspirin on hemostasis, and hemorrhagic complications associated with aspirin therapy in urologic surgery were reviewed.

Aspirin and Urology.—The hemorrhagic effect of aspirin appears to be more important in urology than in other surgical specialties, for several reasons. Aspirin has been found to have a greater antithrombotic effect in male than in female patients. In addition, patients with urologic problems are often elderly and are more likely to be taking aspirin daily for cardiovascular or cerebrovascular disease. Research has shown that bleeding is more frequent and the need for transfusions is increased after prostatectomy in patients taking aspirin before surgery. In patients undergoing transurethral resection of the prostate, aspirin not only may increase postoperative bleeding but also cause excessive perioperative bleeding, thereby prolonging the duration of surgery. Aspirin is probably a risk factor in other urologic procedures, including the biopsy of prostate or kidney, transurethral resection of bladder tumors, and percutaneous lithotripsy. Hemostasis depends greatly on a normal coagulation system in these procedures. Urologists must identify patients at potential risk for excessive bleeding during and after surgery through patient history of preoperative aspirin ingestion. Aspirin treatment should be discontinued at least 7 days before invasive urologic procedures. Desmopressin is useful for correcting bleeding complications associated with aspirin.

Conclusions.—Aspirin appears to increase the risk of hemorrhagic complications in surgery. Urologists in particular need to be aware of this. Studies have shown that aspirin may play a role in bleeding complications after prostatectomy, prostate biopsy, and extracorporeal shock-wave lithotripsy. More controlled clinical trials are needed to determine the bleeding complications associated with aspirin therapy in patients undergoing urologic surgery.

▶ There are many reports in the literature to the effect that aspirin can increase postoperative bleeding and the need for blood transfusions. The procedures include cardiothoracic surgery, hip surgery, tonsillectomy, cholecystectomy, and prostatectomy. Aspirin-induced complications have also been alleged after head injuries, prostate biopsy, and extracorporeal shockwave lithotripsy.

It seems prudent (and important, in view of the many folks on aspirin for prophylaxis or treatment) to stop aspirin for at least a week before any invasive procedure.

L. Lasagna, M.D.

Depot Medroxyprogesterone in the Management of Benign Prostatic Hyperplasia
Onu PE (Makurdi Gen Hosp, Nigeria)
Eur Urol 28:229–235, 1995   11–2

Background.—Recognition of benign prostatic hyperplasia (BPH) as an androgen-dependent process has prompted development of medical treatment strategies to decrease bladder outlet obstruction. Recent studies have suggested that progressive decrease in prostatic volume accompanies chronic decrease in intraprostatic dihydrotestosterone. Effective treatment of BPH might therefore be provided by a compound such as medroxyprogesterone acetate, which inhibits luteinizing-hormone release, decreases plasma testosterone synthesis, and inhibits 5 α-reductase. The safety and efficacy of use of high-dose medroxyprogesterone acetate (depot medroxyprogesterone) for improving symptoms of BPH was examined.

Methods.—Eighty men (mean age, 66 years) with BPH received either depot medroxyprogesterone or placebo in a double-blind, randomized trial. The depot preparation was administered to allow continuous release of the progestational drug for 12 weeks (150 mg, 1 IM injection). Follow-up continued for 12 months; comprehensive clinical examinations and laboratory tests were performed at baseline and at the end of follow-up. Testosterone was measured by radioimmunoassay. The study was completed by 29 patients receiving placebo and 39 patients receiving the treatment.

Results.—After 3 months (the duration of effect of the depot medroxyprogesterone) prostate volume was reduced by 25% among treated patients and 3% among patients receiving placebo. Serum testosterone levels reached castration values in treated patients within 3 days; levels in controls were unchanged. Maximum urinary flow rates among treated patients increased by 3.7 mL/sec over those of patients receiving placebo. Patients receiving placebo showed no significant decrease in total urinary symptom scores, but scores for treated patients decreased by 4.9 points. Irritative symptoms also decreased only in treated patients. After 3 months, reversal occurred in urinary symptoms and urodynamic changes, but status was still significantly improved over baseline. Prostate size returned to pretreatment levels within 18 to 36 weeks. A significant number of treated patients reported impotence, decreased libido, and decreased ejaculate volume, but no hot flashes were reported. Side effects ceased in the fifth or sixth month for all treated patients.

Conclusion.—Depot medroxyprogesterone induces a significant sustained decrease in serum testosterone levels and a decrease in prostatic volume and urinary symptoms in men with BPH, resulting in increased urinary flow rates. When potency is a secondary consideration, treatment of prostatic obstruction with depot medroxyprogesterone is both safe and effective.

▶ Aging men frequently have urinary symptoms as a consequence of BPH that is androgen-dependent. Finasteride can help by decreasing intraprostatic dihydrotestosterone, but significant benefits are not experienced by all patients receiving this inhibitor, so better remedies deserve to be searched for.

These authors consider depot medroxyprogesterone to be more effective, easier to administer, and much cheaper than finasteride. The drawbacks are decreased libido and sexual performance. Interesting idea.

L. Lasagna, M.D.

A Multicenter, Randomized, Double-blind, Placebo-controlled Study to Evaluate the Safety and Efficacy of Terazosin in the Treatment of Benign Prostatic Hyperplasia
Elhilali MM, Ramsey EW, Barkin J, et al (McGill Univ, Montreal; Univ of Manitoba, Winnipeg; Univ of Toronto; et al)
Urology 47:335–342, 1996   11–3

Introduction.—Surgical treatment of benign prostatic hyperplasia (BPH) is costly and is associated with a significant incidence of postoperative complications, treatment failures, and reoperations. Some patients are too high risk or are unwilling to undergo surgical management. Effective nonsurgical management of BPH would be desirable. α-Adrenoceptors are abundant in the bladder neck and trigone. Several small trials have indicated that selective α-blockers increase maximum and average flow rate, decrease residual volume, and improve obstructive symptoms in BPH. Terazosin is a long-acting α_1-blocker that has been shown to provide significant improvements in urodynamic parameters and obstructive and irritative symptoms. The safety and efficacy of terazosin in the treatment of BPH was evaluated in a prospective, multicenter, randomized, double-blind, placebo-controlled trial.

Methods.—A total of 224 patients with BPH from 11 different treatment sites were randomly assigned to receive 24 weeks of active terazosin treatment or placebo. The patients were evaluated regularly for treatment response.

Results.—One hundred thirty-four of the patients were evaluable. Peak and mean urinary flow rates were significantly increased in patients treated with terazosin, compared to patients treated with placebo. In 36% of terazosin-treated patients, there was an increase in unadjusted peak flow rate of more than 30%, compared to 21% in the placebo group. Patients in the treatment group experienced significant improvements in obstructive and irritative symptoms, compared to the placebo group. A total of 83 adverse effects were reported by 42 patients in the placebo group, compared to 120 adverse effects reported by 51 patients in the terazosin group. Most of the adverse effects for both groups were considered to be mild or moderate. Four of 17 patients in the treatment group and 2 of 7 patients in the placebo group who reported hypotension-related adverse effects were eliminated from the trial. Significantly larger changes in blood pressure from baseline to final visit were observed for the treatment group, compared to the placebo group. There were no significant changes from baseline to final visit in hematology, blood chemistry, urinalysis, hepatic function, or renal function for either group.

Conclusion.—Terazosin was found to be safe and effective in relieving the signs and symptoms of BPH. It can be considered a viable alternative in the treatment of BPH.

▶ Pharmacotherapeutics is really quite a derivative science. It has to depend on the establishment of basic principles; in this case, the location of α_1-adrenoceptors. Of course, it also has to depend on many other things, such as developments in pharmaceutical chemistry and the pathophysiology of various diseases. Other studies published this year have shown that terazosin was superior to finasteride and to placebo in the treatment of BPH. Of course, the other drug, finasteride, specifically inhibits steroid 5α-reductase, which converts testosterone into the very potent androgen 5α-dihydrotestosterone. It helps some patients with BPH, but may have other important effects as well.

M. Weintraub, M.D.

Ameliorative Effect of Allopurinol on Nonbacterial Prostatitis: A Parallel Double-Blind Controlled Study
Persson B-E, Ronquist G, Ekblom M (Univ Hosp, Uppsala, Sweden; Uppsala Univ, Sweden)
J Urol 155:961–964, 1996
11–4

Background.—Nonbacterial prostatitis is a common, benign disease that causes genital and pelvic pain, urgency to void, and sensitivity to cold. It is typically recurrent and each episode lasts several months. Its cause is not clear, but urine reflux has been implicated. The effect of allopurinol treatment on the symptoms of nonbacterial prostatitis and on the concentrations of urate in prostatic secretions was studied in a randomized, double-blind, placebo-controlled trial.

Methods.—Fifty-four patients with nonbacterial prostatitis were randomly assigned to 1 of 3 treatment groups: placebo only twice daily, 300 mg of allopurinol in the morning and placebo in the evening, or 300 mg of allopurinol in the morning and again in the evening. Treatment was continued for 8 months. Blood, urine, and prostatic secretion samples were obtained on days 30, 140, 240, and 330 and were analyzed for urate and creatinine concentrations. The prostatic symptoms were subjectively evaluated daily. A physician rated the pain on rectal examination.

Results.—Thirty-four patients completed the study. Allopurinol treatment was associated with decreasing urate concentrations in relation to creatinine concentrations in serum, urine, and prostatic secretion during the first 25 days of treatment in a dose-dependent fashion. The subjective discomfort ratings were significantly lower in the treatment groups than in the placebo group, as were the pain grading scores assigned by the physician. The treatment groups had significantly less pain at the post-treatment visit as well.

Conclusion.—Allopurinol treatment of nonbacterial prostatitis results in positive effects on both biochemical values and symptoms. The findings supported a causal relationship between urine reflux and an inflammatory reaction in the prostate gland.

▶ Actually, the link between the theory, the open label test of a drug, and the proof by a clinical trial should be supported in every way. One imagines that a crucial part of this study—the identification of appropriate patients—was done well. However, even if some mistakes were made, the effects were robust enough to withstand the errors. I think that the investigators used the area under the curve to calculate the subjective improvement scores. This is relatively difficult because, given the type of manipulations that the investigators had to perform to measure the amount of urate in the urine and in the prostate, they had to carry out what is, in effect, a treatment of the prostatitis by digital massage. So, in fact, the actual differences are probably much greater. For example, if the investigators could have used a no-treatment group, it would have led to a greater difference from allopurinol.

M. Weintraub, M.D.

Oral Fluconazole Compared With Bladder Irrigation With Amphotericin B for Treatment of Fungal Urinary Tract Infections in Elderly Patients

Jacobs LG, Skidmore EA, Freeman K, et al (Albert Einstein College of Medicine, Bronx, NY)

Clin Infect Dis 22:30–35, 1996   11–5

Background.—Because of the common use of antibiotics, corticosteroids, and bladder catheters, the incidence of funguria has increased dramatically in the elderly population. Bladder irrigation with amphotericin B is the standard therapy. However, this treatment involves the use of an indwelling bladder catheter for 2–4 days, which is uncomfortable, requires intensive nursing attention, and may increase the risk of bacteriuria. New oral triazole antifungal agents have been developed and may be useful in treating funguria. The efficacy and safety of oral fluconazole and amphotericin B bladder irrigation was compared in older patients with funguria.

Methods.—A total of 109 hospitalized patients older than age 65 years with funguria were randomly assigned to treatment with a 5-day course of either amphotericin B bladder irrigation (59 patients) or oral fluconazole (50 patients). Urine cultures were tested for fungal growth 2 days and 1 month after treatment.

Results.—Two days after treatment, funguria was eradicated in 96% of the patients treated with amphotericin B bladder irrigation and in 73% of the patients treated with oral fluconazole, a statistically significant difference. At 1 month after study entry, urine specimens were available from 61 patients and indicated a sustained cure in 42% of the patients treated with amphotericin B bladder irrigation and 34% of the patients treated with oral fluconazole, a nonsignificant difference. The 1-month mortality rate was significantly greater in the amphotericin B group than in the fluconazole group (=1% vs. 22%). There were only 5 minor, mild adverse effects of fluconazole treatment.

Conclusion.—Both drugs had good clinical efficacy in the treatment of funguria in elderly patients. Because of the invasiveness of bladder irrigation, oral fluconazole is recommended as the initial treatment for funguria, with amphotericin B bladder irrigation used when patients do not respond to fluconazole.

▶ Even if this study had only shown that fluconazole was essentially equivalent to or slightly worse than amphotericin B, I would have said, "Go for it!" The work involved had to be more with amphotericin B. The mortality figures—although hard to interpret in frail, elderly sick folks, even if statistically significant—have to tell us something. At least they give us a clue that fluconazole taken by mouth was safer than amphotericin instilled in the bladder. Even if we do not understand that funguria has all the attributes of a real infection and it can be serious, initial oral treatment with fluconazole appears preferable.

M. Weintraub, M.D.

Contraceptive Efficacy of Testosterone-Induced Azoospermia and Oligozoospermia in Normal Men

World Health Organization Task Force on Methods for the Regulation of Male Fertility (World Health Organization, Geneva)
Fertil Steril 65:821–829, 1996   11–6

Background.—Reversible male contraceptive methods would permit a man to participate in controlling a couple's fertility. Hormonal methods—based on the reversible suppression of gonadotropin secretion, which would reduce sperm production enough to restrict fertility—are closest to serviceable implementation in men. The fertility of normal men who had either severe oligozoospermia or azoospermia as a result of weekly IM injections of T enanthate was investigated in a prospective, multicenter, noncomparative contraceptive efficacy study.

Participants and Methods.—Three hundred ninety-nine normal, healthy, fertile men aged 21–45 years from 15 centers in 9 countries participated. All participants requested a male contraceptive method and began receiving weekly IM injections of 200 mg T enanthate. The suppression phase of the study began at the first IM injection and continued until entry criteria for the efficacy phase were met (consistent azoospermia or oligozoospermia, which was defined as 3 consecutive specimens at 2-week intervals with sperm concentrations under the oligozoospermia threshold). All participants were required to meet efficacy phase criteria within 6 months; those failing to do so were discontinued because of nonsuppression. The efficacy phase began at the date of the third qualifying semen sample. During this 12-month phase, weekly T enanthate injections were continued, but all other contraceptive methods were stopped. The incidence of pregnancies occurring during the efficacy phase was determined.

Results.—Among men with oligozoospermia ($0.1–3 \times 10^6$ sperm per milliliter), 4 pregnancies were documented during 49.5 person-years. Among men with azoospermia, no pregnancies occurred during 230.4 person-years. Pregnancy rates were 8.1 per 100 person-years for oligozoospermia and 0.0 per 100 person-years for azoospermia or 1.4 per 100 person-years for oligozoospermia and azoospermia combined. An association between pregnancy rates and sperm concentration was noted. In 8 men, insufficient suppression of spermatogenesis was documented, and in 4, failure to achieve suppression was noted. Injections were discontinued because of personal reasons in 50 men, dislike of the injection schedule in 21 men, and medical reasons in 35 men. No serious treatment-related adverse effects were noted. After discontinuing the injections, testis size, hormones, and clinical chemistry variables all returned to baseline. There were no observed changes in blood pressure, and no evidence of hepatotoxicity was noted. Thirty-three couples went on to achieve pregnancy after injections were stopped.

Conclusions.—This male hormonal contraceptive regimen resulted in sustained suppression of spermatogenesis to the point of azoospermia or severe oligozoospermia in 98% of the participants. Men who have persistent oligozoospermia, however, are more likely to experience significant failure rates. The treatment is reversible and is associated with few short-term side effects. A hormonal contraceptive for men is thus an achievable goal. New hormonal regimens that would allow more convenient delivery and better spermatogenesis suppression are needed.

▶ As good as these results are (and they are pretty good), the schedule of inducing oligozoospermia, which took several months and didn't even occur in many of the men, made this technique too cumbersome and difficult. One thing that's really interesting is why the testosterone didn't induce oligozoospermia in all the candidates. Some men even did not have suppression of spermatogenesis. In the long run, this technique is probably not going to work. It just lays the potential for other forms of testosterone (microspheres and implants) to be studied more effectively. However, even then, the men may not achieve oligozoospermia, and someone ought to find out why.

M. Weintraub, M.D.

Complementary Effects of Propranolol and Nonoxynol-9 Upon Human Sperm Motility
White DR, Clarkson JS, Ratnasooriya WD, et al (MRC Reproductive Biology Unit, Edinburgh, Scotland; Ojai, Calif)
Contraception 52:241–247, 1995   11–7

Purpose.—Nonoxynol-9, currently the most widely used spermicide, is a surfactant and so may have difficulty in making contact with spermatozoa. A form of the β-blocker propranolol—which lacks β-blocking ability but retains local anesthetic properties—has been investigated as an alternative vaginal contraceptive. Two propranolol compounds were studied for their effects on human sperm motility in vitro, along with non-oxynol-9.

Findings.—All 3 compounds studied—nonoxynol-9, DL-propranolol, and D-propranolol—produced complete cessation of sperm movement in vitro. Efficacy was greater still when nonoxynol-9 and propranolol were used in combination, suggesting a possible complementary interaction. Propranolol's effects on sperm motility were associated with an influx of calcium, but this did not appear to be its primary mechanism. Doses of propranolol that were too low to affect motility did inhibit sperm-oocyte fusion.

Conclusions.—Nonoxynol-9 and propranolol appear to have complementary effects on the motility of human spermatozoa. The mechanism of these effects is uncertain, but the 2 compounds likely affect different components of membrane function. The addition of propranolol to spermicidal preparations could permit a lower dose of nonoxynol-9, possibly reducing the detergent-mediated side effects of the latter agent while retaining its anti-AIDS potential.

▶ The use of propranolol to enhance the effectiveness of nonoxynol-9 is a very attractive possibility. It is difficult to study the effects of nonoxynol-9 without doing clinical trials with pregnancy as the end point. Researchers are studying this area, however; so perhaps we will be able to see the combination studied with some nonpregnancy outcome as the measure of success.

M. Weintraub, M.D.

Effect of Raising Endogenous Testosterone Levels in Impotent Men With Secondary Hypogonadism: Double Blind Placebo-controlled Trial With Clomiphene Citrate
Guay AT, Bansal S, Heatley GJ (Lahey Clinic, Burlington, Mass; Brown Univ, Providence, RI)
J Clin Endocrinol Metab 80:3546–3552, 1995   11–8

Background.—Both sexual function and the level of circulating androgens decline with age in men. However, there is some experimental evidence that restoring androgen levels with exogenous testosterone does not improve sexual function. The effects of exogenous testosterone administration on the levels of circulating testosterone, libido, and erectile function were studied in men with secondary hypogonadism, defined as a low free testosterone level with a compensatory increase in luteinizing hormone (LH) secretion.

Methods.—Seventeen men with secondary hypogonadism received either clomiphene citrate or placebo for 8 weeks, then received the other drug for 8 weeks after a 2-week washout period. The serum levels of LH, follicle stimulating hormone (FSH), total testosterone, and free testosterone were measured at the end of each month of treatment within 2 hours of drug administration. Nocturnal penile tumescence and rigidity testing were performed at baseline and at the end of each treatment phase. At each of these times, the patients also completed a questionnaire with items regarding sexual satisfaction and the frequency of sexual activity.

Results.—Compared with the placebo phase, the clomiphene phase was characterized by significant increases in all of the serum hormone levels. However, there were no significant differences between treatment phases in any of the subjective parameters of sexual response as revealed by the questionnaires or in nocturnal tumescence and rigidity as measured by the RigiScan. In addition, the patients could not accurately identify whether they were receiving clomiphene or placebo. In secondary analyses of patient subgroups, younger patients did show improved parameters of sexual function and improved nocturnal penile tumescence and rigidity with clomiphene treatment.

Conclusion.—Although younger patients without chronic diseases may have improved sexual function with clomiphene citrate, androgens should not be administered routinely, as sexual dysfunction and reduced testosterone levels are more often not causally related.

▶ Well, who could have predicted it? The levels of LH and FSH increased dramatically in the clomiphene group, but the actual performance or satisfaction of sexual function was really unchanged. In addition, the secondary analysis done in the younger vs. the older men failed, as well. We frequently see physiologic measures of drug effect go one way and the clinical effects go another way. Hence, the need for clinical trials. Many statisticians and clinicians would say that by performing such an analysis, the investigators were really on a fishing expedition preparing hypotheses to be tested in the next study. The real problem may have been that the periods of treatment were too short in this study; a 2-week treatment period followed by a crossover to the other treatment might not be enough.

M. Weintraub, M.D.

The Antiandrogen Withdrawal Syndrome: Experience in a Large Cohort of Unselected Patients With Advanced Prostate Cancer
Small EJ, Srinivas S (Univ of California, San Francisco)
Cancer 76:1428–1434, 1995   11–9

Objective —Discontinuing flutamide has proved effective in some patients with hormone-resistant prostatic cancer. The results of withdrawing flutamide in 107 consecutive men with metastatic prostate cancer in whom progressive disease developed while they were receiving the drug were studied. In addition to antiandrogen therapy, the patients had undergone orchiectomy or received a luteinizing hormone–releasing hormone agonist.

Observations.—Three of the 82 evaluable patients had at least an 80% decrease in serum prostate-specific antigen, and 9 others had a 50% or greater decrease in prostate-specific antigen, for an overall response rate of 15%. The median duration of response was 3 months, although some patients responded for longer than a year. Whether or not concomitant treatment was given did not influence the response to flutamide withdrawal. Patients who responded had received flutamide for a longer time than nonresponders (21.5 vs. 12.0 months), but the difference was not statistically significant. Patients who responded to drug withdrawal lived longer after the start of treatment for metastatic disease (44.5 vs. 35.0 months), but this difference also was not significant.

Implication.—Antiandrogen withdrawal should be tried before starting treatment for hormone-resistant prostate cancer.

▶ Why withdrawal of the antiandrogen flutamide should, in some patients, lead to substantial decreases in serum prostate-specific antigen is not at all clear. It has been hypothesized that a mutation in the hormone-binding domain of the androgen receptor allows antiandrogens to act as partial agonists. This theory is supported by the fact that the longer the treatment with flutamide, the more likely is it that antiandrogen withdrawal will result in prostate-specific antigen decrease.

L. Lasagna, M.D.

Sertraline-Associated Syndrome of Inappropriate Antidiuretic Hormone: Case Report and Review of the Literature
Bradley ME, Foote EF, Lee EN, et al (State Univ of New Jersey, Piscataway; Lehigh Valley Hosp, Allentown, Pa)
Pharmacotherapy 16:680–683, 1996   11–10

Background.—Selective serotonin reuptake inhibitors first became available for the treatment of depression in 1987. However, the syndrome of inappropriate antidiuretic hormone (SIADH) has been associated with their use in some patients.

> *Case Report.*—Woman, 78, was admitted for work-up of chronic, intermittent diarrhea of 1 year's duration. She was treated for dehydration and had no recurrence of diarrhea after admission, but she showed depressive symptoms. On the second hospital day she began receiving sertraline (Zoloft, Roerig, New York, NY) at a dosage of 50 mg/day. The woman's serum sodium level, which was 134 mEq/L on admission and 136 mEq/L on hospital day 3, decreased to 119 mEq/L by hospital day 5. She became encephalopathic with myoclonus. Laboratory tests showed a urinary sodium of 125 mEq/L, a urine osmolality of 474 mOsm/kg, and a plasma osmolality of 262 mOsm/kg. The findings of concentrated urine in the presence of hyponatremia and clinical symptoms in the absence of concurrent orthostatic hypotension, edema, or dehydration indicated a diagnosis of SIADH. On the sixth hospital day, sertraline was discontinued and the patient was treated with sodium chloride, demeclocycline, and fluid restriction. The patient's condition improved and she was discharged on hospital day 17.

Discussion.—During the episode of hyponatremia, the patient was also receiving nizatidine, levothyroxine, thiamine, calcium carbonate, magnesium oxide, and ceftriaxone, none of which has been associated with SIADH. Selective serotonin reuptake inhibitors have been associated with SIADH, although the mechanism involved is unclear. Determination of causality is confounded by the fact that patients with psychiatric disorders show potential for excessive water intake, and by the fact that the average age of patients experiencing this phenomenon is more than 70 years. Controlled studies considering these factors are needed.

▶ I wish I knew why so many drugs, including oral antidiabetic agents, drugs used for the treatment of cancer, psychotropic agents, sedatives, and others, as well as diseases, including the cancers that produce antidiuretic hormone, encephalitis, or meningitis and pulmonary diseases, cause antidiuretic hormone to be secreted in excess. Somebody really ought to sit down and work out the mechanism by which this is accomplished and see if there is not some commonality between the drugs, at least, as well as the diseases, to explain why all these things result in inappropriate antidiuretic hormone.

M. Weintraub, M.D.

Safety of Pamidronate in Patients With Renal Failure and Hypercalcemia
Machado CE, Flombaum CD (Mem Sloan-Kettering Cancer Ctr, New York)
Clin Nephro 45:175–179, 1996   11–11

Purpose.—Hypercalcemia is a potentially life-threatening problem for cancer patients. One commonly used treatment for hypercalcemia of malignancy is pamidronate (APD), but there is concern about possible nephrotoxicity with bisphosphonate drugs. The safety and efficacy of APD treatment for hypercalcemia in patients with underlying renal insufficiency were evaluated.

Methods.—The retrospective study included 31 patients at 1 cancer center who received APD treatment while they had renal insufficiency, defined as a serum creatinine level of 1.5 mg/dL or greater. The patients received a total of 33 courses of APD in doses ranging from 60 to 90 mg. Data on changes in renal function and the occurrence of adverse effects were gathered from the medical records.

Results.—With APD treatment, 91% of patients had improvement or resolution of their hypercalcemia. Just 1 patient, who died on the third hospital day, failed to respond to APD. There was a temporary decline in renal function during 8 courses of APD; however, the increases in serum creatinine either occurred before treatment or resulted from other causes. No adverse systemic effects of APD treatment were noted.

Conclusions.—Pamidronate treatment appears to be safe for use in patients with hypercalcemia of malignancy and underlying renal disease. No systemic or renal toxic side effects are noted when ADP is given over 24 hours and with adequate hydration.

▶ The investigators retrospectively evaluated the safety and effectiveness of APD in patients with serious hypercalcemia and renal insufficiency. In the introduction to this paper, the authors review several nonspecific forms of treatment and their adverse effects. They include saline infusion (volume overload), mithramycin (drug accumulation and toxicity), gallium nitrate (nephrotoxicity), and calcitonin (tachyphylaxis). Each of the toxicities are important and not shared with APD. Like other bisphosphonates, APD would be useful in the hypercalcemia of carcinoma because it inhibits osteoclast-mediated bone reabsorption, which often leads to increased serum calcium. In addition to the treatment outlined in this particular study, the current hot use of bisphosphonates is for treating osteoporosis with drugs such as aldronate. Although bisphosphonates have been around for many years, we are still discovering more things about their use in treating heterotopic bony calcifications and other diseases.

M. Weintraub, M.D.

12 Infectious Diseases

Vancomycin Use in a University Medical Center: Comparison With Hospital Infection Control Practices Advisory Committee Guidelines
Evans ME, Kortas KJ (Univ of Kentucky, Lexington)
Infect Control Hosp Epidemiol 17:356–359, 1996   12–1

Background.—The incidence of vancomycin-resistant enterococci is increasing. To reduce this incidence, the Hospital Infection Control Practices Advisory Committee (HIC-PAC) has prepared guidelines for the appropriate use of vancomycin. These guidelines were compared with actual practice in a tertiary-care university hospital.

Methods.—The hospital records of all patients receiving vancomycin during a 1-month period were reviewed. The reasons for prescribing vancomycin were compared with the 5 HIC-PAC guidelines for the appropriate use of vancomycin.

Results.—There were 101 prescriptions for vancomycin during the 1-month study period. The reasons stated for vancomycin prescription complied with HIC-PAC guidelines in 35 patients. Of these 35 patients, 28 had serious infections that were presumed caused by β-lactam–resistant gram-positive microorganisms. Subsequently, cultures proved the presence of β-lactam–resistant bacteria in 8 of 18 patients.

Vancomycin was prescribed for reasons inconsistent with HIC-PAC guidelines in 66 patients. Empirical vancomycin therapy was begun in 44 patients from whom the appropriate cultures were not obtained. Nineteen of the patients were immunocompromised. Prophylactic vancomycin was given to 6 patients undergoing routine surgical procedures not involving the implantation of prosthetic materials or a device. Two children with *Clostridium difficile* colitis were treated with oral vancomycin because they could not tolerate the taste of oral metronidazole. Empirical treatment with vancomycin was also begun in 1 patient with a history of methicillin-resistant *Staphylococcus aureus* (MRSA) infection and in 1 patient with presumed pneumococcal meningitis, who also received cefotaxime. Other unsanctioned reasons for vancomycin treatment included prophylaxis during stem-cell infusion, the placement or pulling of deep intravascular lines, and for an open head wound in an unconscious trauma patient with an unknown drug allergy history.

Conclusions.—The majority of vancomycin prescriptions were not consistent with the HIC-PAC guidelines. However, the review revealed 3 additional clinical situations that may be appropriate indications for vancomycin use: in combination with cefotaxime in patients with presumed *Streptococcus pneumoniae* meningitis, in pediatric patients with *C. difficile* colitis who cannot swallow metronidazole tablets, and in patients with a known MRSA infection. It is suggested that limiting prescription rights for vancomycin to experienced, fully trained physicians is necessary to improve the use of vancomycin.

▶ One of the depressing things about academic medical centers is the difficulty in getting hospital staff to comply with practice guidelines. The only truly effective way to force "proper" antibiotic prescribing is to require such prescribing to be done *only* by (as this article says) "a select group of experienced physicians who are trained fully in the use, as well as the misuse" of antibiotics.

L. Lasagna, M.D.

Once-Daily Aminoglycoside Dosing: Impact on Requests and Costs for Therapeutic Drug Monitoring
Nicolau DP, Wu AHB, Finocchiaro S, et al (Hartford Hosp, Conn)
Ther Drug Monit 18:263–266, 1996   12–2

Background.—Recently, many investigators have studied the use of once-daily aminoglycosides (ODA). In October 1992, a facility-wide ODA program was implemented in an 850-bed community-teaching hospital.

Methods and Findings.—Adults prescribed aminoglycosides after that date were converted automatically to the ODA program, which involved administering a fixed 7-mg/kg IV dose of gentamicin or tobramycin for 60 minutes every 24 hours or more in patients with creatinine clearances of more than 60 mL/min. In the first phase of implementation, therapeutic drug monitoring (TDM) was performed by random serum concentration and nomogram use. In the second phase, serum drug level assessments were eliminated in patients with normal renal function. When fully implemented, the program resulted in a 40% reduction in the request for gentamicin and tobramycin serum levels compared with historic ordering patterns for conventional aminoglycoside dosing regimens. The incidence of nephrotoxicity also was decreased from 3% to 5% with conventional aminoglycoside dosing to 1.2% during phase 1 and 1.3% during phase 2. Eliminating TDM requests totaling 300 for gentamicin and 50 for tobramycin per month was estimated to save the institution more than $100,000 a year.

Conclusions.—The ODA approach appears to be effective and safe. Reducing the required serum aminoglycoside levels with this ODA dosing method is estimated to result in a substantial cost savings.

▶ This abstracted paper is about eliminating therapeutic drug monitoring requests for patients who are receiving ODA dosing. If you can perform these changes in a systematic way across all patients, that is really very helpful. Too often, physicians order a whole series of peak-and-trough blood levels that really do not aid the patients very much.

M. Weintraub, M.D.

Transmission of Multidrug-Resistant *Mycobacterium tuberculosis* During a Long Airplane Flight
Kenyon TA, Valway SE, Ihle WW, et al (Ctrs for Disease Control and Prevention, Atlanta, Ga)
N Engl J Med 334:933–938, 1996   12–3

Introduction.—A state health department notified the Centers for Disease Control and Prevention (CDC) about a foreign visitor who had died of complications of multidrug-resistant pulmonary tuberculosis. Before diagnosis, the patient had flown from Honolulu to Chicago and from Chicago to Baltimore and had returned 1 month later. An investigation of the passengers and flight crew exposed to the patient was conducted.

Methods.—The passengers and members of the flight crews were notified about their possible exposure to tuberculosis, advised to have a skin test, and asked to report the results and complete a questionnaire requesting demographic and epidemiologic information. The contacts who reported positive tuberculin skin tests or conversions were then interviewed regarding other risk factors for tuberculosis.

Results.—Of the 925 passengers and crew members notified, 802 reported the results of a tuberculin skin test. Eleven contacts on the first 2 flights had positive tuberculin skin tests; all had other risk factors and none had been seated near the patient. Two of the 3 contacts with positive tuberculin skin tests on flight 3 had other risk factors, and none had conversion. The patient with no other risk factors had been seated 3 rows away from the patient. Fifteen contacts on flight 4 had positive tuberculin skin tests, and 4 had conversions. Of these, 6 contacts, including the 4 with conversions, had no other risk factors and had been seated in the same cabin section as the patient. Four of these contacts had been seated within 2 rows of the patient, and the other 2 reported visiting friends seated near the patient.

Discussion.—*Mycobacterium tuberculosis* may be transmitted from passenger to passenger or to flight crew members on commercial aircraft. Based on this and 5 other investigations of possible transmission of *M. tuberculosis* on aircraft, the CDC made recommendations that the notification of passengers and flight crews regarding possible exposure to tuberculosis be based on the flight duration, the infectiousness of the patient, and seating proximity to the patient.

▶ I used to joke when I was discussing noncompliance and say that I hoped the person sitting next to me on the bus had taken his antituberculous therapy that morning. However, I never thought that if I took a long airplane flight, a person with multidrug-resistant tuberculosis would or could infect me. This is one of the risks of modern life and modern travel. We should ask our patients with a recent conversion of a tuberculosis skin test if he or she has taken a long airplane flight.

M. Weintraub, M.D.

Comparison of Characteristics of Patients and Treatment Outcome for Pulmonary Nontuberculous Mycobacterial Infection and Pulmonary Tuberculosis

Jarad NA, Demertzis P, Jones DJM, et al (London Chest Hosp)
Thorax 51:137–139, 1996   12–4

Background.—Nontuberculous mycobacteria are ubiquitous in soil, tap water, and animals. Many exposures are asymptomatic, but clinically significant infections do occur, with widely ranging severity. Affected patients often have clinical and radiographic signs indistinguishable from those of tuberculosis and so are often treated with isoniazid, rifampicin, and pyrazinamide before the culture results are obtained. However, nontuberculous mycobacteria are often resistant to these medications. Patients with tuberculous and nontuberculous mycobacterial infections were studied retrospectively to identify differentiating patient characteristics.

Methods.—The case notes, chest radiographs, and microbiological results of 70 patients with nontuberculous mycobacterial infections and 221 patients with *Mycobacterium tuberculosis* infections (controls) seen over a 7-year period were reviewed. Data were collected on patient characteristics, patterns of resistance to first-line drugs, and relapse.

Results.—The infecting nontuberculous mycobacteria included *Mycobacterium xenopi* in 23 patients, *Mycobacterium kansasii* in 19, *Mycobacterium fortuitum* in 14, *Mycobacterium chelonae* in 5, *Mycobacterium malmoense* in 3, *Mycobacterium gordonae* in 2, *Mycobacterium avium intracellulare* in 2, and *Mycobacterium scrufulacium* and *Mycobacterium bovis* in 1 each. Compared to the patients with tuberculosis, those with nontuberculous mycobacterial infections were older and more likely to be Caucasian. There was pre-existing lung disease or AIDS in 74% of the patients with nontuberculous mycobacteria but only 16.7% of the patients with tuberculosis. There was resistance to first-line drugs in 90% of the patients with nontuberculous mycobacteria and 3.2% of the patients with tuberculosis. However, susceptibility to rifampicin and ethambutol was found in all the *M. kansasii* and all but 1 of the *M. xenopi* isolates. Although all patients with tuberculosis were treated, some patients with nontuberculous mycobacteria were not treated because of a lack of clinical or radiographic signs, or because of the presence of advanced underlying lung disease. Of the 70 patients with nontuberculous mycobacteria, 29 were treated and 9 died. Among cases diagnosed before 1991, relapse occurred in 6 of the 10 patients with *M. xenopi*, 1 of the 5 patients with *M. kansasii*, and 11 of the 157 patients with tuberculosis.

Conclusions.—Nontuberculous mycobacterial infection should be suspected in older Caucasian patients with pre-existing lung disease. Combination treatment with rifampicin and ethambutol is recommended for suspected nontuberculous mycobacterial infections, although a prospective study is needed to determine the efficacy of this approach. Infection with *M. xenopi* has a high relapse rate.

Risk Factors for Hepatotoxicity From Antituberculosis Drugs: A Case-Control Study
Pande JN, Singh SPN, Khilnani GC, et al (All India Inst of Med Sciences, New Delhi)
Thorax 51:132–136, 1996   12–5

Background.—Short-course chemotherapy with rifampicin and isoniazid is an effective therapy for tuberculosis but is associated with hepatotoxicity. The mechanism of and risk factors for this hepatotoxicity are unclear. Risk factors for hepatitis in patients undergoing short-course chemotherapy for tuberculosis were assessed in a prospective, case-control study.

Methods.—The cases were 86 consecutive patients in whom hepatitis developed as a result of short-course antituberculosis therapy. All were negative for the various markers of viral hepatitis. The control subjects were 406 consecutive patients at the same clinic who received short-course chemotherapy without the development of hepatitis. The potential risk factors analyzed were age, sex, body mass index, history of alcohol intake, acetylator status, and serum proteins.

Results.—Patients in the case group were older than those in the control group. They also had lower serum levels. The case patients were more likely to have a history of high alcohol intake, had radiologic evidence of more extensive disease, and were more likely to be "slow acetylators." The other risk factors were similar between the groups.

Conclusions.—In patients receiving short-course chemotherapy for tuberculosis, risk factors for hepatotoxicity include advanced age, hypoalbuminemia, high alcohol intake, slow acetylator phenotype, and extensive disease. The development of hepatitis after exposure to antituberculous drugs may be more likely in patients with 1 or more of these risk factors. These findings await confirmation in large, prospective studies.

▶ The authors of the first paper (Abstract 12–4) indicate that we should be thinking more about nontuberculous *Mycobacterium,* especially in older people and in those with preexisting lung disease or AIDS. Not only should we be thinking of it, we should be treating it with rifampicin and ethambutol, without other medications. In the second paper (Abstract 12–5), the toxicity of rifampicin, ethambutol, and other medications is considered, at least as it pertains to hepatic toxicity. Unfortunately, the authors were unable to comment on the development of hepatitis in all the drug regimens containing rifampicin and isoniazid, rather than just rifampicin and ethambutol. Still, the development of drug-induced hepatitis has its risk factors, including drinking large amounts of alcohol and having a low serum albumin concentration, a slow acetylator phenotype, and extensive disease.

M. Weintraub, M.D.

Use of Predicted Risk of Mortality to Evaluate the Efficacy of Anticytokine Therapy in Sepsis

Knaus WA, for the rhIL-1ra Phase III Sepsis Syndrome Study Group (George Washington Univ, Washington, DC; Duke Univ, Durham, NC; Synergen, Boulder, Colo; et al)
Crit Care Med 24:46–56, 1996   12–6

Background.—Infection is an important cause of morbidity and mortality in severely ill hospital patients. Death is usually the result of an overwhelming response to infection or to multiple organ system failure, both of which can be attributed to the effects of intrinsic biological responses, which is now called the systemic inflammatory response. Although these responses are beneficial in moderation, they can contribute to organ dysfunction and death if excessive or prolonged. Therefore, anticytokine agents aimed at the modification of this response are being developed. One problem is distinguishing those patients whose systemic inflammatory response is appropriate from those whom it places at increased risk of death. The application of the Predicted Risk of Mortality model to a phase III clinical evaluation of a novel anticytokine treatment, recombinant human interleukin-1-receptor antagonist (rhIL-1ra) was reported.

Study Design.—Sixty-three centers in 8 countries participated in a phase III, double-blind, placebo-controlled multicenter clinical trial of anticytokine therapy for sepsis. The study group consisted of 893 sepsis patients; 302 were randomized to placebo, 298 to treatment with 1.0 mg/kg/h, and 293 to treatment with 2.0 mg/kg/h rhIL-1ra for 72 hours. An independent, sepsis-specific log-normal regression model that predicts the risk of mortality over 28 days was applied to all patients in the study group (Fig 2). The trial data were also analyzed by the Acute Physiology Score of Acute Physiology and Chronic Health Evaluation II (APACHE II) and the Acute Physiology Score of APACHE III.

Results.—There was a significant increase in survival time for all patients treated with rhIL-1ra, but patients with a Predicted Risk of Mortality of less than 24% did not significantly benefit from this therapy. Retrospective analysis of time-to-death data indicated that treatment with rhIL-1ra decreased the risk of death in the first 2 days for patients with at least a 24% Predicted Risk of Mortality, but not in those with less than a 24% Predicted Risk of Mortality. The Predicted Risk of Mortality model projected a 28 day mortality rate of 35% for placebo patients and a 34% rate was actually observed. The model also accurately stratified patients along a full age of risk. There was a wide distribution of patient risk for

Percent of Patients

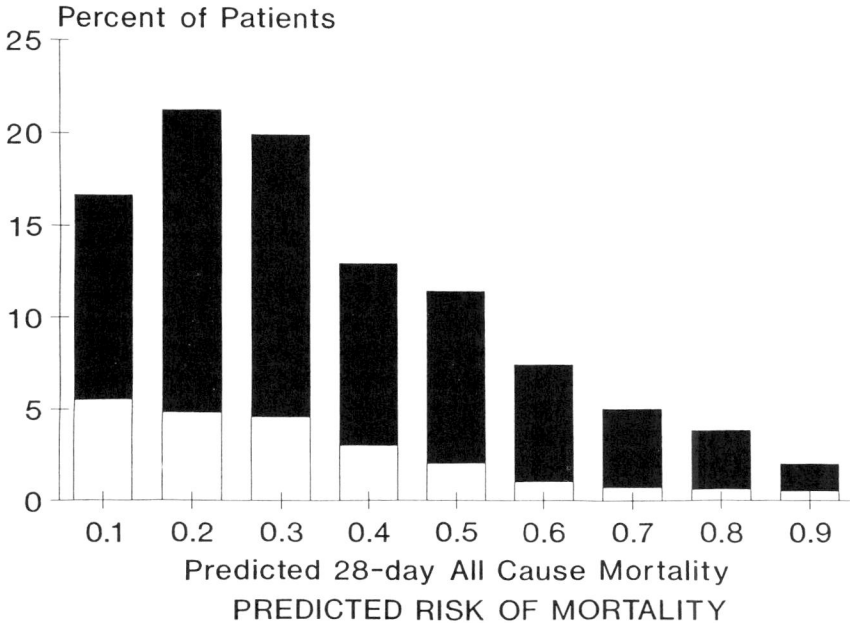

PREDICTED RISK OF MORTALITY

FIGURE 2.—Distribution of baseline predicted risk for all 713 patients meeting predefined criteria for shock, which are defined as a systolic blood pressure of ≤90 mm Hg, mean arterial pressure of ≤70 mm Hg, or a decrease in systolic blood pressure of ≥40 mm Hg, or the use of vasopressors to maintain blood pressure (excluding dopamine of <5.0 µg/kg/min), which persisted despite adequate fluid resuscitation. The *open portions of the bar* represent patients without shock ($n = 180$), and the *solid portions* represent patients with shock ($n = 713$). (Courtesy of Knaus WA, for the rhIL-1ra Phase III Sepsis Syndrome Study Group: Use of predicted risk of mortality to evaluate the efficacy of anticytokine therapy in sepsis. *Crit Care Med* 24:46–56, 1996).

28-day mortality among all patients and within patient subgroups, such as those with shock and organ dysfunction. Two alternate risk models were also used, and the Acute Physiology Score of APACHE III revealed a significant survival benefit of rhIL-1ra treatment in the study group.

Conclusion.—Through the use of an appropriate analytic model, such as the Predicted Risk of Mortality model, a significant increase in survival time was observed in patients with sepsis syndrome who were treated with the novel anticytokine, rhIL-1ra. There was a direct relationship between a patient's entry Predicted Risk of Mortality and treatment effectiveness. Assessment of individual risk may be useful to analyze clinical benefit of new therapies for sepsis and to monitor outcome.

▶ The problem with sepsis is to make the diagnosis, and make it accurately, before the onset of therapy. Still, as shown in Figure 2, most patients had sepsis and were reasonable candidates for this intervention. This study used an interesting outcome criteria called the Predicted Risk of Mortality to measure whether the anticytokine therapy with rhIL-1ra worked. The prediction of serious outcomes is a critical issue. The use of APACHE III had been considered the best system, although it is always difficult to ascribe to individual patients the accuracy that one obtains for groups and, in fact, the accuracy level is not so great. Another problem is that this Predicted Rate of Mortality was applied to a subset of patients and it hasn't been applied, or even tested, in other very sick patients. Still, it's an important step for people who work with very ill patients and seek some standard against which to test pharmacotherapy.

M. Weintraub, M.D.

Effects of Pentoxifylline on Circulating Cytokine Concentrations and Hemodynamics in Patients With Septic Shock: Results From a Double-blind, Randomized, Placebo-controlled Study

Zeni F, Pain F Vindimian M, et al (Bellevue Hosp, CHU Saint-Etienne, France)
Crit Care Med 24:207–214, 1996 12–7

Background.—Despite advances in treatment, mortality from septic shock remains high. Pentoxifylline, a methylxanthine derivative, may be of benefit in septic patients by increasing circulation and decreasing release of tumor necrosis factor (TNF), a central mediator of toxicity. To examine whether continuous infusion of pentoxifylline alters serum cytokine concentrations, a prospective, randomized, double-blind, placebo-controlled study was performed.

Methods.—Sixteen patients with septic shock were randomly assigned to receive either 1 mg/kg of pentoxifylline or placebo. At 0, 3, 6, 12, 18, 24, and 48 hours, TNF, interleukin-6 (IL-6), and interleukin-8 (IL-8) serum concentrations were assessed. Pulmonary artery catheter–derived hemodynamics also were assessed.

Results.—In the 8 patients with septic shock in the treatment group, serum concentrations of TNF were significantly lower than in the 8 patients in the placebo group. Serum concentrations of IL-6 and IL-8 were not significantly different between the 2 groups. There were no adverse reactions. There were 5 deaths in the treatment group and 4 deaths in the placebo group.

Conclusions.—Although pentoxifylline was well tolerated and reduced serum TNF concentrations in patients with septic shock, it had no effect on the mortality rate in this small study group. A larger trial will be required to determine whether pentoxifylline can improve outcome in patients with septic shock.

▶ It is always interesting to me how chemicals with one action can be shown to have many actions once we find out about them. The examples are so numerous that they almost do not bear mentioning, but included are thalidomide, which has actions in leprosy, graft-versus-host reaction, and Behçet's syndrome, and verapamil, which has an effect on multiple-drug-resistant cancer, angiotensin-converting enzyme inhibitors, and heart failure. And the list goes on and on. Thus, we come to pentoxifylline, which in animals decreases the release of TNF, which seems to be related somehow to the toxicity of septic shock. Of course, the treatment of septic shock involves 3 areas. First is the elimination of infection after it has been identified. Second is making sure that important organ systems have adequate blood flow and their function is maintained. Third involves attacking the pathologic factors causing the shock.

Unfortunately, despite an effect of pentoxifylline, a methylxanthine-like caffeine that lowered the production of TNF in this small (8 patients per group) study, there was no effect on septic shock. Oh, well, back to the drawing board.

M. Weintraub, M.D.

Corticosteroid Treatment for Sepsis: A Critical Appraisal and Meta-analysis of the Literature
Cronin L, Cook DJ, Carlet J, et al (McMaster Univ, Hamilton, Ontario, Canada; St Joseph's Hosp, Hamilton, Ontario, Canada; St Joseph's Hosp, Paris; et al)
Crit Care Med 23:1430–1439, 1995   12–8

Background.—Despite improved management of critically ill patients, mortality remains high among those with severe infection, sepsis, and septic shock. Corticosteroid treatment for these patients has been widely investigated, but with inconsistent results. A meta-analysis of clinical trials evaluated the effect of corticosteroid treatment on mortality and other adverse events.

Methods.—Published and unpublished research on corticosteroid treatment in patients with sepsis and septic shock were identified with computer and manual searches. The 9 relevant, randomized, controlled trials were scored for methodologic quality. The data were combined to estimate the relative risk of mortality and of adverse treatment reactions.

Results.—The studies had methodologic quality scores ranging from 4 to 12. There were trends toward increased mortality rates in patients with sepsis or septic shock in association with corticosteroid treatment in studies with both good and poor methodologic quality. Among only patients with septic shock, corticosteroid treatment had no effect on mortality in the studies overall, whereas in studies with good methodologic quality, corticosteroid treatment was associated with greater mortality. Although corticosteroid treatment was not associated with an increased incidence of secondary infection, there was a trend toward increased mortality from secondary infections in patients treated with corticosteroids. A trend toward increased gastrointestinal bleeding was evident in patients treated with corticosteroids. Additional reported adverse treatment effects included increased blood urea nitrogen and bilirubin values and adult respiratory distress syndrome.

Conclusions.—Corticosteroids do not improve survival in patients with severe infection and have significant adverse effects. It is recommended that future clinical trials of immune-modulating agents be methodologically rigorous, as methodology may have a profound effect on the results.

▶ After all these years and a whole lot of studies, there is still no reason to give steroids to patients with severe infection, sepsis, or septic shock. Can we move on to other approaches?

L. Lasagna, M.D.

Is It Time to Reposition Vasopressors and Inotropes in Sepsis?
Rudis MI, Basha MA, Zarowitz BJ (Wayne State Univ, Detroit; Henry Ford Health Sciences Ctr, Detroit)
Crit Care Med 24:525–537, 1996   12–9

Background.—Patients with sepsis syndrome and the systemic inflammatory response syndrome typically have diffuse, ineffective tissue and cellular oxygen utilization, peripheral vasodilation, myocardial depression, and hemodynamic collapse. Much research has compared the efficacy of vasopressor and inotropic agents in increasing hemodynamic stability and survival among such patients. The literature on the current use of vasopressors and inotropes in the treatment of sepsis and sepsis syndrome was reviewed.

Methods.—All relevant English and French language studies on hemodynamic support with selected vasopressors and inotropic drugs published between 1975 and 1994 were identified in a Medical Literature Analysis and Retrieval System On-Line (MEDLINE) search. The analysis focused on prospective, randomized, controlled comparative studies. When data were limited, however, open-label, observational, and comparative studies as well as case series were assessed.

Findings.—Larger than usual doses of epinephrine, norepinephrine, and phenylephrine consistently increased hemodynamic values. Oxygen transport values appeared to rise more reliably with epinephrine than with norepinephrine. Dobutamine, 2.5–6 µg/kg/min, raised oxygen transport variables and hemodynamics to predetermined goals in only 30% to 70% of the patients. There was no advantage to greater infusion rates.

Conclusions.—There is not enough evidence to support goal-directed vasopressor or inotrope treatment in patients with sepsis syndrome. However, vasopressor treatment used earlier in sepsis syndrome may be more promising. Large, comparative, controlled studies are needed to assess mortality and development of multiple organ system dysfunction.

▶ We seem to be better at explaining septic shock than treating it. Even prompt and appropriate empiric antibiotics and supportive therapy work in less than half of such patients at best. And other measures such as antiendotoxins, interleukin receptor antagonists, tumor necrosis factor inhibitors, and nitric oxide synthase inhibitors have not looked very promising.

This review of the literature on vasopressors and inotropes summarizes the present unsatisfactory state of affairs.

L. Lasagna, M.D.

Vaccination Levels in Los Angeles Public Health Centers: The Contribution of Missed Opportunities to Vaccinate and Other Factors
Wood D, Pereyra M, Halfon N, et al (RAND Corp, Santa Monica, Calif; Cedars-Sinai Med Ctr, Los Angeles; Centers for Disease Control and Prevention, Atlanta, Ga)
Am J Public Health 85:850–853, 1995   12–10

Background.—American preschool children have low levels of measles immunization, particularly for those in poor, inner-city areas. Factors linked to this problem include poor access to care and high rates of missed opportunities to vaccinate, but the true contribution of these factors to immunization rates is unknown. To assess immunization coverage rates and contributing factors, a study of preschool children in Los Angeles County public health centers was conducted.

Methods.—The study sample comprised a random sample of 752 records of children 2 years of age enrolled at 5 public health centers. The records were abstracted to determine the children's immunization coverage rates and the contribution of missed opportunities to vaccinate, among other factors.

Results.—Just 27% of the children had up-to-date vaccination status. Factors associated with being up-to-date with vaccinations included the number of missed opportunities to vaccinate and the number of well-child visits. Fifty-two percent of all visits represented missed opportunities to vaccinate. Many of these missed opportunities involved minor illness diagnoses and inaccurate assessment of the child's immunization status by nurses.

Conclusions.—Children enrolled in Los Angeles public health clinics have low immunization rates. Factors contributing to those problems including missed opportunities to vaccinate and having too few well-child visits. Steps to improve vaccination rates may include reducing clinic barriers and improving patient follow-up through tracking systems.

Is Underimmunization a Marker for Insufficient Utilization of Preventive and Primary Care?
Rodewald LE, Szilagyi PG, Shiuh T, et al (Univ of Rochester, NY; Ctrs for Disease Control and Prevention, Atlanta, Ga)
Arch Pediatr Adolesc Med 149:393–397, 1995   12–11

Background.—There is renewed interest in underimmunization of young children and the possible interventions to correct this problem. Strategies that seek to increase the number of sites at which immunizations could be given, regardless of access to comprehensive primary care, run the risk of fragmenting the provision of health services. Underimmunization was studied as a marker for the lack of current and future preventive and acute primary care.

Methods.—The historical cohort study included 1,178 infants and children, 12 to 30 months of age, who were patients at an urban primary care center. The children's records were reviewed to determine their immunization status; anemia, tuberculosis, and lead-screening status; and clinic usage history. Any instance in which a recommended screening was missed by more than 3 months past the standard age was regarded as a screening delay. Screening delay was used as a dependent variable in logistic regression analysis, with predictor variables of immunization status, well-child attendance status, and number of acute care visits.

Results.—At 1 year of age, more than one third of the infants were less than fully immunized. Underimmunized children, compared with fully immunized children, were at greater risk for delay in screening for anemia, with a relative risk (RR) of 7.5; tuberculosis, RR, 1.7; and blood lead level, RR, 2.1. As immunization delay increased, so did the risk of screening delay. The underimmunized children had 47% fewer preventive health care visits than the fully immunized children and 50% more missed appointments. On logistic regression predicting anemia screening delay at 1 year old, the effect of underimmunization was independent of the effect of utilization, with an odds ratio of 7.7.

Conclusions.—Underimmunization is a strong and independent indicator of inadequate preventive and acute primary care in young children. New interventions to increase intervention rates may also be able to target children at risk of inadequate health supervision. As long as immunizations are not separated from primary care, efforts to increase immunization could improve other aspects of primary care as well.

▶ The 2 papers reviewed and abstracted here (Abstracts 12–10 and 12–11) as well as another paper[1] all found similar problems with the vaccination levels being less than optimal. The authors believed that we all missed opportunities in vaccinating the children when we had our hands on them, either in the neonatal ICU or in a public health center. However, the paper from Rochester (Abstract 12–11) states that one should not try to immunize children when they come for an emergency department visit. The authors believe that the immunization has to be unattached to primary care. Children participating in large immunization campaigns may be at risk for not having their primary care needs addressed.

Looking at all of the literature that comes in to the 1997 YEAR BOOK OF DRUG THERAPY allows one to see that 4 different journals (*Archives of Pediatrics and Adolescent Medicine, Canadian Medical Association Journal*, the *American Journal of Public Health,* and *Infection Control and Hospital Epidemiology*) address the same issue in a slightly different way. Nobody questions that we are not doing as good a job as we could be in immunizing children and adults (including adult health care workers). In many cases, it is as though a light went on all over the world and people started investigating.

To improve vaccination rates, we will just have to do better with our immunizations.

M. Weintraub, M.D.

Reference

1. Meleth S, Dahlgren LS, Sankaran R, et al: Vaccination status of infants discharged from a neonatal intensive care unit. *Can Med Assoc J* 153:415–419, 1995.

Knowledge and Attitudes of Healthcare Workers About Influenza: Why Are They Not Getting Vaccinated?

Heimberger T, Chang H-G, Shaikh M, et al (Centers for Disease Control and Prevention, Atlanta, Ga; New York State Dept of Health, Albany; Middletown Psychiatric Ctr, Middletown, NY)
Infect Control Hosp Epidemiol 16:412–414, 1995   12–12

Objective.—Health care workers (HCWs) are an important potential source of influenza transmission to elderly patients, and annual influenza vaccination is recommended for HCWs who have contact with high-risk patients. However, the vaccine acceptance rate among HCWs remains low. Reasons for this low acceptance rate were explored in a survey study.

Methods.—An anonymous questionnaire regarding knowledge of influenza and attitudes about influenza vaccination was distributed to 1,293 HCWs. The study was performed at a chronic care psychiatric facility at which an influenza outbreak had recently occurred. The response rate was 71%.

Results.—Factors predicting current influenza vaccination status were having received a vaccine previously, with a relative risk (RR) of 69.7; age 50 years or older, RR, 2.4; and knowing that influenza vaccine does not cause influenza, RR, 2.3. Nonmedical HCWs and nonmedical employees were twice as likely to have been vaccinated as medical personnel.

Conclusions.—Health care workers have low rates of influenza vaccination. Fear of side effects and avoidance of medications are the most common reasons for not receiving vaccination. Influenza vaccination rates might be increased through educational measures to address misconceptions and through more vigorous administrative efforts to vaccinate health care employees.

▶ This year, several football players did not compete in the play-off games heading to the Super Bowl because of serious cases of influenza, even though the teams had influenza vaccination programs. These players refused to be vaccinated even though it could have been done for free and the physician was there to give the vaccine. The authors studied HCWs, who should know better than football players the value of vaccines and in particular the value of the vaccine for influenza. The best thing was the program for increasing influenza vaccination by attacking the roadblocks for vaccination. Unfortunately, the most stringent plan for increasing vaccinations asked the employees to sign an informed consent if they chose not to be vaccinated. In addition to frightening employees, this does leave them open to legal implications if their jobs were changed or if they did get sick. Still, other parts of the plan seem applicable and worth investigating.

M. Weintraub, M.D.

Prevalence and Incidence of Adult Pertussis in an Urban Population
Nennig ME Shinefield HR, Edwards KM, et al (Kaiser Permanente Pediatric Vaccine Study Ctr, Oakland, Calif; Vanderbilt Univ, Nashville, Tenn)
JAMA 275:672–1674, 1996   12–13

Background.—Although pertussis vaccine is effective and readily available, the prevalence of pertussis has increased nationally. The prevalence of adult pertussis was prospectively investigated, and its importance in the epidemiology of pertussis was considered.

Methods.—A total of 153 patients older than 18 years referred for cough persisting for at least 2 weeks and 154 randomly selected controls with no history of cough during the previous 3 months were studied. Patients and controls completed a brief questionnaire on the onset of symptoms, the duration of cough, past history of pertussis and immunization, and current cough treatment. Serum samples were obtained, and pertussis toxin antibodies were assayed with an enzyme-linked immunosorbent assay.

Results.—Of the 153 patients referred for persistent cough, 12.4% had an elevated pertussis toxin antibody level. The incidence was estimated to be 176 cases per 100,000 person-years. Of the 19 patients with pertussis, 9 (47%) had a history of childhood immunizations and 2 (11%) had a history of whooping cough in childhood, whereas the immunization status was uncertain in 4 patients (21%).

Conclusions.—Pertussis is more common in adults than has been previously reported, making adult pertussis a substantial public health threat. Therefore, pertussis immunization after the age of 7 years should be considered, to reduce the risk of transmission from infected adults to infants and children.

▶ Pertussis cases have increased in the United States despite the availability of an effective vaccine. The incidence seems to peak every 3 or 4 years. Although a large proportion of such cases occur in infants, there has been a shift toward an increased number of cases in individuals aged 15 years or older. Adult pertussis is a very real problem, and booster doses of acellular pertussis vaccine after 7 years of age may be a wise public health move.

L. Lasagna, M.D.

Evaluating New Vaccines for Developing Countries: Efficacy or Effectiveness?

Clemens J, Brenner R, Rao M, et al (Natl Inst of Child Health and Human Development, Bethesda, Md)
JAMA 275:390–397, 1996   12–14

Background.—Vaccination is a key part of primary health care in the developing world, and there is pressure to expand the range of vaccines offered. However, the availability of more new vaccines raises important questions about their clinical evaluation. The challenge is to determine whether the costs of purchasing and administering a new vaccine are justified by its preventive benefits. The potential value of an effectiveness rather than an efficacy approach to evaluating new vaccines was reviewed.

The Contemporary Evaluation Sequence.—Conventionally, vaccines are first tested for safety and immunogenicity in a low-risk population, phase I; then tested in the target population, phase II; then studied for safety and clinical protection in randomized, clinical trials of the target population, phase III. This sequence focuses on measuring the vaccine's efficacy by assessing its performance under idealized conditions. As a result, it may actually contribute to uncertainty about whether the vaccine achieves a suitable balance between costs and benefits. In this way, efficacy studies can hinder rational decision-making about whether to introduce a new vaccine.

Vaccine Effectiveness Trials.—As an alternative to studies of vaccine efficacy, studies of vaccine effectiveness may offer a more pragmatic approach. In these studies, the vaccine's performance is evaluated under the actual conditions of a public health program. The effectiveness approach gathers data on the direct and indirect effects of the vaccine while comprehensively addressing outcomes that are important from the public health perspective. A few prospective effectiveness trials of vaccines have been performed in both developed and developing countries. These studies can have a major impact on public health policy, as 1 study did in disproving the notion that measles vaccine would not improve the survival of young children in less developed settings.

Discussion.—Effectiveness trials may be a very useful tool for evaluating new vaccines for use in the developing world. By testing vaccines under the ordinary conditions of a public health program, effectiveness studies may accelerate the introduction of effective new vaccines by resolving debates about their costs vs. benefits. Effectiveness trials can provide a rational basis for triaging new vaccines and thus may help in attracting research funding from international agencies.

▶ These authors raise an important question—granted that a vaccine should be studied under the most favorable conditions possible, so as to avoid a type II statistical error (concluding erroneously that the vaccine doesn't work). We nevertheless need to know how good the vaccine is "in real life," i.e., under the conditions that prevail in ordinary public health programs.

Read this article in its entirety if the topic interests you; it's terrific.

L. Lasagna, M.D.

The Effectiveness of Vaccination Against Influenza in Healthy, Working Adults
Nichol KL, Lind A, Margolis KL, et al (Veterans Affairs Med Ctr, Minneapolis; Hennepin County Med Ctr, Minneapolis; Univ of Minnesota, Minneapolis; et al)
N Engl J Med 333:889–893, 1995   12–15

Objective.—A randomized, double-blind, placebo-controlled trial to evaluate the effects of vaccination against influenza in a low-risk population was performed.

Background.—Influenza affects all age groups, although most deaths occur in the elderly. The average of annual attack rates is 10% to 20%. Millions of days are lost from work annually because of influenza. Vaccination is recommended for individuals at high risk for complications of influenza, as well as those who want to avoid illness.

Methods.—The influenza vaccine or placebo was administered to 841 healthy, working adults between 18 and 64 years. Outcome measures included upper respiratory illness, days of work lost, and use of health care services.

Results.—Research subjects who received the influenza vaccine had 25% fewer episodes of upper respiratory illness, 43% fewer days of work lost, and 44% fewer visits to a physician's office. Estimated cost savings was about $47.00 per person.

Discussion.—There are considerable benefits to healthy, working adults from vaccination against influenza. These benefits are both health-related and economic. Differences in serious complications of influenza between study groups were not evaluated. These findings may have important implications for working adults.

▶ Although no age group is immune to attacks of influenza, most flu-related deaths occur in the elderly. The study abstracted asks whether vaccination against influenza can be recommended to healthy, working adults younger than 65 years of age. The answer is a resounding yes! Vaccination in such people is cost-effective and decreases the risk of discomfort.

L. Lasagna, M.D.

The Efficacy of Influenza Vaccine in Elderly Persons: A Meta-analysis and Review of the Literature

Gross PA, Hermogenes AW, Sacks HS, et al (Hackensack Med Ctr, NJ; New Jersey Med School, Newark; Mt Sinai Med Ctr, New York; et al)
Ann Intern Med 123:518–527, 1995   12–16

Background.—Influenza viruses in elderly individuals can still be fatal or cause serious complications. Research on the efficacy of influenza vaccines in the elderly has yielded inconsistent findings. However, several studies have reported a decreased incidence of pneumonia and mortality with these vaccines. A meta-analysis of published studies on influenza vaccine efficacy in the elderly was performed.

Methods.—A MEDLINE search was conducted to identify cohort observational studies with mortality assessments. Other types of studies also were reviewed.

Findings.—In the 20 cohort studies included in the meta-analysis, the pooled estimates of vaccine efficacy were 56% for preventing respiratory illness, 53% for preventing pneumonia, 50% for preventing hospitalization, and 68% for preventing death. In 3 recent case-control studies, vaccine efficacy ranged from 32% to 45% for preventing hospitalization for pneumonia, from 31% to 65% for preventing hospital deaths from pneumonia and influenza, from 43% to 50% for preventing hospital deaths from all respiratory conditions, and from 27% to 30% for preventing deaths from all causes. The 1 randomized, double-blind, placebo-controlled trial reviewed demonstrated a 50% or greater reduction in influenza-related disease. The 2 recent cost-effectiveness studies reviewed confirmed that influenza vaccine effectively decreases influenza-related morbidity and mortality and results in important cost savings per year per vaccinated individual.

Conclusions.—Many studies confirm that influenza vaccine decreases the risks of pneumonia, hospitalization, and death among the elderly during influenza epidemics when the vaccine strain used is similar to the epidemic strain. Thus, immunization against influenza is an essential part of care for the elderly.

▶ Except for those rare individuals who have significant adverse reactions after flu shots, the great majority of elderly individuals would profit from annual injections of influenza vaccine.

L. Lasagna, M.D.

Early Immunization With Inactivated Poliovirus Vaccine in Premature Infants

Linder N, Yaron M, Handsher R, et al (Tel Aviv Univ, Israel; Chaim Sheba Med Ctr, Tel Hashomer, Israel; Meir Gen Hosp, Kfar Saba, Israel)
J Pediatr 127:128–130, 1995   12–17

Background.—Although the American Academy of Pediatrics Committee on Infectious Diseases recommends that premature infants be immunized against poliomyelitis at the chronological age of 2 months, immunization actually takes place later. As many as half of premature infants may lack immunity against poliovirus.

Study Plan.—The protective immunity conferred by inactivated polio vaccine (IPV) was evaluated in 80 premature newborns whose gestational ages ranged from 30 to 35 weeks and who weighed at least 1,000 g at birth. Thirty-nine study infants received IPV at age 5 to 10 days as well as routine immunization at age 2 months. The 41 control infants did not receive an early dose of IPV.

Results.—Eighty-six percent of all infants had protective antibody titers of 1:8 or greater against all poliovirus types. At age 1 month, 97% of study infants but only 71% of controls had protective titers against poliovirus 3. At age 3 months the respective figures were 97% and 79%. The best 1-month serologic responses were in infants who, at birth, had the lowest titers of antibody against all poliovirus types.

Conclusion.—Premature infants may safely receive IPV shortly after birth, and early immunization will reduce susceptibility to infection, especially by poliovirus 3.

▶ Some infants unfortunately contract poliomyelitis before they have a chance to be vaccinated. Premature infants are particularly at risk because they tend to have low titers of maternal antibody. On the other hand, such low titers seem to predispose vaccinated infants to a better antibody response to polio vaccine.

Preterm infants have been previously reported[1, 2] to respond adequately to both Salk and Sabin vaccines at 2 months of age, and Pagano et al.[3] long ago reported a good response to oral polio vaccine given soon after birth. This article suggests that early poliovirus vaccination is practical, safe, and effective.

L. Lasagna, M.D.

References

1. Smolec P, et al: Antibody response to oral polio vaccine in premature infants. *J Pediatr* 103:917–919, 1983.
2. *J Pediatr* 120:686–689, 1992.
3. Pagano JS, Cornely D, Plotkin SA: The response of premature infants to infection with attenuated poliovirus. *Pediatrics* 29:794–807, 1962.

Reporting Vaccine-associated Paralytic Poliomyelitis: Concordance Between the CDC and the National Vaccine Injury Compensation Program
Weibel RE, Benor DE (Natl Vaccine Injury Compensation Program, Health Resources and Services Administration, Rockville, Md; US Dept of Health and Human Services, Rockville, Md)
Am J Public Health 86:734–737, 1996   12–18

Background.—The National Vaccine Injury Compensation Program, a federal "no-fault" system, was established to compensate persons who were injured or who died as a result of certain immunizations. Persons who acquire paralytic poliomyelitis either after they receive a polio vaccine other than inactivated polio vaccine or from another person who received oral poliovirus vaccine are eligible for compensation under certain conditions. Cases of poliomyelitis are also reported to the Centers for Disease Control (CDC). Concordance between the CDC and the national compensation program was investigated.

Methods and Findings.—Of 118 cases of vaccine-related paralytic poliomyelitis, 18 were initially reported only to the compensation program, and 50 only to the CDC. The other 50 cases were reported to both. The annual incidence of these cases, as determined from data from both systems, ranged from 6 to 13 a year. An increase of 1.4 cases per year was observed when initial reports only to the compensation program were included in the data analyzed.

Conclusions.—The National Vaccine Injury Compensation Program receives additional reports of cases of vaccine-related paralytic poliomyelitis. This program provides important supplemental data on the incidence of vaccine-associated paralytic poliomyelitis.

▶ A decade ago, the United States created a federal "no-fault" system to provide compensation to persons harmed by specific immunizations. It was intended to facilitate such compensation and obviate the need for long, drawn-out, and expensive litigation. Although health care providers are legally required to report adverse reactions to vaccines, there is no penalty for failure to do so. Vaccine-related poliomyelitis is rare, but the risk is not zero. It is paradoxical that the only polio to be seen in the western hemisphere is that transmitted by vaccines, which have eliminated all wild virus problems for more than 4.5 years. Maybe we need to stop using oral polio vaccine and incorporate inactivated polio vaccine into diphtheria-pertussis-tetanus vaccine.

L. Lasagna, M.D.

The Prevalence of Drug-resistant *Streptococcus pneumoniae* in Atlanta
Hofmann J Cetron MS, Farley MM, et al (Ctrs for Disease Control and Prevention, Atlanta, Ga; Emory Univ, Atlanta, Ga)
N Engl J Med 333:481–486, 1995   12–19

Introduction.—In asymptomatic individuals, pneumococci adhere to but do not enter human endothelial cells. However, when endothelial cells are activated with thrombin or tumor-necrosis factor, bacterial entry is increased by 20- to 40-fold. The involvement of platelet-activating factor (PAF) has been suggested by the strong inhibition of pneumococcal entry into activated endothelial cells in the presence of a specific PAF-receptor antagonist. The molecular elements of pneumococcal entry into endothelial cells were studied.

Methods.—Mechanisms involved in pneumococcal attachment were studied in both activated and resting cells with molecular analyses and in animal models.

Results.—The PAF receptor was involved in pneumococcal adherence only in activated cells, suggesting a cognate ligand for the PAF receptor in virulent pneumococci. Phosphorylcholine in the cell wall was suggested as the pneumococcal ligand by the reduction of pneumococcal binding when choline was replaced with ethanolamine or cells were incubated with purified cell wall fragments, antiphosphorylcholine antibody, or 2% choline. Cells transfected with PAF-receptor complementary DNA showed strong pneumococcal adherence, which was reduced in ethanolamine-exposed bacteria and attenuated by exogenous PAF and PAF-receptor antagonists. Phospholipase C was activated by ligation of the PAF receptor by PAF, which was not reduced by pneumococcal ligation with the PAF receptor. Activation-dependent adherence or pneumococcal entrance into the pulmonary epithelium and the progression to overt pneumonia in rabbits after pulmonary epithelial activation by exogenous interleukin-1 was significantly attenuated in rabbits given PAF-receptor antagonist.

Conclusions.—The presentation of the PAF receptor in activated cells plays a crucial role in facilitating progression from asymptomatic colonization to bacteremia.

▶ *Streptococcus pneumoniae* causes more than $4 billion in health care–related expenditures annually in the United States, but until recently, antibiotic treatment was generally very effective.

This present study documents still another area of the country where drug-resistant strains of this organism are now commonly found. This growing problem points up the need for increased vaccination of the public against such infections—and for new choices of antibiotics. These authors suggest a combination of an extended-spectrum cephalosporin plus vancomycin for suspected pneumococcal meningitis, but they doubt the need for vancomycin in less serious infections.

L. Lasagna, M.D.

Moving?

I'd like to receive my *Year Book of Drug Therapy* without interruption.
Please note the following change of address, effective:

Name: _____

New Address: _____

_____

City: _____ State: _____ Zip: _____

Old Address: _____

_____

City: _____ State: _____ Zip: _____

Reservation Card

Yes, I would like my own copy of *Year Book of Drug Therapy*. Please begin my subscription with the current edition according to the terms described below.* I understand that I will have 30 days to examine each annual edition. If satisfied, I will pay just $79.95 plus sales tax, postage and handling (price subject to change without notice).

Name: _____

Address: _____

City: _____ State: _____ Zip: _____

Method of Payment

○ Visa   ○ Mastercard   ○ AmEx   ○ Bill me   ○ Check (in US dollars, payable to Mosby, Inc.)

Card number: _____ Exp date: _____

Signature: _____

LS-0909

*Your *Year Book* Service Guarantee:

When you subscribe to the *Year Book*, we'll send you an advance notice of future volumes about two months before they publish. This automatic notice system is designed to take up as little of your time as possible. If you do not want the *Year Book*, the advance notice makes it quick and easy for you to let us know your decision, and you will always have at least 20 days to decide. If we don't hear from you, we'll send you the new volume as soon as it's available. And, of course, the *Year Book* is yours to examine free of charge for 30 days (postage, handling and applicable sales tax are added to each shipment.).

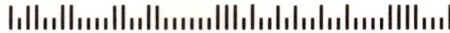

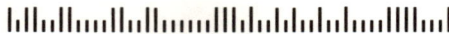

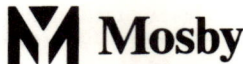

Mosby

Dedicated to publishing excellence

Impaired Antibody Responses to Pneumococcal Polysaccharide in Elderly Patients With Low Serum Vitamin B$_{12}$ Levels

Fata FT, Herzlich BC, Schiffman G, et al (Univ of New York, Brooklyn)
Ann Intern Med 124:299–304, 1996   12–20

Purpose.—Polyvalent pneumococcal polysaccharide vaccine is indicated for the prevention of pneumococcal infection in individuals older than 65 years and in patients with certain chronic diseases. For unknown reasons, about one fourth of immunocompetent elderly people do not respond to type 3 capsular polysaccharide vaccination. Depletion of vitamin B$_{12}$, or cobalamin, was evaluated as a possible explanation for this impaired antibody response.

Methods.—The controlled, prospective cohort study included 15 hospitalized elderly patients with low serum vitamin B$_{12}$ levels and 15 controls. The patients and controls were matched for age and diagnosis. All received a subcutaneous injection of 0.5 mL of the 23-polyvalent pneumococcal polysaccharide vaccine. Before and 4 weeks after vaccination, the patients' serum antibody titers to 12 pneumococcal serotypes were determined by radioimmunoassay.

Results.—The patients with low vitamin B$_{12}$ levels had a lesser difference between the geometric mean of the vaccine antibody titers before and after vaccination than did the control group. This was so for all 12 serotypes tested. Vitamin B$_{12}$ status was an independent predictor of antibody response after controlling for mean corpuscular volume and age. Furthermore, the increase in antibody titer was independently predicted by erythrocyte mean corpuscular volume.

Conclusions.—Elderly patients with vitamin B$_{12}$ depletion demonstrate impaired antibody responses to the 23-polyvalent pneumococcal polysaccharide vaccine. The next step is to find out whether vitamin B$_{12}$ treatment can enhance specific immunoglobulin synthesis, thus improving the clinical efficacy of the pneumococcal vaccine. Until this question is answered, there are insufficient grounds for giving vitamin B$_{12}$ to patients with subclinical vitamin B$_{12}$ deficiency in an effort to increase antibody responsiveness.

▶ No one really knows why almost a fourth of otherwise seemingly healthy oldsters don't respond with antibodies to type 3 pneumococcal capsular polysaccharide.

The authors of this study have wondered whether a possible explanation for at least some of these failures may be related to suboptimal nutrition, because 7% to 15% of elderly individuals have low serum B$_{12}$ levels. The results of this study confirm their suspicion, and now we need to find out whether B$_{12}$ supplementation can solve the problem.

L. Lasagna, M.D.

Neisseria Meningitidis With Decreased Susceptibility to Penicillin in Saskatchewan, Canada

Blondeau JM, Ashton FE, Isaacson M, et al (Univ of Saskatchewan, Saskatoon, Canada; Lab Centre for Disease Control, Ottawa, Ont, Canada)
J Clin Microbiol 33:1784–1786, 1995   12–21

Objective.—Strains of *Neisseria meningitidis* with decreased susceptibility to penicillin have appeared in many parts of the world, but moderately penicillin-resistant *N. meningitidis* has been rare in North America. An outbreak of meningococcal disease in Saskatoon, Saskatchewan, Canada, caused by *N. meningitidis* with decreased susceptibility to penicillin, was investigated.

Findings.—Field studies identified 11 patients infected with *N. meningitidis* with decreased susceptibility to penicillin, all from Saskatoon or the surrounding area. A possible epidemiologic link was found in just 3 of the 11 patients, 9 of whom were children aged 5 years or younger. All of the isolates were serogroup C, electrophoretic type 15. The infecting strains had penicillin minimum inhibitory concentration of 0.12 to 0.25 µg/mL, compared with less than 0.05 µg/mL for fully susceptible strains. The results of pulsed-field gel electrophoresis showed that all of the decreased-susceptibility isolates had identical genomic fingerprints. Strains from patients with *N. meningitidis* infection from other parts of Saskatchewan were susceptible to penicillin and of varying genomic fingerprints.

Conclusions.—A moderately penicillin-resistant strain of *N. meningitidis* appears to be prevalent in Saskatoon. The findings underscore the need for comprehensive monitoring of meningococci for the emergence of penicillin resistance, as well as resistance to other antibiotics.

▶ A lot of countries are plagued with meningococci that are moderately resistant to penicillin. Although this study records an outbreak of meningococcal disease in Canada, the United States has had the problem for at least 5 years.

L. Lasagna, M.D.

Pneumocystis carinii Pneumonia in Patients Without Acquired Immunodeficiency Syndrome: Associated Illnesses and Prior Corticosteroid Therapy

Yale SH, Limper AH (Mayo Clinic, Rochester, Minn)
Mayo Clin Proc 71:5–13, 1996   12–22

Background.—Corticosteroids have been found to predispose patients with malignancies to the development of *Pneumocystis carinii* pneumonia (PCP). Data on the frequency, dosage, and duration of corticosteroid treatment in other patient groups before PCP development are lacking. The clinical spectrum of immunosuppressive conditions and systemic corticosteroid treatment associated with the development of PCP were reported.

Methods.—One hundred sixteen consecutive patients without AIDS were studied retrospectively. All had been seen at 1 center for an initial episode of PCP between 1985 and 1991.

Findings.—Thirty percent of the patients had hematologic malignancy; 25% had organ transplantation; 22.4% had inflammatory disorders; 12.9% had solid tumors; and 9.5% had miscellaneous conditions. Systemic corticosteroid treatment had been given to 90.5% of the total group within 1 month of PCP diagnosis. The median daily corticosteroid dose was the equivalent of 30 mg of prednisone, although as little as 16 mg of prednisone per day had been given to 25% of the patients. Corticosteroid treatment had been given for a median of 12 weeks before pneumonia developed. In 25% of the patients, however, PCP developed after 8 weeks or less of corticosteroid treatment. Forty-three percent of the patients had respiratory failure. Thirty-four percent of the patients with PCP died in the hospital.

Conclusions.—Premorbid corticosteroid treatment is probably not the only factor contributing to the development of PCP in these patients. However, systemic corticosteroid treatment, even in moderate doses, had been given to most patients in the month preceding PCP onset. In patients requiring prolonged systemic corticosteroid treatment, PCP prophylaxis should be considered.

▶ This is a reminder that AIDS isn't the only condition that increases the risk of pneumonia caused by *P. carinii*. Systemic corticosteroid therapy is another cause, even in moderate doses.

Alternate-day or inhaled corticosteroids seem okay. The authors quite rightly suggest we should at least consider the possibility of anti–*P. carinii* prophylaxis.

L. Lasagna, M.D.

Randomised Comparison of Ganciclovir and High-Dose Acyclovir for Long-Term Cytomegalovirus Prophylaxis in Liver-Transplant Recipients

Winston DJ, Wirin D, Shaked A, et al (Univ of California, Los Angeles)
Lancet 346:69–74, 1995   12–23

Background.—Several different approaches have been tried in attempts to prevent cytomegalovirus (CMV) infection in solid-organ transplant recipients, including CMV immune globulin, high-dose acyclovir, and short-course ganciclovir. Still, rates of CMV-related morbidity and mortality remain high. Long-term ganciclovir and high-dose acyclovir were compared for prophylaxis against CMV disease in liver transplant patients.

Methods.—The controlled trial included 250 patients undergoing liver transplantation. They were randomized to receive either long-term ganciclovir or a standard prophylactic regimen of high-dose acyclovir. Ganciclovir was given IV in a dose of 6 mg/kg/day from day 1 to day 30, then at the same dose on Monday through Friday until day 100. Acyclovir was given IV at a dose of 10 mg/kg every 8 hours from day 1 until hospital discharge, then orally 800 mg 4 times a day until day 100. Cultures, serologic and laboratory tests, and tissue biopsies were performed to monitor for the development of CMV infection, CMV disease, and drug toxicity.

Results.—The CMV infection rate through the first 120 days after transplantation was 38% in the acyclovir group vs. 5% in the ganciclovir group. Ten percent of the patients receiving acyclovir had symptomatic CMV disease as compared with just 1% of those receiving ganciclovir. The CMV infection rate in CMV antibody–positive patients was 37% with acyclovir vs. 4% with ganciclovir; in CMV antibody–negative patients, the rates were 42% and 11%, respectively. On multivariate analysis, ganciclovir treatment was the most significant protective factor against CMV infection and disease. The 2 prophylactic regimens were relatively well tolerated, with comparable rates of leukopenia, thrombocytopenia, renal failure, and other adverse events.

Conclusions.—Long-term ganciclovir treatment prevents virtually all CMV infection and disease in liver transplant recipients. Toxicity is about the same as with standard acyclovir prophylaxis. Long-term ganciclovir provides protection throughout the period of greatest risk for CMV disease with an agent that has greater anti-CMV activity than previously used treatments.

▶ Very few investigators can make the kind of statement that these people did at the end of their study. It says, and I quote, "CMV can be almost completely eliminated as a significant pathogen in liver transplant patients by the long-term administration of ganciclovir." In addition to making that broad and very welcome statement, the investigators did a number of very interesting things with their data, including a multivariate analysis. They tried to determine factors that might influence CMV disease, as well as the results of prophylactic therapy. Many of the factors that were important were related to the type of transplant, such as an increase in ABO mismatch or using cyclosporine as prophylaxis against rejection instead of tacrolimus. Having many episodes of documented rejection increases CMV disease as well. It sometimes seems that patients receiving a transplant just have the pharmacy shelves emptied and all the medications poured into them. That's why we really have to be very careful as to the proof of the value of the prophylactic and therapeutic medicines that are used for transplants.

M. Weintraub, M.D.

Famciclovir for the Treatment of Acute Herpes Zoster: Effects on Acute Disease and Postherpetic Neuralgia: A Randomized, Double-blind, Placebo-controlled Trial

Tyring S, and the Collaborative Famciclovir Herpes Zoster Study Group (Univ of Texas, Galveston; St John Hosp, Nassau Bay, Tex; St Louis Univ, Mo; et al)

Ann Intern Med 123:89–96, 1995   12–24

Background.—Acyclovir has been the only antiviral agent approved for the treatment of acute herpes zoster, even though its effect on postherpetic neuralgia is controversial. A new drug, famciclovir, was approved in June 1994 for the treatment of patients with herpes zoster. It has been shown to be well absorbed, with activity against varicella-zoster virus, herpes simplex virus types 1 and 2, and Epstein-Barr virus. In vitro comparisons have shown that famciclovir and acyclovir have similar potency, but famciclovir has a more favorable half-life in cells infected with varicella-zoster virus. The clinical efficacy and safety of famciclovir in the treatment of acute herpes zoster and its effect on postherpetic neuralgia were evaluated in a double-blind, placebo-controlled, multicenter trial.

Methods.—A total of 419 adult, immunocompetent patients with uncomplicated herpes zoster were randomly assigned to treatment with 500 mg of famciclovir (138 patients), 750 mg of famciclovir (135 patients), or placebo (146 patients) 3 times daily for 7 days. Their lesions and pain were evaluated daily during treatment and for 7 days after treatment, then weekly until all of the lesions had lost their crusts, and then monthly for 5 more months. Efficacy analyses, based on intention to treat, included comparisons of the time to full lesion crusting; duration of viral shedding; time to resolution of vesicles, ulcers, crusts, and acute pain; and duration of postherpetic neuralgia.

Results.—Patients treated with famciclovir had shorter times to full crusting and to resolution of vesicles, ulcers, and crusts than did patients in the placebo group. Patients in the famciclovir groups stopped shedding virus approximately twice as quickly as the patients in the placebo group. Overall, no significant differences were found in the median time to acute pain resolution, but in patients with severe rash, pain resolved significantly more quickly in the famciclovir groups than in the placebo group. Famciclovir treatment, at either dose, was associated with significant reductions in the duration of postherpetic neuralgia, particularly among patients older than 50 years of age, in whom postherpetic neuralgia is most likely. The patients tolerated famciclovir well, with adverse events comparable to those experienced in the placebo group.

Conclusions.—Famciclovir given 3 times a day for 7 days was safe and effective, accelerating lesion healing and reducing the duration of viral shedding and postherpetic neuralgia. No dose-response differences were found in the efficacy or safety of 500-mg and 750-mg doses.

▶ Acute herpes zoster can be a dreadful ailment, and the persistent postherpetic neuralgia suffered by many patients (especially the elderly) can be maddening. Although antidepressants with or without an antipsychotic drug (as in the combination Triavil) often can help (and sometimes cure) this neuralgia, it would be even better to prevent the neuralgia or at least to cut down its duration.

Famciclovir seems, in this trial, not to have affected the occurrence of postherpetic neuralgia (which occurred in slightly fewer than half of the patients), although the duration of this disabling complication was significantly reduced.

L. Lasagna, M.D.

Biotherapeutic Agents: A Neglected Modality for the Treatment and Prevention of Selected Intestinal and Vaginal Infections

Elmer GW, Surawicz CM, McFarland LV (Univ of Washington, Seattle)
JAMA 275:870–876, 1996   12–25

Background.—Crude mixtures of microorganisms have long been used to treat infections. The potential of "biotherapeutic agents"—microorganisms with therapeutic properties—for preventing and/or treating certain intestinal and vaginal infections was evaluated.

Methods.—In a search of the MEDLINE database, relevant articles published from 1966 to September 1995 were identified. All placebo-controlled studies of biotherapeutic agents in humans were reviewed.

Findings.—Biotherapeutic agents have been used successfully in the prevention of antibiotic-associated diarrhea and acute infantile diarrhea. Such agents have also been successful in the treatment of recurrent *Clostridium difficile* disease and other various diarrheal illnesses. Limited evidence suggests that *Lactobacillus acidophilus* may prevent candidal vaginitis. Few adverse effects have occurred. However, only small numbers of patients or volunteers were included in many of these studies.

Conclusion.—The use of selected microorganisms appears to be effective in preventing and treating certain intestinal infections. Such therapy may also be beneficial in treating vaginal infections. Additional research on the potential of biotherapeutic agents is warranted.

▶ Actually, the use of biotherapeutic agents—microorganisms of a specific type—may become a new and valuable therapeutic modality. We need to have larger and better clinical trials of these whole organisms. There may be a more major role for biotherapeutic agents in bone marrow transplant and immunosuppressed patients.

M. Weintraub, M.D.

Doxycycline Compared With Azithromycin for Treating Women With Genital *Chlamydia trachomatis* Infections: An Incremental Cost-Effectiveness Analysis

Magid D, Douglas JM Jr, Schwartz JS (Univ of Washington, Seattle; Denver Dept of Health; Univ of Pennsylvania, Philadelphia)
Ann Intern Med 124:389–399, 1996   12–26

Background.—The traditional first-line therapy for cervical chlamydial infection is doxycycline, given twice daily for 7 days. The success of this treatment is dependent on the patients' compliance. Azithromycin, given as a single 1-g dose, has recently been shown to be an effective therapy for cervical chlamydial infection, but it is more expensive than 1 course of doxycycline. The health outcomes, costs, and incremental cost-effectiveness of the 2 therapies were compared in women with uncomplicated cervical infection with *Chlamydia trachomatis*.

Methods.—A decision model was constructed to calculate health outcomes and costs of hypothetical cohorts of women with uncomplicated cervical chlamydial infections treated with either doxycycline, 100 mg twice daily for 7 days, or azithromycin in a single 1-g dose (Fig 1). The risk for adverse antibiotic reactions, pelvic inflammatory disease and its sequelae, and the sequelae of chlamydia in new sexual partners and neonates were evaluated for both treatment strategies. Probability estimates, based on a literature review and expert survey, were calculated in relation to a range of epidemiologic and clinical variables, including various levels of compliance. The direct medical costs resulting from infection sequelae were estimated for each medical outcome. Incremental cost-effectiveness ratios of the 2 interventions were calculated, with 1 intervention more

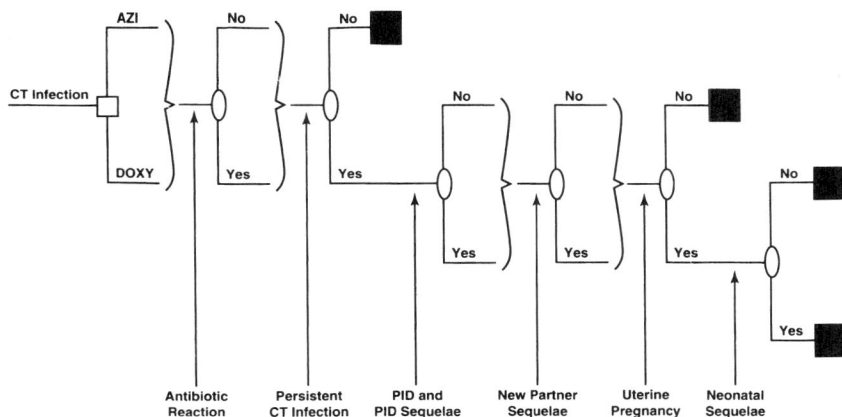

FIGURE 1.—Decision tree for the azithromycin (*AZI*) and doxycycline (*DOXY*) treatment strategies. The *open square* at the left indicates the initial decision about treatment. The *open ovals* denote possible clinical events, and the *solid squares* indicate outcomes. *Abbreviations: CT, Chlamydia trachomatis* infection; *PID*, pelvic inflammatory disease. (Courtesy of Magid D, Douglas JM Jr, Schwartz JS: Doxycycline compared with azithromycin for treating women with genital *Chlamydia trachomatis* infections: An incremental cost-effectiveness analysis. *Ann Intern Med* 124:389–399, 1996.)

effective and more expensive than the other using multivariate sensitivity analyses.

Results.—Estimates of health outcomes indicated that the azithromycin strategy was associated with fewer infectious sequelae and complications, resulting in a cost per patient of $39.51, compared with the cost per patient of $69.07 with the doxycycline strategy. There was an incremental cost-effectiveness of $521 per prevented major complication. These results were relatively insensitive to univariate sensitivity analysis. With multivariate analysis, making the doxycycline maximally effective, the azithromycin strategy was still more effective and less expensive as long as the base cost difference was $9.80 or less.

Conclusions.—Azithromycin therapy is more cost-effective than doxycycline therapy, because of the fewer associated major and minor complications. The azithromycin strategy was shown to be robustly superior after sensitivity analyses. However, the adoption of this strategy may be limited by the current fragmented health care system, in which prevention and sequelae costs may be borne by separate providers.

▶ I wish that people would stop doing modeling exercises, such as this, without any clinical trial adapted to the excellent model that they propose for choosing between doxycycline and azithromycin.

M. Weintraub, M.D.

The Treatment of Bacterial Vaginosis With a 3 Day Course of 2% Clindamycin Cream: Results of a Multicentre, Double Blind, Placebo Controlled Trial
Ahmed-Jushuf IH on behalf of B V Investigators Group (Nottingham City Hosp, England; Gen Hosp, Birmingham, England; Royal Liverpool Univ, England)
Genitourin Med 71:254–256, 1995   12–27

Objective.—Patients with symptomatic bacterial vaginosis (BV) were recruited for a study of the safety and efficacy of treatment with a 3-day course of intravaginal 2% clindamycin cream. Oral metronidazole, the therapy of choice for almost 20 years, has high relapse rates and unpleasant side effects.

Patients and Methods.—Study participants were 221 premenopausal women 18 years or older who received a diagnosis of BV on the basis of clinical and laboratory findings. In a double-blind fashion, 107 were randomly assigned to 20 g 2% clindamycin cream and 114 were randomly assigned to placebo cream. Response to therapy was assessed at 1 and 4 weeks.

Results.—Treatment and follow-up visits were completed by 141 (63.8%) of the women. The active treatment and placebo groups were comparable in age, ethnicity, history of genital infections, and other recorded variables. At 1 week, 75% of the clindamycin group but only 13%

of the placebo group were classified as improved. At 4 weeks, the success rate was 41% in the clindamycin group compared with 4% in the placebo group. One fourth of patients who were improved at 1 week were reported to have a recurrence of BV at 4 weeks. Clindamycin cream was associated with only mild side effects that resolved spontaneously.

Conclusion.—Clindamycin cream (2%), administered for 3 days via disposable applicator, was significantly more effective than placebo in treating BV. Recurrence rates were similar to those reported for oral metronidazole, but clindamycin was quite well tolerated.

▶ Bacterial vaginosis is mysterious but common. It is characterized by a fishy-smelling vaginal discharge, increased vaginal pH, a mixed bacterial flora, and "clue cells" (vaginal epithelial cells covered with polymorphic bacteria).

Oral metronidazole has been the treatment of choice for close to 20 years but is not ideal. Clindamycin taken orally seems to work, and this study indicates that it can work for at least some affected women when applied intravaginally for 3 days. This report thus replicates an earlier study that was similarly favorable.[1]

L. Lasagna, M.D.

Reference

1. Dhar J, Arya OP, Timmins DJ, et al: Treatment of bacterial vaginosis with a three day course of 2% clindamycin vaginal cream: A pilot study. *Genitourin Med* 70:121–123, 1994.

Azithromycin Compared With Amoxicillin in the Treatment of Erythema Migrans: A Double-Blind, Randomized, Controlled Trial
Luft BJ, Dattwyler RJ, Johnson RC, et al (State Univ of New York, Stony Brook; Univ of Minnesota, Minneapolis; Kaiser Permanente, Rocky Hill, Conn; et al)
Ann Intern Med 124:785–791, 1996   12–28

Background.—Both amoxicillin and azithromycin have shown excellent activity against *Borrelia burgdorferi* in open trials. To assess their relative efficacy, relief of the acute manifestations and their sequelae were compared in patients with erythema migrans treated with either a 20-day course of amoxicillin or a 7-day course of azithromycin in a large, multicenter, double-blind, randomized trial.

Methods.—Adult patients with erythema migrans were stratified by the presence or absence of flu-like symptoms, then randomly assigned to treatment with either azithromycin, 500 mg once daily for 7 days, or amoxicillin, 500 mg 3 times daily for 20 days. The azithromycin group was given placebo twice daily for 7 days, then 3 times daily for the next 13 days. The patients were examined at baseline and 8, 20, 30, 90, and 180 days after treatment began. Their response was assessed with clearance of erythema migrans and relief of symptoms. Blood samples were obtained during examinations for *B. burgdorferi* serologic testing.

Results.—Of the 217 evaluable patients, a complete response was achieved on day 20 by 88% of the amoxicillin group compared with 76% of the azithromycin group. All of the patients treated with amoxicillin had at least a partial response within the first 20 days, whereas 3 patients treated with azithromycin had no response or worsened in the first 20 days. A complete response in the azithromycin group was more common among seropositive than seronegative patients. Relapse within 6 months occurred in 16% of the azithromycin group and only 4% of the amoxicillin group. Relapse was significantly predicted by a partial response. Adverse events occurred in 35% of the azithromycin group and 24% of the amoxicillin group.

Conclusions.—Amoxicillin was significantly more effective than azithromycin for complete resolution of erythema migrans and prevention of relapse within 6 months. Further study is needed to determine the long-term efficacy of these treatments. The relationship between complete response to azithromycin therapy and humoral response to *B. burgdorferi* suggests that an early immune response may help limit early disease, or that there is a synergistic association between humoral response and azithromycin.

▶ This was a very well-done study. It was a little risky because it was a "double-dummy" study, which means that people had to receive a placebo to make the dosing schedules equal. It is unfortunate that there was some bias against azithromycin because it really is easier to take a dose of medication once or twice a day rather than trying to take a medication 3 times a day, which means a middle-of-the-day dose. Still, amoxicillin with its more complicated schedule was shown to be more effective. In some clinical trials, other interesting information is developed. These investigators also answered questions about the natural history of erythema migrans, Lyme disease, as well as its clinical presentation and the enzyme-linked immunosorbent assay for serologic testing.

M. Weintraub, M.D.

Trimethoprim-Sulfamethoxazole (Co-Trimoxazole) for the Prevention of Relapses of Wegener's Granulomatosis
Stegeman CA, for the Dutch Co-Trimoxazole Wegener Study Group (Univ Hosp, Groningen, The Netherlands)
N Engl J Med 335:16–20, 1996   12–29

Introduction.—There is a strong association between active Wegener's granulomatosis and the presence of antineutrophil cytoplasmic antibodies. There is a possible role of microbial organisms in recurrent Wegener's granulomatosis, as evidenced by reports of beneficial effects of treatment with trimethoprim and sulfamethoxazole (co-trimoxazole). The efficacy of co-trimoxazole in preventing relapses in patients with Wegener's granulomatosis in remission was evaluated in a prospective, double-blind, placebo-controlled, multicenter trial.

Methods.—Eighty-one patients with Wegener's granulomatosis in remission were randomized to receive co-trimoxazole (800 mg of sulfamethoxazole and 160 mg of trimethoprim) or placebo twice daily for 24 months. Patients were excluded if significant side effects developed or creatinine clearance persistently fell below 30 mL/min. Serum antineutrophil cytoplasmic antibodies were measured. Patients were evaluated every 3 months.

Results.—Forty-one patients received co-trimoxazole and 40 received placebo. Eight of the patients receiving co-trimoxazole were unable to continue treatment because of side effects, which resolved with cessation of treatment. Two patients in the placebo group were dropped; 1 had recurrent urinary tract infections and 1 withdrew consent. One patient in the placebo group died of myocardial infarction. There was no evidence of active Wegener's granulomatosis in this patient at autopsy. The median level of treatment compliance was 98% for patients in both groups. At 24-month follow-up, 82% and 60% of patients, respectively, in the co-trimoxazole and placebo groups were in remission (Fig 1). Patients in the treatment group had a significantly lower annual number of infectious episodes. Patients in the treatment group had significantly fewer respiratory tract infections, compared to the placebo group (76% vs. 86%). Seven patients in the placebo group and 4 patients in the treatment group had relapses within 6 months after a respiratory tract infection. Treatment with co-trimoxazole and the presence of antineutrophil cytoplasmic antibodies at baseline were significantly correlated with disease-free survival.

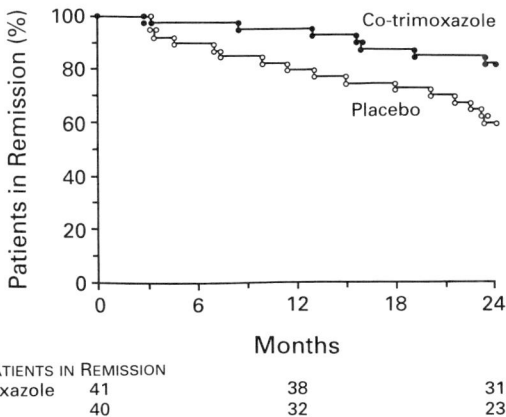

NO. OF PATIENTS IN REMISSION
Co-trimoxazole	41	38	31
Placebo	40	32	23

FIGURE 1.—Disease-free interval from the start of co-trimoxazole or placebo treatment to relapse in patients with Wegener's granulomatosis. The difference in the disease-free interval between the co-trimoxazole group and the placebo group was statistically significant (by the log-rank test) at 24 months (relative risk of relapse, 0.40; 95 percent confidence interval, 0.17 to 0.98). (Courtesy of Stegeman CA, for the Dutch Co-Trimoxazole Wegener's Study Group: Trimethoprim-sulfamethoxazole (co-trimoxazole) for the prevention of relapses of Wegener's granulomatosis. *N Engl J Med* 355:16–20, copyright 1996, Massachusetts Medical Society. Reprinted by permission of *The New England Journal of Medicine.*)

Conclusion.—Prolonged treatment with co-trimoxazole was associated with a reduction in the number of relapses in patients with Wegener's granulomatosis. This reduction was particularly evident in relapses involving the upper airways. It is possible that this treatment approach exerts its protective effect by preventing infections.

▶ Wegener's granulomatosis may be one of those cancers that is really an infectious disease. Actually, many diseases are now seen to have an infectious origin. Certainly, peptic ulcer disease meets the criteria in at least 60% of cases. Or, perhaps, the granulomatous disease is a response to an infectious trigger. Another potential mechanism is that trimethoprim suppresses folic acid metabolism and so does sulfamethoxazole, acting on a different step in the process. In this case, the drug may have some sort of immunosuppressant property as well. This really excellent clinical trial substantiates much of the evidence from open-label studies. The adverse effects of co-trimoxazole may not be as important in clinical treatment as they are in a clinical trial. Now what we have to do is to check the dose, the duration of therapy, and the method of giving the medication. It seems pretty exciting to me.

M. Weintraub, M.D.

Azathioprine for Long-term Maintenance of Remission in Autoimmune Hepatitis
Johnson PJ, McFarlane IG, Williams R (King's College Hosp, London)
N Engl J Med 333:958–963, 1995   12–30

Background.—Although most patients with autoimmune hepatitis respond to prednisolone therapy, which usually is combined with azathioprine, a majority will relapse when treatment is withdrawn. Maintenance treatment with azathioprine is attractive because it will avoid serious toxicity from prolonged steroid therapy. None of 25 patients maintained on 2 mg/kg daily relapsed during a 1-year follow-up period.

Study Plan.—These 25 patients now have been followed up for 10 years, and 47 others have been maintained on azathioprine. When maintenance treatment began, the patients had been in complete remission for a year or longer while receiving 5–15 mg/kg of prednisolone and 1 mg/kg of azathioprine daily. Steroid therapy was gradually withdrawn, and the daily dose of azathioprine was increased to 2 mg/kg. Patients who remained asymptomatic and continued to have normal serum globulin and aspartate aminotransferase levels were considered to be in remission.

Results.—Sixty of the 72 patients (83%) remained in remission for a median of 67 months while on azathioprine alone. Only 3 of 48 follow-up liver biopsies, taken from 42 patients, showed more than mild inflammation. Thirty-two patients lost body weight after steroid treatment ended, and 26 lost their cushingoid facies. Four patients had evidence of myelosuppression, but 2 of them continued in remission when steroid therapy was resumed. In a majority of patients given azathioprine for longer than 2 years, lymphopenia developed. Only 1 of 9 deaths was a result of liver failure.

Conclusion.—Once autoimmune hepatitis has been in complete remission for a year on combined steroid–azathioprine treatment, steroid therapy may be withdrawn and patients can be maintained on a higher dose of azathioprine alone.

▶ We're able to keep autoimmune hepatitis in remission in most patients, but cures are rare. Because corticosteroids taken for a prolonged period of time put one at risk for both cosmetic and more severe complications, it is appropriate to ask whether nonsteroid immunosuppression is attainable with azathioprine alone. The answer seems to be—at least for some patients—yes.

L. Lasagna, M.D.

Treatment of Hepatitis C Virus in Elderly Persons With Interferon α
Van Thiel DH, Friedlander L, Caraceni P, et al (Baptist Med Ctr of Oklahoma, Oklahoma City; West Penn Hosp, Pittsburgh, Pa)
J Gerontol 50A:M330–M333, 1995   12–31

Introduction.—Hepatitis C virus (HCV) infection is more common in adults than children and more common in older adults than younger adults. However, because of fear that older adults will be less likely to tolerate the side effects of interferon-α (IFN) therapy, few older adults with HCV infection are treated. The effectiveness and tolerance of IFN treatment in elderly patients with HCV infection were assessed.

Methods.—The study included 25 patients infected with HCV who were older than 65 years. All patients were positive for HCV antibody and requested treatment for their HCV infection. They received 5 megaunits (MU) of IFN given subcutaneously 3 times weekly for 6 months. They were compared with 25 younger adults whose mean age was 44 years and who were matched for sex and histologic disease. Patients who had a normal serum alanine aminotransferase (ALT) level after 6 months were considered complete responders, and those whose ALT level decreased by more than 50% but remained in the abnormal range were considered partial responders.

Results.—Laboratory studies found no biochemical differences between the older and younger patients after 6 months of IFN treatment, and there was no significant difference in the response rates: 48% for the elderly patients and 41% for the younger adults. None of the elderly patients stopped taking IFN treatment during the study period, and the untoward effects of treatment were similar in type and severity between the 2 groups.

Conclusions.—Interferon-α treatment can be successfully administered to elderly patients with HCV infection. Response rates are similar to those achieved in younger adult patients. The untoward effects of IFN treatment are no different for elderly patients as compared with younger adult patients.

▶ Interferon-α is the only FDA-approved therapy for HCV and works as well in the elderly as in younger adults. There is no good scientific basis for denying such therapy to older patients.

L. Lasagna, M.D.

13 Neoplastic Diseases

Fludarabine Phosphate: A DNA Synthesis Inhibitor With Potent Immunosuppressive Activity and Minimal Clinical Toxicity
Goodman ER, Fiedor PS, Fein S, et al (Columbia Univ, New York)
Am Surg 62:435–442, 1996   13–1

Purpose.—The vidarabine derivative fludarabine phosphate works by inhibition of DNA synthesis to selectively eliminate normal and malignant mononuclear cells. This drug is selective for lymphocytes and other mononuclear cells because it acts only on cells that are rich in the enzyme deoxycytidine kinase. Fludarabine's effects on various immune functions were evaluated in vitro and in vivo in a move toward developing fludarabine's potential as an immunosuppressive agent.

Findings.—In fludarabine-treated cultures, mononuclear cells were depleted within 24 hours, with CD4 and CD8 T cells being more sensitive than CD20 B cells or CD34 bone marrow precursors. Elimination of cells from culture was further enhanced by mitogenic activation of lymphocytes. Fludarabine produced greater than 90% inhibition of phytohemagglutinin-induced T-cell proliferation and greater than 95% inhibition of mixed lymphocyte reactions.

In monkeys and baboons, 5 days of fludarabine treatment produced T-cell and B-cell lymphopenia. The only apparent side effect was transient neutropenia. Monkeys pretreated with fludarabine before ABO-compatible skin allografting had graft survival of 16 days, compared with 8 days for control animals (Figs 7 and 8). Further studies of secondary allotransplantation into presensitized recipients also demonstrated longer graft survival in animals pretreated with fludarabine.

Conclusion.—Fludarabine is a promising and powerful immunosuppressive agent. Although several problems remain, fludarabine targets both activated T and B cells and has low clinical toxicity. Fludarabine is likely to be used as a safe lympholytic agent, possibly replacing azathioprine in combination rejection prophylaxis regimens.

▶ Fludarabine monophosphate was first found to have significant activity in non-Hodgkin's lymphoma and chronic lymphatic leukemia. Because it is halogenated, it is resistant to degradation by adenosine deaminase but is active only after it is metabolized to the triphosphate form. Undesirable

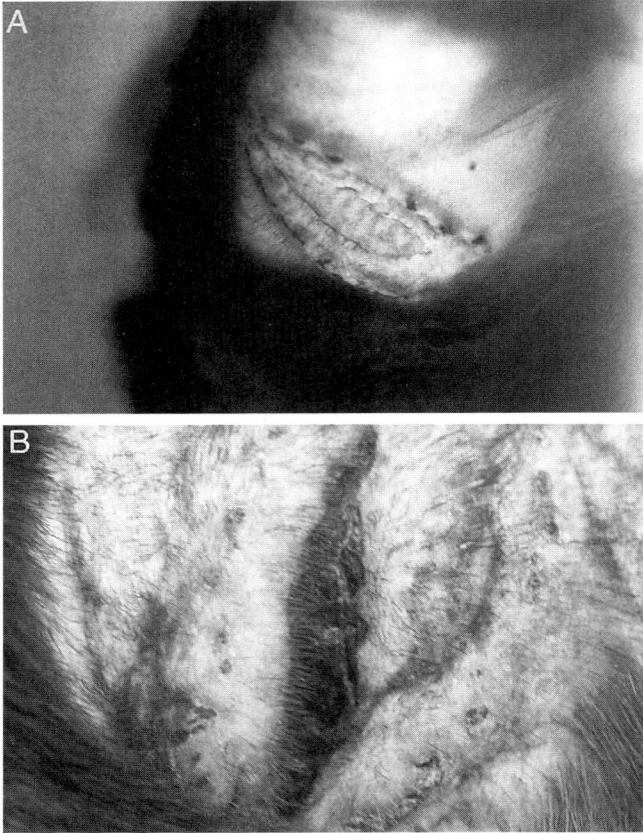

FIGURE 7.—Photographs of ABO-compatible Cynomolgus monkey skin allografts taken 8 days after transplantation. **A,** recipient pretreated with fludarabine. **B,** recipient pretreated with saline. (Courtesy of Goodman ER, Fiedor PS, Fein S, et al: Fludarabine phosphate: A DNA synthesis inhibitor with potent immunosuppressive activity and minimal clinical toxicity. *Am Surg* 62:435–442, 1996.)

effects include drops in circulating T and B cells, malaise, nausea, diarrhea, and transient myelosuppression. I would venture the guess that fludarabine will be used more often in the future, both as part of combination chemotherapy and as monotherapy in treating lymphomas, and also to prevent graft rejection.

L. Lasagna, M.D.

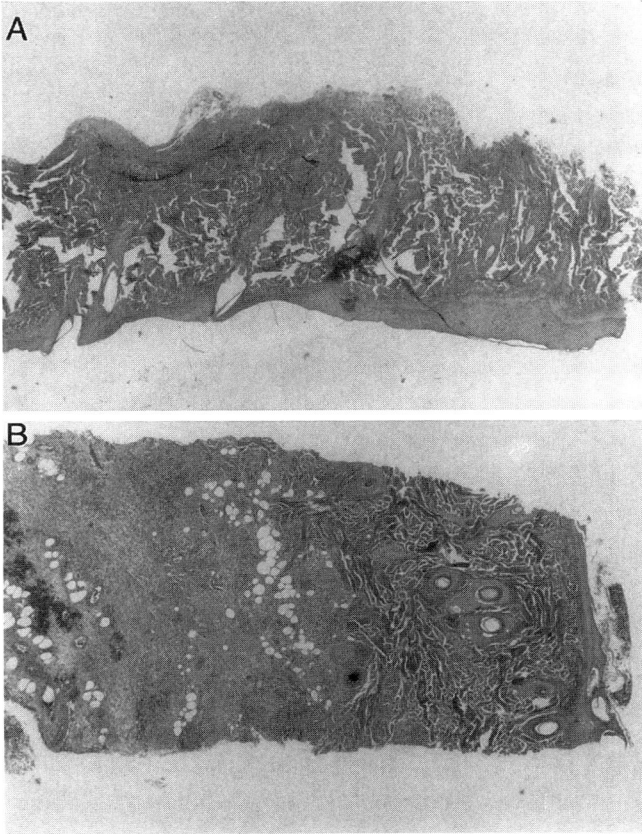

FIGURE 8.—**A** and **B**, hematoxylin and eosin-stained sections of biopsies of grafts shown in Fig 7 (biopsies also performed on eighth day after transplantation). (Courtesy of Goodman ER, Fiedor PS, Fein S, et al: Fludarabine phosphate: A DNA synthesis inhibitor with potent immunosuppressive activity and minimal clinical toxicity. *Am Surg* 62:435–442, 1996.)

Combination Finasteride and Flutamide in Advanced Carcinoma of the Prostate: Effective Therapy With Minimal Side Effects

Fleshner NE, Trachtenberg J (Univ of Toronto)
J Urol 154:1642–1646, 1995   13–2

Background.—Animal research suggests that the combination of fluta-mide and finasteride suppresses the rat ventral prostate to the same degree as luteinizing hormone–releasing hormone agonist plus flutamide. Because these 2 drugs do not reduce serum testosterone levels, they should be useful in the treatment of prostate cancer.

Methods.—The combination of finasteride and flutamide was given to 22 patients with stages C and D1 carcinoma of the prostate. All were sexually active. Patients were followed up for a mean of 22 months.

Findings.—Initially, the average prostate-specific antigen level was 42.9 ng/mL. The mean prostate-specific antigen level at 3 months was 3.6 ng/mL and at 6 months was 2.9 ng/mL. These outcomes appeared to be durable at 24 months. Eighty-six percent of the men maintained sexual function. The main complaint about sexual function was dry ejaculation, reported by 71%. Other side effects were minimal. Thirty-three percent reported diarrhea, and 19% had gynecomastia.

Conclusions.—Until a randomized trial of finasteride and flutamide combination therapy can be performed, this treatment should be reserved for patients who are relatively young and sexually active. Further research on this combination should compare its efficacy with that of standard forms of androgen deprivation treatment and include psychological testing, quality-of-life scales, and survival.

▶ Most prostate cancer patients treated with hormonal therapy become impotent. In addition to loss of libido, there are psychosocial disturbances, muscle wasting, anemia, malaise, hot flashes, and osteoporosis.

Fleshner and Trachtenberg speculated that by selectively blocking dihydrotestosterone, the major hormone affecting prostatic tissue, they might treat prostate cancer effectively with minimal side effects and a better quality of life.

The results are encouraging, even if, on average, the prostate-specific antigen levels are somewhat higher than with standard therapy.

L. Lasagna, M.D.

Estrogens in the Treatment of Prostate Cancer
Cox RL, Crawford ED (Univ of Colorado, Denver)
J Urol 154:1991–1998, 1995   13–3

Background.—Estrogens have long been used in the treatment of metastatic prostate carcinoma. The efficacy and complications of this treatment were studied.

Methods and Findings.—The literature on estrogen treatment of prostate cancer was extensively reviewed. Estrogen treatment is generally successful in patients with advanced prostate cancer. A dose of 1 mg of diethylstilbestrol daily continues to be a medical alternative to bilateral orchiectomy in cases of advanced cancer of the prostate. However, patients given this dose must be monitored carefully, with assays of testosterone level obtained if the response is suboptimal. Adjustments should be made if a castrate level has not been achieved with this dose. High doses of this agent—3 mg or higher—are associated with a prohibitively high risk of cardiovascular death. Low doses of diethylstilbestrol have been associated with nonlethal toxicities, such as gynecomastia and edema. Also, the efficacy of diethylstilbestrol has not been compared with that of combined androgen blockade or luteinizing hormone–releasing hormone analogue alone.

Conclusions.—Estrogen therapy is at least as effective as orchiectomy or a luteinizing hormone–releasing hormone analogue in the treatment of metastatic prostate cancer. Additional studies of orally and parenterally administered estrogens are needed to determine whether their toxicity can be reduced and their efficacy increased cost-effectively.

▶ Metastatic prostate cancer is all too common, and a source of considerable misery and, ultimately, death. For more than 55 years, estrogen therapy has been an effective and relatively inexpensive therapy for this malignancy and a medical alternative to bilateral orchiectomy or luteinizing hormone–releasing hormone analogues, although high doses of diethylstilbestrol carry a prohibitively high risk of cardiovascular death. Even at low doses, however, gynecomastia and edema may be seen.

Controlled trials are needed to compare estrogen alone with estrogen in combination with anti-estrogens.

L. Lasagna, M.D.

Advances and Trends in Hormonal Therapy for Advanced Prostate Cancer
Debruyne FMJ, Dijkman GA (Univ Hosp, Nijmegen, The Netherlands; Ignatius Hosp, Breda, The Netherlands)
Eur Urol 28:177–188, 1995   13–4

Introduction.—Prostate cancer is a major cause of cancer-related death. Prostate cancer growth is stimulated by androgens, mainly testosterone, so the initial therapy for patients with advanced prostate cancer is hormonal. Surgical castration is still regarded as the "gold standard" for hormonal treatment of prostate cancer, although psychological factors make this treatment unacceptable for most patients. The current state of hormonal treatment for advanced prostate cancer was reviewed.

Available Treatments.—Medical castration provides the hormonal equivalent of surgical castration, but without the psychological trauma. This may be achieved with luteinizing hormone–releasing hormone analogues, antiandrogens, and estrogens, although estrogens are infrequently used because of their cardiovascular and feminizing side effects. Complete androgen ablation appears to depend on blocking androgens of both testicular and adrenal origin. Thus, adding antiandrogen therapy to medical or surgical castration to achieve combined androgen blockade (CAB) may be an appropriate treatment approach for advanced prostate cancer. Three independent trials have demonstrated substantial advantages of CAB over castration in terms of time to progression and survival. The evidence suggests that CAB is most beneficial for patients with minimal metastatic disease.

Other hormonal therapy approaches under investigation include the enzyme 5α-reductase inhibitors, the steroidal antiandrogen chlormadinone acetate, and the trypanocidal drug suramin. For patients with non-metastatic prostate cancer, there is growing interest in the use of neoadjuvant or adjuvant hormonal therapy, used along with prostatectomy or radiotherapy. Intermittent androgen withdrawal therapy is being investigated as well. As more hormonal treatments for prostate cancer become available, patients are likely to become increasingly involved in making treatment decisions.

Summary.—A number of different hormonal approaches are available for the management of advanced prostate cancer, and the range of options will continue to grow. This trend will allow physicians and patients greater choice in selecting the best therapy and should improve the quality of life for patients with prostate cancer.

▶ Having therapeutic options is always desirable. Androgen blockade (by surgery, drugs, or both) obviously helps most patients with advanced prostate cancer achieve a significant tumor response, and this approach has been accepted for over half a century.

Because androgens are derived from both the testes and the adrenals, surgical castration may be less effective than such medical alternatives as luteinizing hormone–releasing hormone analogues, steroidal antiandrogens, and nonsteroidal antiandrogens, either alone or in combination with castration.

L. Lasagna, M.D.

Cardiac and Vascular Morbidity in Women Receiving Adjuvant Tamoxifen for Breast Cancer in a Randomised Trial
McDonald CC, For the Scottish Cancer Trials Breast Group (Univ of Edinburgh, Scotland; Argyll and Clyde Health Board, Paisley, Scotland; Internatl Med College, Kuala Lumpur, Malaysia)
BMJ 311:977–980, 1995   13–5

Background.—Tamoxifen is an estrogen antagonist widely used for adjuvant and prophylactic treatment of breast cancer. Although an optimal treatment period has not been established, 5 years of treatment is demonstrably better than 2 years, and it is possible that the best therapy would be lifelong treatment. Previous studies have shown that tamoxifen not only aids in the prevention of recurrent breast cancer, but also has a protective effect against myocardial infarction. The effect of tamoxifen on nonfatal myocardial infarction and other cardiovascular disease was evaluated.

Patients and Methods.—The Scottish adjuvant tamoxifen trial comprised 1,312 women with primary operable breast cancer. These women were randomly selected to receive either tamoxifen for 5 years or no adjuvant therapy. Women receiving tamoxifen were then offered the option of continuing treatment after 5 years. In patients with evidence of disease relapse, tamoxifen use was either discontinued among women in the treatment group or started among those in the control group. Analyses therefore also considered risk according to actual tamoxifen use.

Results.—Primary analysis of treatment by intent-to-treat criteria showed a reduced risk for cardiovascular heart disease among women receiving tamoxifen. Hazard ratios indicated that tamoxifen was beneficial (hazard ratio > 1), although when admission for myocardial infarction and other ischemic disease was examined, this did not reach statistical significance. Additionally, an increase in thromboembolic events was noted among women receiving tamoxifen. When adjusted for actual tamoxifen use, statistical significance was observed for both current use and any past use of tamoxifen with respect to myocardial infarction. Of the latter 2 categories, current use of tamoxifen offered the most protection. A statistically significant increase in thromboembolic events also was found among current users of tamoxifen.

Conclusion.—Although there is an increased risk of thromboembolic events in women taking tamoxifen, the benefit achieved through reduction in myocardial infarction is greater.

▶ Tamoxifen plays an important role in cancer chemotherapy as adjuvant treatment of breast cancer. Its success has prompted some to suggest that perhaps women with this disease should take the drug for life, and that perhaps it should be taken prophylactically to prevent breast cancer.

Such long-term usage has quite reasonably led to the question of whether it is harmful to take tamoxifen for many years. The answer seems to be that the drug may rarely be associated with a risk of pulmonary embolism, but it seems to reduce the risk of myocardial infarction.

L. Lasagna, M.D.

Does Knowledge Guide Practice? Another Look at the Management of Non–Small-Cell Lung Cancer
Raby B, Pater J, Mackillop WJ (Queen's Univ, Kingston, Ont, Canada; Natl Cancer Inst of Canada Clinical Trials Group, Kingston, Ont, Canada; Kingston Regional Cancer Centre, Ontario, Canada; et al)
J Clin Oncol 13:1904–1911, 1995   13–6

Background.—Recent studies of the treatment efficacy in patients with non–small-cell lung cancer (NSCLC) may be expected to reduce the variation in treatment recommendations for such patients. The current beliefs of Canadian physicians regarding the appropriate role of chemotherapy and radiotherapy in the management of NSCLC were surveyed.

Methods.—Three hundred thirty surveys were mailed to a random sample of respirologists, thoracic surgeons, radiation oncologists, and medical oncologists. The respondents were asked to estimate the prognosis in each of 3 cases described and to give treatment recommendations. The survey response rate was 74%.

Findings.—Treatment recommendations showed wide variation. After complete resection for stage II NSCLC, no adjuvant therapy was recommended by 68% of the respondents, radiotherapy by 28%, chemotherapy by 1%, and radiotherapy and chemotherapy by 3%. Seventeen percent of the respondents recommended no active therapy for an asymptomatic patient with stage IIIb NSCLC; 16% recommended radiation and chemotherapy, and 2% recommended chemotherapy only. Eighty percent of respondents recommended no active treatment and 20% recommended chemotherapy for an asymptomatic patient with a stage IV NSCLC. There was a wide range in beliefs about the natural history of NSCLC and its response to therapy. Three fourths of the respondents thought that adjuvant radiotherapy did not prolong survival in patients with stage II disease, and the remainder thought it did. Thirty percent believed that adding chemotherapy to radiotherapy in patients with stage III disease increased survival, whereas 70% believed it did not. Fifty-five percent thought that chemotherapy increased median survival in patients with stage IV disease, whereas 45% thought it did not. Physicians' beliefs regarding treatment efficacy were highly correlated with their recommendations.

Conclusion.—Despite recent findings on the treatment of NSCLC, Canadian physicians still do not agree on the role of radiotherapy and chemotherapy in patients with this disease. The new knowledge appears to have had little effect on physicians' beliefs and practice variations.

Chemotherapy for Non–Small Cell Lung Cancer
Carbone DP, Minna JD (Univ of Texas, Dallas)
BMJ 311:889–890, 1995   13–7

Background.—Because the absolute survival benefits observed for chemotherapy in patients with non–small-cell lung cancer (NSCLC) are relatively small, large numbers of patients are needed to confidently draw conclusions. The results of a recently published meta-analysis of updated data on 9,387 patients with NSCLC were discussed.

Chemotherapy for NSCLC.—Fifty-two randomized clinical trials comparing chemotherapy with no chemotherapy were analyzed by Albertini et al. Early, locally advanced, and advanced disease were represented. In patients with early disease treated with surgery and chemotherapy, the addition of alkylating agents (in vogue 10 years ago) resulted in a 15% increase in mortality. However, patients in several subgroups given more modern regimens containing cisplatin had significant survival benefits. Although the benefits were significant statistically, their clinical effects were only modest. However, if chemotherapy were administered to the appropriate patients, tens of thousands would be alive at 1 year who would not otherwise be. Identifying the subset of patients responsive to chemotherapy could markedly improve the risk-benefit ratio of chemotherapy in the entire population.

Conclusion.—Continued studies of newer, even more active agents may be beneficial in the treatment of NSCLC. However, such agents must be selected carefully. Taxanes, new antimetabolites, and antitubulin agents are among the promising new drugs. Studies to determine whether particular molecular characteristics of tumors can identify subsets of patients likely to benefit from chemotherapy are also needed.

▶ Put together, these 2 papers (Abstracts 13–6 and 13–7) show that doctors do not know about chemotherapy and radiation therapy for the treatment of NSCLC and, if they do, they may not be convinced of their efficacy in actual practice. In some cases, you would have to say that the doctors have a point because the median survival was prolonged by only 1.5 months. However, fewer people died who had received chemotherapy with cisplatin, and some people responded well to radiation therapy. I am not convinced that the doctors who answered the questionnaire were entirely wrong. They could have made a judgment that chemotherapy or radiation therapy is not really valuable for patients with NSCLC. In any case, these Canadian doctors were not as aggressive in their treatment as physicians in the United States.

These papers illustrate some of the problems that teachers of medical students and medical practitioners face. Sometimes the problems are geographical; sometimes they are accidental, such as having a practitioner with strong beliefs one way or the other; sometimes they are cultural, as in the United States physicians and the Canadian doctors; and sometimes they are just related to whether or not there is a good cancer center with excellent physicians nearby. Sometimes it may be that the patient requests the therapy and the doctor just goes along with it. That may be an important determinant of future practice decisions, but health organizations will have their say.

M. Weintraub, M.D.

Randomized Double-blind Placebo-controlled Trial of Cisplatin and Etoposide Plus Megestrol Acetate/Placebo in Extensive-stage Small-Cell Lung Cancer: A North Central Cancer Treatment Group Study
Rowland KM Jr, Loprinzi CL, Shaw EG, et al (North Central Cancer Treatment Group, Rochester, Minn; Mayo Clinc and Mayo Found, Rochester, Minn; Duluth Community Clinical Oncology Program, Minn; et al)
J Clin Oncol 14:135–141, 1996   13–8

Background.—Advanced small-cell lung cancer has a high response rate to combination chemotherapy with cisplatin and etoposide, but is rarely cured, resulting in a median survival of 8–10 months. Food intake, appetite, and quality of life have been found to be powerful prognostic indicators in these patients. Treatment with megestrol acetate can decrease nausea and vomiting, thereby increasing food intake and appetite. The effect of treatment with megestrol acetate during chemotherapy cycles on quality of life and survival in patients with advanced small-cell lung cancer was examined in a randomized, double-blind, placebo-controlled trial.

Methods.—Over a 3-year period, 243 patients were randomly assigned to receive either 800 mg/day of megestrol acetate or placebo during chemotherapy. All patients underwent four 3-day cycles of cisplatin and etoposide chemotherapy. The patients were assessed for response after completing all 4 cycles. They completed a questionnaire regarding quality of life, appetite, nausea, emesis, taste, satiety, edema, and perception of actual and desired weight change monthly during chemotherapy and every 4 months after chemotherapy. Survival was calculated by the Kaplan-Meier method.

Results.—There was an overall response rate of 74%. The placebo group had a statistically significantly higher overall response rate than the treatment group (80% vs. 68%), but the rates of complete response were similar. The 2 groups had similar 1-year survival rates, but there were more frequent earlier deaths in the megestrol acetate group. The placebo group had a better quality of life at baseline, but there was little change in the quality of life in either group throughout the study. Patients receiving megestrol acetate reported less nausea and vomiting. There was objective evidence of less nausea, vomiting, and anorexia and better edema-free weight gain in this group. The treatment group had 11 grade 3 and 4 thromboembolic events, compared with only 2 in the placebo group. Although there was greater myelosuppression in the placebo group, there were fewer septic deaths.

Conclusion.—Although megestrol acetate reduced the nausea, vomiting, and weight loss in these patients with extensive-stage small-cell lung cancer during chemotherapy, it had no effect on either quality of life or survival. It cannot be recommended for routine use because of the lack of survival benefit and the increased incidence of thromboembolic phenomena.

▶ Who said negative trials aren't published? Actually, one reason for the publication of negative trials, as in this case, is the amount of time and money spent on the study and the number of patients involved in proving whatever points there are to prove. The investigators used a very appropriate caveat for megestrol acetate in pointing out that it would probably help patients with cancer anorexia/cachexia, which are really troublesome.

M. Weintraub, M.D.

Chemotherapy in Non-Small Cell Lung Cancer: A Meta-analysis Using Updated Data on Individual Patients From 52 Randomised Clinical Trials
Stewart LA, for the Non-Small Cell Lung Cancer Collaborative Group (Cambridge, England)
BMJ 311:899–909 1995
13–9

Background.—Although cytotoxic chemotherapy is used routinely in patients with small cell lung cancer, its value in patients with non–small cell lung cancer has not been established definitively. The efficacy of cytotoxic chemotherapy in such patients was further explored in a meta-analysis including 52 studies conducted worldwide.

Methods and Findings.—Data were obtained from published and unpublished randomized clinical trials. A total of 9,387 patients, 7,151 of whom died, had been enrolled in these studies. Patient survival was the outcome measure. In all comparisons including modern chemotherapeutic regimens containing cisplatin, results favored chemotherapy. Outcomes reached conventional levels of significance when radical radiotherapy and supportive care were used. The hazard ratio in comparisons of surgery without and with chemotherapy was 0.87. A hazard ratio of 0.87 was also documented in trials comparing radical radiotherapy without and with chemotherapy. Comparisons of supportive care without and with chemotherapy yielded a 0.73 hazard ratio. The drugs essential for achieving these effects could not be identified. Patient subgroups showed no difference in effect sizes. In all older studies except for those of radical radiotherapy, the use of long-term alkylating agents tended to be associated with detrimental effects. In the adjuvant surgical comparison, this effect was significant.

Conclusions.—Modern chemotherapeutic regimens may be beneficial in patients with non–small cell lung cancer of all stages. Further research is needed to confirm this possibility, to assess the value of short-term chemotherapy, and to compare different chemotherapeutic regimens.

▶ This meta-analysis looked at randomized, controlled trials using chemotherapy for small cell carcinoma. One could say that there has been 30 years of treatment of small cell carcinoma and it is still not clear whether such treatment was helpful or harmful. This study goes a long way toward telling us that chemotherapeutic regimens have a role in treating such cancers, that the overall odds of chemotherapy helping in small cell carcinoma appear to be definite. Certainly more work is needed to improve the quality of the meta-analysis. We always worry that trials were left out because the results were bad and they weren't published, or that the treatments used were surpassed before the study could be finished, or that studies were excluded because of many other reasons. The meta-analysis also tells us that we need better chemotherapy. Certainly, we should be explaining to patients the risks and benefits that occur with treatment. We should promise the patient that we will stop therapy when it does not seem to be working.

M. Weintraub, M.D.

Long-Term Use of Nonsteroidal Antiinflammatory Drugs and Other Chemopreventors and Risk of Subsequent Colorectal Neoplasia

Peleg II, Lubin MF, Cotsonis GA, et al (Univ of Iowa, Iowa City; Emory Univ, Atlanta, Ga; Grady Mem Hosp, Atlanta, Ga)
Dig Dis Sci 41:1319–1326, 1996   13–10

Introduction.—There is mounting evidence from animal and human trials that the use of aspirin and other nonsteroidal anti-inflammatory drugs (NSAIDs) may provide a chemopreventive effect against colorectal cancer. Some trials have reported equivocal results. The relation between dispensed aspirin, NSAIDs, steroidal anti-inflammatory drugs (SAIDs), acetaminophen, calcium, psyllium, and multivitamin preparations, and the risk for subsequent colorectal adenoma and adenocarcinoma was investigated.

Methods.—The records of all patients diagnosed with incident adenocarcinoma from July 1, 1987 to December 31, 1992, and of all patients diagnosed with incident histologically proven colorectal adenoma from August 1, 1990 to March 1, 1993, were reviewed for the use of aspirin, nonaspirin NSAIDs, SAIDs, acetaminophen, calcium, psyllium, and multivitamins. Each of the patients was matched with 2 control subjects who were free of cancer or colorectal adenoma. Records of control subjects were reviewed for the same drug use information. Duration of drug use and cumulative dose were calculated for all research subjects. The risk of colorectal adenoma and adenocarcinoma with the use of the aforementioned drugs was calculated.

Results.—There were 113 consecutive patients with an incident diagnosis of colorectal adenoma and 93 consecutive patients with a diagnosis of colorectal adenocarcinoma. Patients with carcinoma were older than patients with adenoma and control subjects. There was a time- and dose-dependent reduction in the risk for adenoma and adenocarcinoma with increasing use of aspirin and nonaspirin NSAIDs. There was a significant decrease in risk after 2 years of NSAID use in doses similar to those advised for the prevention of cardiovascular disease or commonly prescribed for the management of musculoskeletal pain. This same risk reduction was not observed with the use of SAIDs. Acetaminophen, calcium, psyllium, and multivitamin use was associated with significant risk reduction.

Conclusion.—Short-term or intermittent recent use of NSAIDs may be enough to provide significant risk reduction of colorectal neoplasia. This is encouraging, because more than 40% of patients aged 60 years and older are thought to have adenomatous lesions. The risk of side effects from these drugs must be considered before considering their chemopreventive benefits.

▶ In a previous comment, I asked a question: "Given the adverse effects of NSAIDs, why would anybody use them?" I postulated that if something new came along, everybody would drop the current medications. Well, I am always willing to be wrong. Studies like this one have been around for a couple of years and perhaps they are quite correct. This may be another reason why we prescribe these NSAIDs. Any new drugs will have to undergo similar testing.

M. Weintraub, M.D.

Aspirin and the Risk of Colorectal Cancer in Women

Giovannucci E, Egan KM, Hunter DJ, et al (Harvard Med School, Boston; Harvard School of Public Health, Boston)
N Engl J Med 333:609–614, 1995   13–11

Introduction.—Research undertaken to study the effect of aspirin use and the risk of colorectal cancer has been inconsistent. The purpose of this study was to establish a correlation between colon and rectal cancers and aspirin usage.

Methods.—Almost 90,000 women in the Nurses Health Study, with no diagnosis nor any family history of colorectal cancer, completed a baseline questionnaire on medication usage and diet. This was followed up every two years with another questionnaire on aspirin and other NSAID usage. Cases of adenomatous polyps of both participants, and their next of kin, were documented. The association between aspirin use and the occurrence of a new colon or rectal cancer over a 12 year period was then analyzed.

Results.—Over the 8 year period of this study, 331 cases of not previously reported colorectal cancer were documented among women in the Nurses Health Study. Individuals who in the initial questionnaire reported themselves as being regular aspirin users (those who took at least 2 aspirins per week) for a 4 year period had a lower risk of cancer development than did nonusers. A drop in risk was observed for women who used aspirin regularly for at least 10 years and this decrease became significant at 20 years of regular aspirin usage. After controlling for other risk factors, women who on 3 consecutive questionnaires (which were filled out every 2 years) reported regular aspirin use, were 38 percent less likely to develop a colorectal cancer. A significant inverse relationship was shown between the intake of 4 to 6 aspirins a week and risk of development of colorectal cancer. These results are even more impressive since over the course of the study, women who did take aspirin had a higher rate of endoscopy.

Discussion.—Results show that in women long-term use of aspirin (10 years or more), at a rate of 4 to 6 tablets per week, decreases the risk of colorectal cancer in women. Endoscopy, which could lead to a possibly earlier detection of tumors, actually showed a decrease in the actual number of colorectal tumors among aspirin users. Possible mechanisms for the action of aspirin in this instance include the inhibition of cyclooxygenase and subsequent inhibition of prostaglandin action, or the inhibition of phospholipase activity. Also, it has been documented that aspirin can modulate levels of prostaglandin levels in the rectal epithelium. This work requires further research, especially since low-dose aspirin has been shown to decrease the incidence of cardiovascular disease.

▶ Colorectal cancer takes a large toll of the United States population annually, and it would be nice to have an impact for the good on this unpleasant disease.

In animal and human studies, both aspirin and newer nonsteroidal anti-inflammatory drugs seem to inhibit colonic carcinogenesis. It is still not clear how much aspirin is needed to decrease the incidence of colorectal cancer, nor for how long it needs to be taken to get benefit. The answers are needed if public health policy is to be optimally constructed.

L. Lasagna, M.D.

Relationship Between 5-Fluorouracil (5-FU) Dose Intensity and Therapeutic Response in Patients With Advanced Colorectal Cancer Receiving Infusional Therapy Containing 5-FU

Gamelin EC, Danquechin-Dorval EM, Dumesnil YF, et al (Centre Paul Papin, Angers, France; Hopital Trousseau, Tours, France; Centre Hospitalier de Nîmes, France; et al)

Cancer 77:441–451, 1996   13–12

Introduction.—Abundant clinical experience attests to the therapeutic efficacy of 5-fluorouracil (5-FU) with leucovorin (LV) in treating metastatic colorectal cancer, but the best way to administer these drugs remains uncertain.

Study Plan.—Forty patients with measurable metastases of colorectal cancer were given weekly 5-FU treatment in the form of a continuous 8-hour infusion. The initial dose was 1 g/m^2, and the dose was increased in increments of 250 mg/m^2 at 3-week intervals and potentiated by 400 mg of LV per m.^{2} Plasma levels of 5-FU were estimated each week by liquid chromatography.

Results.—Six patients had a complete, and 12, a partial response 3 months after treatment, for an overall response rate of 45%. Nine patients had a minor response, 9 had stable disease, and 4 progressed. The overall median survival time was 14 months. Fifty-five percent of patients were living 1 year after treatment, and 51% were living without disease. Plasma 5-FU levels reached approximately 2 g/L as early as the second dose level (1,250 mg/m^2). High drug levels predicted an objective response and better survival, but not to a significant degree. Acute toxicity correlated with a plasma 5-FU level greater than 3 g/L but not with the administered dose.

Conclusion.—The metabolism of infused 5-FU is variable in patients with metastatic colorectal cancer, regardless of the dose administered, suggesting that the dose be individually adjusted.

▶ The history of 5-FU has been plagued by variability in response, across patients and across clinics. This article suggests that some of the variability is explicable by polymorphic 5-FU metabolism and that optimal individual therapy requires attention to the achievement of effective plasma levels of the drug both to increase efficacy and decrease toxicity.

L. Lasagna, M.D.

Randomized Trial of Interferon Maintenance in Multiple Myeloma: A Study of the National Cancer Institute of Canada Clinical Trials Group

Browman GP, Bergsagel D, Sicheri D, et al (Queen's Univ, Kingston, Canada)
J Clin Oncol 13:2354–2360, 1995   13–13

Background.—Studies of the benefit of interferon (IFN) maintenance in patients with myeloma have yielded conflicting results. The National Cancer Institute of Canada Clinical Trials Group initiated a randomized trial in 1987 comparing IFN maintenance with observation in patients with myeloma who had responded to melphalan–prednisone (MP) induction treatment.

Methods.—Of 482 patients enrolled in the study, 176 responded to MP and were randomly assigned to the IFN or control groups. All patients had symptomatic clinical stage I, II, or III multiple myeloma. Melphalan–prednisone was stopped after a stable response plateau of the monoclonal protein was achieved. Interferon was continued until relapse and restarted on subsequent MP response. Eighty-five patients underwent IFN maintenance, and 91 were observed. The median follow-up time was 43 months.

Findings.—The median survival duration was 43 months for patients receiving IFN and 35 months for those in the control group. After adjustment for chance imbalances in baseline prognostic factors, primarily performance status, the median survival duration was 44 months for the IFN group and 33 months for the control group. Patients given IFN also had a better progression-free survival rate from randomization to first relapse. Fifty-eight percent of the patients had to decrease their IFN dose because of toxicity. Eighty-four percent of these patients were able to return to their initial dose, and 14% had to discontinue IFN therapy.

Conclusions.—In patients with multiple myeloma who respond to MP, IFN maintenance treatment improves progression-free and overall survival. However, the toxicity is substantial. Patients must weigh this disadvantage against the potential benefits of increased response duration and survival.

▶ The use of MP for induction therapy in cases of multiple myelomas has been going on for a number of years. The response in cases of myelomas has not been terrific. That's why these investigators tried IFN-α-2b to prolong the survival of patients without disease progression. Despite side effects, the IFN group did better. There was one really mind-boggling aspect of this study. The Canadian patients, unlike previous patients, did better when receiving IFN compared with those who did not respond to induction therapy. One could suggest a number of explanations, but it may be beyond explanation at this time. That's what happens when you do clinical trials: Sometimes you get a very surprising effect and it's beneficial, and sometimes you get a very surprising effect and it's detrimental. We don't always believe the beneficial effects. We frequently make the investigators, or preferably another group of investigators, do another study to confirm the findings.

M. Weintraub, M.D.

Efficacy of Pamidronate in Reducing Skeletal Events in Patients With Advanced Multiple Myeloma

Berenson JR, for the Myeloma Aredia Study Group (Univ of California, Los Angeles; St Thomas Hosp, Nashville, Tenn; Univ of Texas, Houston; et al)
N Engl J Med 334:488–493, 1996   13–14

Introduction.—The osteolytic bone destruction occurring in patients with multiple myeloma can cause pain, pathologic fractures, spinal cord compression, and hypercalcemia. These complications are related to an increase in osteoclastic activity mediated by the release of osteoclast-stimulating factors by myeloma cells. Pamidronate or other bisphosphonates may be given to reduce bone resorption through inhibition of osteoclastic activity. The ability of pamidronate to reduce skeletal complications of multiple myeloma was evaluated in a randomized, double-blind, placebo-controlled trial.

Methods.—The study included 392 patients with stage III multiple myeloma and at least 1 osteolytic lesion. Before randomization, the patients were stratified in terms of whether they were receiving first-line or second-line antimyeloma chemotherapy. They were then assigned to receive either placebo or pamidronate, 90 mg as a 4-hour IV infusion every 4 weeks for 9 cycles, in addition to their antimyeloma chemotherapy. The patients were evaluated monthly for skeletal events, i.e., pathologic fracture, irradiation of or surgery on bone, and spinal cord compression. Other outcomes monitored included hypercalcemia, either symptomatic or a serum calcium concentration of 12mg/dL or greater; bone pain; analgesic use; performance status; and quality of life.

Results.—One hundred ninety-six patients in the pamidronate group and 181 in the placebo group were evaluable for efficacy. Twenty-four percent of patients receiving pamidronate had skeletal events, compared with 41% of those receiving placebo. The difference was significant in patients receiving first- or second-line antimyeloma chemotherapy. Pamidronate treatment was associated with a significant decrease in bone pain with no downward change in performance status or quality of life. There were no significant differences in the rate of radiologic progression of osteolytic lesions, metabolic tumor and bone markers, or survival. Pamidronate caused few adverse effects requiring cessation of treatment.

Conclusions.—Pamidronate appears to be an effective adjunctive therapy for patients with advanced multiple myeloma. It reduces the occurrence of skeletal complications while reducing pain and improving quality of life. The treatment is safe, well tolerated, and improves patients' comfort and well-being.

▶ Patients with multiple myeloma run a substantial risk of skeletal complications because of secreted factors that stimulate osteoclastic activity. Because biphosphonates inhibit osteoclastic activity, their use should lead to less bone resorption, with less bone pain and less deterioration in performance. This study provides evidence that the theory is borne out in real life.

L. Lasagna, M.D.

Phase II Trial of Fludarabine Monophosphate as First-line Treatment in Patients With Advanced Follicular Lymphoma: A Multicenter Study by the Groupe d'Etude des Lymphomes de l'Adulte

Solal-Céligny P, Brice P, Brousse N, et al (Hôpital Saint-Louis, Paris)
J Clin Oncol 14:514–519, 1996   13–15

Background.—No conventional chemotherapy regimens are curative in the treatment of follicular non-Hodgkin's lymphoma (NHL). However, a new agent, fludarabine (FAMP), has been shown to have activity against chronic lymphocytic leukemia and in selected patients with low-grade NHL. The efficacy and safety of FAMP was therefore investigated in previously untreated patients with follicular NHL in a multicenter, phase-II trial.

Methods.—Forty-nine untreated patients with stage II, III, or IV follicular NHL with high tumor burden were treated with FAMP. The dosage was 25 mg/m^2/day by IV infusion over 30 minutes for 5 days at 4-week intervals for a maximum of 9 cycles. Response was assessed every 3 cycles. Toxicity was assessed, with a full blood count obtained weekly during the first 3 cycles and then preceding each cycle. Progression-free and relapse-free survival were calculated, as was the time to treatment failure.

Results.—Of the 49 patients, a complete response occurred in 37% and a partial response occurred in 28%, for an overall response rate of 65%. Response occurred within the first 3 cycles. The entire group had a median progression-free survival of 13.6 months, a relapse-free survival of 15.6 months, and a time to treatment failure of 9 months.

Twenty-two patients had at least grade 3 granulocytopenia, occurring in 48 of 334 cycles. No serious infections occurred. Three patients had thrombocytopenia during 4 cycles. Two patients had treatment-related acute paralytic brachial neuritis involving the circumflex nerve. Treatment had to be discontinued in 9 patients because of bone marrow toxicity, peripheral neuropathy, interstitial pneumonitis, or hepatitis.

Conclusions.—Fludarabine is effective against follicular lymphoma, with moderate toxicity. However, as a single agent, it is no more effective than other standard chemotherapy regimens. Therefore, further trials should evaluate its effectiveness in combination with alkylating agents or other drugs.

▶ Fludarabine has been a welcome addition to the oncologic armamentarium. A purine nucleoside analogue with a seemingly unique mode of action, it was developed in a search for more active relatives of cytarabine. The trick was to add a fluorine atom to adenine arabinoside. The drug is given IV, is rapidly dephosphorylated, and then undergoes active transport into cells, where it is rephosphorylated to its sole active derivative. This derivative ultimately leads to cell death by inhibiting DNA and RNA synthesis. Although fludarabine has been mostly studied in chronic lymphocytic leukemia, it has worked well in patients with non-Hodgkin's lymphoma, many of whom had been heavily pretreated.

This report is a pleasure to read, because it shows that for some patients with lymphoma, fludarabine can be a first-line treatment and can be effective when used alone. Toxicity can be a problem, but it was mild in most of these patients.

L. Lasagna, M.D.

Non-Hodgkin's Lymphoma in Patients With Rheumatoid Arthritis Treated With Low Dose Methotrexate
Usman AR, Yunus MB (Univ of Illinois College of Medicine at Peoria)
J Rheumatol 23:1095–1097, 1996   13–16

Introduction.—Rheumatoid arthritis (RA) is effectively treated with low-dose methotrexate (MTX). Two patients with non-Hodgkin's lymphoma (NHL) associated with MTX therapy for RA were described, and other published cases were reviewed.

> *Case 1.*—Man, 66, had a 15-year history of RA, which had been treated with nonsteroidal anti-inflammatory drugs (NSAIDs), aurothioglucose, penicillamine, cyclophosphamide, and prednisone. Treatment was begun with MTX, 7.5 mg/wk, and reduced to 5 mg/wk after 29 months, when RA activity was mild. Four months later, he was hospitalized with fever, chills, and weight loss. He had lymphadenopathy and hepatosplenomegaly. High-grade, large-cell NHL was diagnosed based on lymph node biopsy findings. Treatment with MTX was discontinued and chemotherapy was begun. The NHL responded to the chemotherapy, but he had a recurrence and died 15 months after the diagnosis.
>
> *Case 2.*—Woman, 75, had a 5-year history of RA, which had been treated with NSAIDs, prednisone, and hydroxychloroquine sulfate. Therapy with MTX was begun at 5 mg/wk. The dose was increased 1 year later to 7.5 mg/wk. After another year the dose was decreased to 5 mg/wk, when her symptoms improved. Five months later, she was hospitalized with generalized lymphadenopathy and night sweats. Lymph node biopsy specimens showed diffuse, large-cell NHL. Methotrexate was discontinued and chemotherapy was initiated. However, she died 19 months after diagnosis.

Literature Review.—Sixteen patients treated with MTX for RA in whom NHL developed have been described in the literature. The patients typically had NHL develop shortly after MTX therapy was initiated, during a time of mild RA activity. Of the 18 patients (which includes the 2 patients, just described), 3 had spontaneous remission and 5 died. Treatment included chemotherapy in 11 patients, radiation therapy in 2, and both in 1. A causal relationship has not been established in the literature.

Conclusions.—Cases of lymphoma seen in patients treated with MTX raise concerns about a possible causal relationship. Further studies are needed to characterize this association.

▶ Low-dose MTX has become increasingly popular (and with good cause) in the treatment of chronic arthritis. This study adds 2 new cases of NHL to the 16 previously reported. Whether a cause-and-effect relationship exists between MTX and this neoplastic process has been debated, and will continue to be.

L. Lasagna, M.D.

Methotrexate-associated Lymphoma in Patients With Rheumatoid Arthritis: Report of Two Cases
Bachman TR, Sawitzke AD, Perkins SL, et al (Univ of Utah, Salt Lake City; Salt Lake City Veterans Affairs Med Ctr, Utah)
Arthritis Rheum 39:325–329, 1996   13–17

Background.—Low-dose methotrexate (MTX) is commonly used to treat rheumatoid arthritis (RA) as well as other rheumatic diseases. Although the oncogenic potential of this agent is low, there have been several reports of lymphoma in patients given MTX for rheumatic diseases. Cases of another 2 patients were reviewed.

Case Reports.—The patients were a man, 65 years, and a woman, 66 years. The first patient had a left inguinal mass with a 40-pound weight loss during the preceding year. The second patient had severe seropositive nodular deforming RA, with pain and swelling of many joints. Large-cell lymphoma of B cell phenotype, developing during MTX treatment, was diagnosed in both patients. Nuclear staining for Epstein-Barr virus was observed within the malignant lymphoid cells by in situ hybridization studies. Methotrexate was discontinued after diagnostic biopsy, and lymphoma was undetectable 4 weeks later in both patients.

Conclusions.—Discontinuation of immunosuppressive agents may be warranted before chemotherapy is considered in patients with RA who have a diagnosis of an Epstein-Barr virus–related lymphoproliferative disorder. Clinicians must maintain a high index of suspicion for lymphoma development in patients with rheumatic diseases treated with MTX.

▶ Because lymphomas can be expected to occur coincidentally in at least an occasional patient with rheumatic diseases, such co-morbidity may not prove anything, although when RA is complicated by Felty's syndrome, a 12-fold increased risk of lymphoma has been reported.[1] Cyclophosphamide or azathioprine treatment may increase the risk of lymphoma, but MTX has generally not been placed in this category. However, other reports have described patients with RA with reversible lymphoma after treatment with MTX.

The 2 cases described in this study support the notion that MTX therapy may lead to lymphoproliferative disorders in patients with RA, perhaps by interfering with the host's immune response to Epstein-Barr virus infection. Stopping the MTX should be tried in such cases, because traditional chemotherapy may not be needed if complete remission occurs after such cessation.

L. Lasagna, M.D.

Reference

1. Gridley G, Klippel J, Hoover R, et al: Incidence of cancer among men with the Felty syndrome. *Ann Intern Med* 120:35–39, 1994.

Female Sex and Higher Drug Dose as Risk Factors for Late Cardiotoxic Effects of Doxorubicin Therapy for Childhood Cancer

Lipshultz SE, Lipsitz SR, Mone SM, et al (Children's Hosp, Boston; Harvard Med School, Boston; Dana-Farber Cancer Inst, Boston)
N Engl J Med 332:1738–1743, 1995   13–18

Background.—Increasingly, survivors of childhood cancer are displaying late cardiotoxic effects from doxorubicin treatment. This cardiotoxicity is often progressive, and symptoms are disabling in some patients. Risk factors for late cardiotoxicity were investigated.

Methods.—One hundred twenty children and adults underwent echocardiography at a mean of 8.1 years after treatment for acute lymphoblastic leukemia or osteogenic sarcoma. Treatment had consisted of 244- to 550-mg cumulative doses of doxorubicin per square meter of body surface area. A cohort of 296 normal subjects served as controls.

Findings.—In the patients, all echocardiographic measurements were abnormal at 2 years or more after the completion of therapy. Abnormalities were more frequent and severe in female patients. A multivariate analysis indicated that depressed contractility was associated with female sex and a greater cumulative dose of doxorubicin, which interacted. A greater rate of doxorubicin administration was independently and significantly associated with increased afterload, left ventricular dilatation, and depressed left ventricular function. A higher cumulative dose was associated with depressed left ventricular function. Younger age at diagnosis was correlated with decreased left ventricular wall thickness and mass and increased afterload. There was also an association between a longer time since the completion of doxorubicin treatment and a decrease in left ventricular wall thickness, as well as an increase in afterload.

Conclusion.—Female sex and a higher rate of administration of doxorubicin were independent risk factors for cardiac abnormalities after doxorubicin treatment for childhood cancer. The prevalence and severity of abnormalities increased with the length of follow-up.

▶ Here is another paper that traces adverse reactions to female gender. However, the very likely relationship to higher dose in the smaller and lighter women and the difference in body composition between the genders play a role.

M. Weintraub, M.D.

Misoprostol Prophylaxis for High-dose Chemotherapy-induced Mucositis: A Randomized Double-blind Study
Dueñas-Gonzalez A, Sobrevilla-Calvo P, Frias-Mendivil M, et al (Instituto Nacional de Cancerologia, Tlalpan, Mexico)
Bone Marrow Transplant 17:809–812, 1996   13–19

Objective.—For patients receiving high-dose chemotherapy for cancer, oral mucositis is an important and sometimes dose-limiting complication. Preliminary studies have suggested that the oral prostaglandin E_1 synthetic analog misoprostol may be helpful in preventing mucositis. Misoprostol was tested as prophylaxis against mucositis in patients receiving high-dose chemotherapy.

Methods.—The randomized, double-blind, clinical trial included 15 consecutive patients with lymphoid or solid neoplasms. They received a total of 16 courses of non-cryopreserved peripheral stem cell transplantation using the ifosfamide, carboplatin, and etoposide regimen. The patients were assigned to receive oral misoprostol, 250 µg 3 times a day, or placebo, beginning 4 days before the start of chemotherapy and continuing for 3 weeks. Both groups received the same supportive care.

Results.—The study was stopped early because the incidence and severity of mucositis were significantly lower in the placebo group. There were no differences in myelosuppression, infections, or other complications.

Conclusions.—As given in this study, oral misoprostol does not appear to be useful in the prevention of oral mucositis in patients receiving high-dose chemotherapy. Further studies of the series E prostaglandins for mucositis are warranted because of their cell cytoprotective and proliferative effects in the gastrointestinal tract mucosa.

▶ This is another one of the negative clinical trials that consumes a fair amount of resources to no avail. This study shows us that doing clinical trials without knowing the answer can really help to define the response to a key question. The theoretical basis for this study seems to be helpful and encouraging. It just did not work.

M. Weintraub, M.D.

14 Neurologic Diseases

Perioperative Administration of Caffeine Tablets for Prevention of Post-operative Headaches
Hampl KF, Schneider MC, Rüttimann U, et al (Univ of Basel, Switzerland)
Can J Anaesth 42:789–792, 1995   14–1

Introduction.—Headache is the major symptom of caffeine withdrawal as well as one of the most frequent, if minor, postoperative complaints after general anesthesia. Postanesthesia headache has generally been ascribed to the effects of the anesthesia itself, but caffeine withdrawal could be a contributing factor in at least some of these patients. The effects of prophylactic caffeine administration on the incidence of headache after surgery were investigated.

Methods.—The prospective, double-blind, placebo-controlled trial included 40 patients scheduled for minor surgical procedures with general anesthesia. The patients were randomly assigned to receive either placebo or caffeine tablets to provide a dose equivalent to their average daily caffeine consumption. Compliance with instructions to abstain from other sources of caffeine was confirmed by blood sampling immediately before the operation and the day after. A standardized headache checklist was administered before anesthesia induction, in the evening after surgery, and on the morning of the first postoperative day.

Results.—Headache was reported on the evening after surgery by 50% of the placebo group and on the next morning by 35%. In contrast, none of the patients receiving caffeine tablets had a headache the evening of surgery, and just 1 had a headache on the first day after surgery. No differences were noted in the other symptoms of caffeine withdrawal.

Conclusions.—Caffeine withdrawal may contribute to the occurrence of headache after surgery. Perioperative caffeine administration may be considered for patients with a high daily caffeine intake and a history of caffeine withdrawal headaches who need surgery. This practice not only may reduce the incidence of postoperative headache but also improve compliance with preoperative fasting guidelines.

▶ How sensible! Caffeine withdrawal has for many years been known to lead to headaches, so why not try to prevent withdrawal headaches postoperatively by giving caffeine tablets? Bravo!

L. Lasagna, M.D.

Neuroleptic Drug Exposure and Treatment of Parkinsonism in the Elderly: A Case-Control Study
Avorn J, Bohn RL, Mogun H, et al (Brigham and Women's Hosp, Boston; Harvard Med School, Boston)
Am J Med 99:48–54, 1995   14–2

Background.—Neuroleptic medications are widely prescribed for the elderly. However, the frequency of treatment for drug-induced parkinsonian syndromes in older adults, especially L-dopa-type drugs (which are more appropriate for treating true idiopathic Parkinson's disease), has not been well documented.

Methods.—The current study included 3,512 patients aged 65–99 years enrolled in a large state Medicaid program. All had recently been prescribed a drug to treat parkinsonian symptoms. A control group consisted of similar enrollees receiving no antiparkinsonian agents. The use of neuroleptic drugs in the 90 days preceding antiparkinsonian drug initiation was investigated in a case–control design.

Findings.—Compared with nonusers, patients given neuroleptic agents were 5.4 times more likely to begin antiparkinsonian agents. Neuroleptic users also had a more than twofold increased risk of starting dopaminergic treatment specific for idiopathic Parkinson's disease, which is usually not appropriate. Dose–response relationships were clearly documented. Thirty-seven percent of dopaminergic drug therapy could be attributed to previous neuroleptic use. In 71% of the patients, the neuroleptic was continued.

Conclusions.—In elderly patients, the use of neuroleptic agents commonly results in extrapyramidal dysfunction. Often this side effect is treated with an additional anticholinergic or dopaminergic agent. The use of the former can result in additional side effects, and the use of the latter suggests that extrapyramidal neuroleptic side effects are being mistaken for idiopathic Parkinson's disease.

▶ We can hope that this will be the last study of such patients. The development of newer neuroleptic agents that do not have the side effects of the current drugs will, one hopes, obviate the development of parkinsonism in elderly patients.

M. Weintraub, M.D.

Management of Patients Receiving Interferon Beta-1b for Multiple Sclerosis: Report of a Consensus Conference
Lublin FD, Whitaker JN, Eidelman BH, et al (Thomas Jefferson Univ, Philadelphia; Univ of Alabama, Birmingham; Univ of Pittsburgh, Pa; et al)
Neurology 46:12–18, 1996   14–3

Objective.—Interferon-β1b was approved for use in the treatment of ambulatory patients with relapsing-remitting multiple sclerosis (MS) in

1993. Because of its recent approval, as well as the initial short supply of the drug, there is limited experience with the use of interferon-β1b. Various aspects of interferon-β1b treatment for patients with MS were reviewed.

Consensus Findings.—The double-blind, placebo-controlled trial that led to the approval of interferon-β1b found that treatment reduced the exacerbation rate by one third. In addition, it decreased MS activity in the brain, as evidenced by MRI scan. Ambulatory patients with relapsing-remitting MS are candidates for treatment with interferon-β1b, which is given at a dosage of 0.25 mg, or 8 million IU, by subcutaneous injection every other day. There is evidence that interferon-β1b may be helpful for a wider range of patients. However, it should only be prescribed when the diagnosis is clinically definite MS or laboratory-supported definite MS. The patient's clinical presentation and MS course provide the basis for deciding whether to give interferon-β1b. Injection-site reactions and flu-like symptoms are common. However, these side effects are manageable and subside after a few months in most patients. Some patients will have increased spasticity. Careful follow-up is indicated for patients with severe depression or suicidal ideation, which should be treated symptomatically. Pregnant and nursing women should not receive interferon-β1b.

Discussion.—Based on the experience to date, the use of interferon-β1b for patients with MS effectively reduces disease progression, as evaluated by MRI. Interferon-β1b is relatively easy to use and does not require changes in the patient's symptomatic treatment. When treatment is started, patient education and support are important in maintaining compliance. Interferon-β1b is the first effective treatment for relapsing-remitting MS, and it increases the MS patient's probability of achieving an improved quality of life.

▶ The original labeling on this treatment for MS reflected the nature and findings of a randomized, controlled, multicenter clinical trial. This pivotal trial was limited as to age groups (18–50 years), ambulatory patients, a relapsing-remitting disease course, and at least 2 acute exacerbations in the previous 2 years.

The year after Betaseron's approval by the Food and Drug Administration, a subcommittee of the American Academy of Neurology recommended a broadening of the indications to include patients older than 50 years, those who were not ambulatory, and patients with relapsing-progressive disease. The sentiment expressed was that any patient with MS who had true exacerbations should be able to receive the drug.

Although Betaseron is not *the* answer to MS and produces transient, nonserious adverse events, its use is reasonably simple to implement and does seem to lead to improved quality of life.

L. Lasagna, M.D.

Thrombolytic Therapy With Streptokinase in Acute Ischemic Stroke: The Multicenter Acute Stroke Trial

Hommel M, and the Europe Study Group (Centre Hospitalier Universitaire de Grenoble, France)
N Engl J Med 335:145–150, 1996   14–4

Purpose.—Early thrombolytic therapy is believed to permit reperfusion of ischemic neurons and to enhance functional recovery in patients with acute ischemic stroke. At the same time, there is the possibility of thrombolysis-associated cerebral bleeding and reperfusion-associated injury. The efficacy and safety of thrombolysis with streptokinase for acute ischemic stroke were evaluated in a multicenter, double-blind, randomized, controlled trial.

Methods.—The study included 310 patients at 48 French and British centers. All had moderate-to-severe acute ischemic stroke in the middle cerebral artery territory. Within 6 hours after the onset of stroke, the patients were treated with streptokinase, 1.5 million U over 1 hour, or placebo. Efficacy was evaluated by a binary criterion comprising mortality and severe disability at 6 months. (A Rankin scale score of 3 or greater was considered to denote severe disability.) Safety was evaluated in terms of mortality at 10 days and cerebral hemorrhage.

Results.—Six-month evaluation showed that 79% of patients receiving streptokinase and 81% of those receiving placebo either had died or had severe disability. However, 10-day mortality was 34% in the streptokinase group vs. 18% in the placebo group (Table 2). The excess deaths with streptokinase resulted from hemorrhagic transformation of ischemic cerebral infarcts. Forty-seven percent of the streptokinase-treated patients

TABLE 2.—Efficacy and Safety Outcomes in the Streptokinase and Placebo Groups

OUTCOME	STREPTOKINASE ($n = 156$)	PLACEBO ($n = 154$)	P VALUE
	no. of patients (%)		
Mortality or Rankin score ≥ 3 at 6 mo	124 (79.5)	126 (81.8)	0.60
Mortality at 10 days	53 (34.0)	28 (18.2)	0.002
Cerebral hemorrhage in hospital			
Symptomatic	33 (21.2)	4 (2.6)	< 0.001
Asymptomatic*	63 (45.3)	57 (41.3)	0.50
Unadjusted mortality			
At 3 mo	70 (44.9)	53 (34.4)	0.06
At 6 mo	73 (46.8)	59 (38.3)	0.13

*Data are based on CT scans from 139 patients in the streptokinase group and 138 in the placebo group. Computed tomography was not performed in 18 patients who died early (12 in the streptokinase group and 4 in the placebo group) or were discharged before CT could be performed (1 in each group); scans were not available or were of insufficient quality in 11 patients (3 in the streptokinase group and 8 in the placebo group); and CT was performed too late (i.e., more than 5 days after enrollment) in 4 patients (1 in the streptokinase group and 3 in the placebo group).

(Reprinted by permission of *The New England Journal of Medicine,* courtesy of Hommel M, and the Europe Study Group: Thrombolytic therapy with streptokinase in acute ischemic stroke: The Multicenter Acute Stroke Trial. *N Engl J Med* 335:145–150. Copyright 1996, Massachusetts Medical Society.)

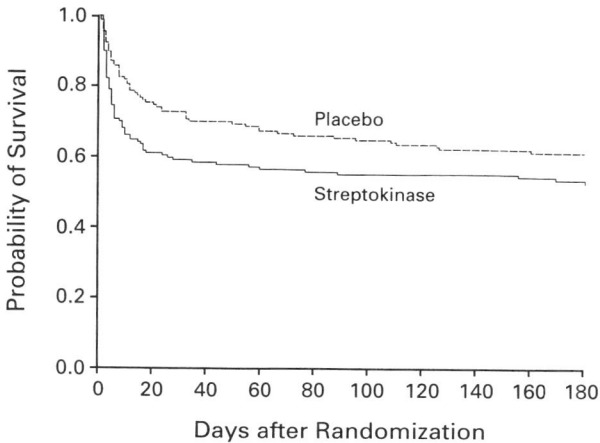

FIGURE 1.—Probability of survival over a period of 6 months among patients with acute ischemic stroke assigned to receive streptokinase or placebo. There were more deaths at 6 months in the streptokinase group than in the placebo group (73 vs. 59; $P = 0.06$ by the log-rank test). (Reprinted by permission of *The New England Journal of Medicine,* courtesy of Hommel M, and The Europe Study Group: Thombolytic therapy with streptokinase in acute ischemic stroke: The Multicenter Acute Stroke Trial. *N Engl J Med* 335:145–150. Copyright 1996, Massachusetts Medical Society.)

were dead at 6 months, compared with 38% of the placebo group (Fig 1). Recruitment for the trial was halted by the Data Monitoring Committee.

Conclusion.—Thrombolytic therapy with streptokinase increases mortality in patients with acute ischemic stroke. This is consistent with the results of most other trials of thrombolytic therapy for stroke; a meta-analysis of all of these trials is being conducted to see whether there is any patient subgroup that can benefit from treatment. Streptokinase should not be a routine treatment for acute ischemic stroke.

▶ Despite the numerical and somatic importance of acute ischemic stroke, the disease lacks an accepted standard treatment. The success of reperfusion in acute coronary occlusion has quite reasonably impelled trials of thrombolytics to see whether a similarly salubrious outcome could be achieved in stroke patients. In the 5 controlled trials to date, only 1 has failed to show an *increased* mortality rate in the thrombolytic group. Too bad.

L. Lasagna, M.D.

Aspirin and Delayed Cerebral Ischemia After Aneurysmal Subarachnoid Hemorrhage
Juvela S (Helsinki Univ)
J Neurosurg 82:945–952, 1995   14–5

Background.—Although aspirin is effective in the secondary prevention of various cardiovascular and cerebrovascular ischemic events in many high-risk patients, it may also increase the risk of hemorrhagic stroke, especially spontaneous intracerebral hemorrhage. Whether aspirin use before or after aneurysmal subarachnoid hemorrhage (SAH) affects the development of ischemic complications or rebleeding is not known. The effects of nonsteroidal anti-inflammatory drugs on the occurrence of delayed cerebral ischemia with fixed neurologic deficit and cerebral infarction on follow-up CT scans were investigated.

Methods and Findings.—Two hundred ninety-one patients were interviewed on their use of aspirin and other drugs before and after hemorrhage. Urine was also screened for salicylates. During a 1-year follow-up, 31 patients (11%) died from initial hemorrhage, and 18 (6%) died from rebleeding within 4 days after hemorrhage. Ninety of the remaining patients (37%) had delayed cerebral ischemia. In 54, delayed cerebral ischemia resulted in a permanent neurologic deficit or death. Eighty-five of the 195 patients undergoing follow-up CT had cerebral infarction not shown on the admission CT scan. Compared with patients who did not have salicylates in their urine on admission, those who did had a 0.4 relative risk of cerebral infarction. This decreased risk was limited to patients who took aspirin before hemorrhage, when the risk of ischemia was 0.21 and that of infarct was 0.18 compared with those who had not taken aspirin. Adjusting for several potential confounding variables did not affect the significance of this reduced risk.

Conclusions.—Aspirin-induced impairment of platelet function at the time of SAH and in the few days after SAH may decrease the risk of ischemic symptoms, particularly cerebral infarction, after aneurysm rupture. Aspirin taken both before and after aneurysm rupture may also increase the risk of rebleeding.

▶ This article illustrates the complex interplay between aspirin, platelets, thromboxane, and intracerebral hemorrhage or SAH. The study revealed that impairment of platelet function at the time of an SAH and during the following few days may reduce the risk of ischemic problems. However, aspirin also increased the risk of rebleeding when taken before or after the aneurysm. This observational study does provide some clues as to a beneficial effect of aspirin. Still, I think it would be foolish to begin treatment in patients with aneurysms because we just don't know the type of hemorrhage, the size of the vessel in which the hemorrhage occurred, and the patient factors that may have made aspirin more or less effective.

M. Weintraub, M.D.

Stroke in Users of Low-dose Oral Contraceptives

Petitti DB, Sidney S, Bernstein A, et al (Kaiser Permanente Med Care Program, Southern California, Pasadena; Kaiser Permanente Med Care Program, Northern California, Oakland)
N Engl J Med 335:8–15, 1996
14–6

Background.—In previous research, the use of oral contraceptives (OCs) has been associated with an increased risk of stroke; however, only OCs containing more estrogen than is now generally used were studied. The relationship between stroke and OC use in a large HMO in which high-estrogen OCs were rarely used was examined.

Methods.—The population-based, case-control study included female patients aged 15 through 44 years who had and had not experienced strokes, fatal and nonfatal. Data on the use of OCs were gathered through interviews.

Findings.—Four hundred eight strokes occurred among 1.1 million girls and women during 3.6 million woman-years, for an incidence of 11.3 strokes per 100,000 woman-years (Table 1). Two hundred ninety-five women with stroke and their matched control subjects were interviewed. Compared with former users and women who had never used OCs, current OC users had an odds ratio of 1.18 for ischemic stroke, after adjustment for other risk factors for stroke. The adjusted odds ratio was 1.14 for hemorrhagic stroke. Current OC use and smoking interacted positively to affect hemorrhagic stroke risk.

TABLE 1.—Types and Subtypes of Strokes

Type	All Strokes	Strokes Included in Our Analysis*
	no. (%)	
Hemorrhagic stroke		
Intraparenchymal	65 (15.9)	44 (14.9)
Subarachnoid†	110 (27.0)	91 (30.8)
Mixed or uncertain	26 (6.4)	16 (5.4)
Venous stroke	6 (1.5)	0
Ischemic infarction		
Cardioembolic	16 (3.9)	13 (4.4)
Caused by arterial dissection	8 (2.0)	6 (2.0)
Other	171 (41.9)	125 (42.4)
Other or unknown	6 (1.5)‡	0
Total	408	295

Note: Because of rounding, percentages may not total 100.

*Strokes were those that occurred in women who were not pregnant, had not undergone hysterectomy, had at least 1 ovary, were interviewed, and had at least 1 matched control and for whom there were complete data on current oral-contraceptive use.

†Includes "pure" intraventricular hemorrhage (8 cases, of which 7 were included in the analysis).

‡Three women were eligible and were interviewed but not included in the analysis.

(Reprinted by permission of *The New England Journal of Medicine*, courtesy of Petitti DB, Sidney S, Bernstein A, et al: Stroke in users of low-dose oral contraceptives. *N Engl J Med* 335:8–15. Copyright 1996, Massachusetts Medical Society.)

Conclusion.—Overall, current low-estrogen OC use does not appear to increase the risk of hemorrhagic stroke. The study confirms that the incidence of stroke among young women is low.

► Thromboembolic events, including strokes, were early identified as a problem in users of the original OCs, but the dose of estrogen has long since been lowered from 80 or 100 µg of estrogen to 30 or 35 µg. The goal behind that change in dose seems to have been achieved. What a pity that there was not better dose-response exploration at the beginning.

L. Lasagna, M.D.

Differential Effect of Aspirin Versus Warfarin on Clinical Stroke Types in Patients With Atrial Fibrillation
Pearce LA, for the Stroke Prevention in Atrial Fibrillation Investigators (Statistics and Epidemiology Research Corp, Seattle)
Neurology 46:238–240, 1996   14–7

Background.—Aspirin has been found to have a differential effect on the prevention of certain clinical types of ischemic stroke. In the Stroke Prevention in Atrial Fibrillation I (SPAF I) study, aspirin prevented noncardioembolic (non-CE) strokes more effectively than CE strokes, compared with placebo. The SPAF II study compared the efficacy and safety of aspirin with that of warfarin in patients with atrial fibrillation.

Methods.—A total of 1,100 patients with atrial fibrillation received either 325 mg of aspirin daily or warfarin adjusted to maintain the International Normalized Ratio at 2 to 4.5. Primary end points were ischemic strokes or systemic emboli.

Findings.—Sixty-three ischemic strokes occurred in 63 patients. At the time of the event, 14 were not taking a study medication. Thus, 49 strokes were analyzed. Warfarin was found to be significantly better than aspirin in preventing CE strokes as well as strokes of uncertain pathophysiology. The 2 agents were equally effective in preventing non-CE strokes.

Conclusion.—Patients with atrial fibrillation at particular risk for CE stroke apparently benefit most from warfarin treatment. It is hoped that the current data will increase interest in defining more reliable clinical markers of pathophysiologic stroke mechanisms and better elucidating the pharmacologic activity of antithrombotic treatments.

► This article contains some very important information valuable to all doctors treating atrial fibrillation. The main study (SPAF I) related that aspirin prevented non-CE strokes more effectively than CE strokes when compared with placebo. This study compared aspirin and warfarin. It showed that, as illustrated in the figure, stroke prevention by the different medications varies by type and treatment.

M. Weintraub, M.D.

Tissue Plasminogen Activator for Acute Ischemic Stroke

Marler JR, for the National Institute of Neurological Disorders and Stroke rt-PA Stroke Study Group (Natl Inst of Neurological Disorders and Stroke, Bethesda, Md)

N Engl J Med 333:1581–1587, 1995   14–8

Background.—Initial trials of thrombolytic therapy for patients with acute ischemic stroke were associated with high rates of intracerebral hemorrhage. These results prompted careful evaluation of the risks and benefits of recombinant human tissue plasminogen activator (t-PA) for cerebral arterial thrombolysis. Recent results have suggested that t-PA treatment is beneficial when given within 3 hours after the onset of stroke. To evaluate the benefits of IV t-PA for patients with ischemic stroke, a 2-part, randomized trial was done.

Methods.—The first part of the trial, which included 291 patients, sought to determine whether t-PA had clinical activity in patients with ischemic stroke. This outcome was defined as a 4-point improvement over baseline in the National Institutes of Health stroke scale score, or by resolution of the neurologic deficit within 24 hours after stroke onset. The second part of the study, which involved 333 patients, was designed to determine whether t-PA treatment had sustained clinical benefit at 3 months. The results were assessed by 4 outcome measures addressing differing aspects of stroke recovery: the Barthel index, the modified Rankin scale, the Glasgow coma scale, and the National Institutes of Health stroke scale. The results of the 2 parts were pooled and stratified to gain a complete picture of the effectiveness of t-PA.

Results.—In the first part of the study, the t-PA and placebo groups were not significantly different in the percentage of patients with neurologic improvement at 24 hours after stroke onset. In the second part, however, patients receiving t-PA had significant improvement on all 4 measures. The results of part 1 predicted long-term clinical benefit in part 2, with a 1.7 global odds ratio for a favorable outcome. Patients in the t-PA group were at least 30% more likely to be left with minimal or no disability at 3 months' follow-up. Six percent of patients in the t-PA group had symptomatic intracerebral hemorrhage within 36 hours after stroke onset, compared with 0.6% of the placebo group. Three-month mortality was 17% for the t-PA group and 21% for the placebo group.

Conclusions.—For patients with acute ischemic stroke, giving IV t-PA within 3 hours after the onset of stroke appears to produce significantly better 3-month clinical outcomes than placebo. This benefit holds even though t-PA treatment carries a higher risk of symptomatic intracerebral hemorrhage. Outcomes are better with t-PA than placebo regardless of the type of stroke diagnosed at baseline.

▶ The positive conclusions of these authors are not shared by everyone. The benefits are not overwhelming, and the risks of increased intracerebral hemorrhage are very real.

L. Lasagna, M.D.

Comparative Cognitive Effects of Phenobarbital, Phenytoin, and Valproate in Healthy Adults

Meador KJ, Loring DW, Moore EE, et al (Med College of Georgia, Augusta)
Neurology 45:1494–1499, 1995   14–9

Background.—Studies of the effects of individual antiepileptic drugs on cognition have produced controversial results. To eliminate the confounding effects of seizures, pre-existing cerebral substrate damage, genetic factors, and the psychosocial influences of epilepsy, the cognitive effects of phenobarbital, phenytoin, and valproate were studied in healthy adults. To eliminate selection bias, a randomized, double-blind, incomplete-block, crossover design was used.

Methods.—Fifty-nine healthy adults with no history of neurologic or psychiatric illness received 2 of the 3 antiepileptic drugs (phenobarbital, phenytoin, and valproate) for 1 month each. Dosages of each agent were tapered off for 3 weeks, and a 2-month washout period separated each treatment phase. Cognitive testing, consisting of 12 tests of 4 neurobehavioral constructs (cognitive and motor speed, memory, other cognitive tasks, and mood and symptoms), was done at baseline, at the end of the first and second treatment phases, and at the end of the first and second washout periods.

Results.—Compared with the nondrug conditions, each of the drugs had significant effects on Choice Reaction Time; P3 Potential; Delayed Recall of the Selective Reminding Test; the Symbol Digit Modalities Test; Stroop (all 3 components); Visual Serial Addition Test; and the anger, vigor, fatigue, and confusion components of the Profile of Mood States (POMS). In comparisons among the drug conditions, phenobarbital treatment resulted in significantly worse performance on Choice Reaction Time, Symbol Digit Modalities Test, the word and color tasks of the Stroop, Visual Serial Addition Test, and the anger component of the POMS.

Conclusions.—Although all 3 antiepileptic drugs had significant cognitive effects, cognitive performance was comparatively worse with phenobarbital than with phenytoin or valproate.

▶ Epilepsy is enough of a handicap without adding drug-induced cognitive impairment. Phenobarbital clearly seems the worst of the commonly used antiepileptics in this regard, with phenytoin, valproate, and carbamazepine being roughly the same.

L. Lasagna, M.D.

Chronic Subdural Hematomas and Seizures: The Role of Prophylactic Anticonvulsive Medication

Sabo RA, Hanigan WC, Aldag JC (Univ of Illinois, Peoria)
Surg Neurol 43:579–582, 1995   14–10

Introduction.—The diagnosis and surgical treatment of chronic subdural hematoma (CSH) have improved significantly over the past 20 years. Reported seizure rates in patients with CSH who have surgery have varied widely, and controversy continues regarding the prophylactic use of anticonvulsive medication (ACM). The prevalence and morbidity of seizures, along with the effects of ACM, were assessed retrospectively in patients undergoing surgery for CSH.

Patients and Findings.—The 6-year review included 98 patients who underwent surgical drainage of CSH. There were 65 males and 33 females. Fifty-five percent of the patients were aged 75 years or older; 77% had a history of head trauma. Six patients had a preexisting seizure disorder. In this group, despite having therapeutic serum levels of ACM, 3 patients experienced seizures. None of these patients died. The overall incidence of seizures in the hospital or during follow-up was 20%.

Forty-six percent of the patients with no previous history of seizure received prophylactic treatment with phenytoin sufficient with therapeutic serum levels. Just 1 of these patients had a seizure, compared with 32% of those who did not receive adequate ACM prophylaxis. Eleven patients died within 1 month after discharge, and 6 of them had a new onset of seizures. Risk of seizures and death was unrelated to the patients' age, sex, history of trauma, Markwalder scores on admission, location of hematoma, or type of surgery. Prophylactic ACM treatment continued for a median of 8 months after hospital discharge, with no further episodes of seizure.

Conclusions.—New onset of seizures may occur in up to one fifth of patients undergoing surgical drainage of CSH. This complication is linked to increased morbidity and mortality. Prophylactic ACM treatment can significantly reduce the risk of seizures in this patient population. It is recommended that phenytoin be administered for 6 months after the diagnosis of CSH.

▶ The ability to better diagnose subdural hematomata has reduced acute mortality but resulted in more survivors capable of having seizures over the long term. These seizures can, in turn, lead to a fatal outcome.
This study makes a good case for prophylactic phenytoin.

L. Lasagna, M.D.

Initiation and Duration of Breast-Feeding in Women Receiving Antiepileptics

Ito S, Moretti M, Liau M, et al (Hosp for Sick Children, Toronto)
Am J Obstet Gynecol 172:881–886, 1995   14–11

Background.—Several first-line antiepileptics are considered compatible with breast-feeding in most instances. These include carbamazepine, phenytoin, and valproic acid. The incidence of breast-feeding initiation, the factors involved in choice of feeding methods, and breast-feeding duration were investigated in a group of women taking anticonvulsant agents for a prolonged period of time.

Methods and Findings.—Thirty-four pregnant epileptic women taking antiepileptic agents and 34 pregnant healthy women, matched by age, were studied. Breast-feeding was chosen as the initial method of infant feeding by 50% of the epileptic women and 85% of the healthy control subjects, a significant difference. Advice from physicians and other sources significantly influenced the decision to begin with breast-feeding. Women taking antiepileptics who breast fed initially stopped breast-feeding at 4.7 months postpartum, significantly sooner than did the control subjects, who stopped breast-feeding at a mean of 9.3 months.

Conclusions.—Women taking antiepileptic agents tend to formula-feed their infants, citing "maternal medication" and "maternal illness" as the main reasons for their choice. Those who do initially breast-feed quit significantly earlier than women who do not take antiepileptic drugs.

► This has been a problem for many years. First of all, one usually advises women who become pregnant while taking antiepileptic drugs to continue taking them. I think that the benefit of staying on drugs is quite clear. There is a risk, but it is relatively small and is better than risking frequent seizures for both mother and child. I don't think we have as much data, however, about breast-feeding. Of course, we know more about whether a drug appears in the breast milk, yet we don't have truly definitive guidelines to help patients. In this study, many mothers chose to breast-feed for less time or to bottle-feed. Of course, the child should be examined more frequently by a pediatrician. Physicians should advise mothers that phenobarbital and ethosuximide make breast-feeding too dangerous for the infant. Other medications may be more acceptable for breast-feeding mothers. We need more information so that we can advise mothers more cogently.

M. Weintraub, M.D.

Effect of Carbamazepine and Valproate on Bone Mineral Density

Sheth RD, Wesolowski CA, Jacob JC, et al (West Virginia Univ, Morgantown; Mem Univ of Newfoundland, St. John's, Canada)
J Pediatr 127:256–262, 1995   14–12

Purpose.—Among the exogenous factors that can have an adverse effect on peak bone mineral density are certain medications. Carbamazepine has been linked to changes in bone metabolism, but the possible effects of valproate on bone have not been determined. If anti-epileptic drugs adversely affect bone mineralization, then many children are at increased risk of involutional osteoporosis. To determine the effects of carbamazepine or valproate on bone mineral density, children taking these drugs were studied.

Methods.—Of the children with uncomplicated idiopathic epilepsy in the study, 13 took carbamazepine and 13 took valproate. All 26 patients had been seizure free for more than 6 months; the mean serum trough level was 6.88 µg/mL in the children taking carbamazepine and 72.04 µg/mL in those taking valproate. They and a group of 27 control children underwent dual-energy x-ray absorptiometry to measure axial and appendicular bone mineral density. The 2 groups were comparable in terms of age, race, geographic area, and calcium intake.

Results.—Axial bone mineral density was 14% lower in the children taking valproate than in the control group, after adjustment for sex and age. The valproate group also had a 10% reduction in bone mineral density at the appendicular site. Children who had been taking valproate for a longer time had a greater reduction in bone mineral density. Bone mineral density values in children taking carbamazepine were not significantly different from those of controls.

Conclusions.—Children with idiopathic epilepsy who are receiving valproate monotherapy appear to have significantly reduced axial and appendicular bone mineral density. As a result, these patients may be at elevated risk of osteoporotic fractures. Bone mineral density does not appear to be reduced in children taking carbamazepine.

▶ A number of antiepileptics have been reported to decrease bone density: phenytoin, primidone, and phenobarbital. Carbamazepine has been reported to alter bone metabolism, but it seemed benign in this study. Valproate, on the other hand, looks as though it should be added to the list of osteopenia producers.

L. Lasagna, M.D.

Multiple Sclerosis: Sexual Dysfunction and Its Response to Medications
Mattson D, Petrie M, Srivastava DK, et al (Univ of Rochester, NY)
Arch Neurol 52:862–868, 1995   14–13

Background.—The comprehensive care of patients with multiple sclerosis (MS) should address sexual dysfunction. The frequency and nature of sexual dysfunction associated with MS and its response to medications were reported.

Methods and Findings.—Sixty-five women and 36 men with MS were included in the study. Sixty-three percent of the patients said their sexual activity had diminished. Thirty-five percent said they had less interest in sex than before their diagnosis. Sexual dysfunction was a problem for 57%, including 78% of the men and 45% of the women. Men reported prominent erectile dysfunction; women, problems with vaginal lubrication; and both sexes, reduced sensation and achievement of orgasm. Sexual dysfunction was associated with urinary problems and a history of therapy for or current depression. Sexual dysfunction was unassociated with disease duration, disease type, disability score, or fatigue. Twenty of the 57 patients reporting sexual dysfunction also said they had marital problems. Forty-three of the 60 patients who discussed sexual problems with their spouses and 4 of the 6 who tried formal counseling said it was useful. Unexpectedly, corticosteroid therapy begun for problems other than sexual dysfunction resulted in improved sexual functioning in many patients.

Conclusions.—Sexual dysfunction occurs commonly in patients with MS. Establishing the frequency and nature of such problems allows issues of sexual dysfunction to be addressed in the care of these patients. Certain treatments may be useful for sexual dysfunction, enhancing patients' quality of life.

▶ Boy, have we come a long way. It used to be that sexual dysfunction was rarely discussed by physicians or ancillary medical personnel and patients. In fact, it was so rarely done and so obviously embarrassing, that a wonderful advertisement for an antihypertensive drug was made illustrating the point. It featured an attractive female doctor taking a general history, not specifically focusing on sexual function, and the man being very diffident and trying to use all sorts of euphemisms. I think everyone agrees that we should take such a history. Also, we should remember that medications of all types can cause sexual dysfunction.

                                                                    M. Weintraub, M.D.

15 Obstetrics and Gynecology

Methotrexate and Misoprostol for Early Abortion: A Multicenter Trial. Acceptability
Creinin MD, Burke AE (Univ of Pittsburgh, Pa; Magee-Womens Hosp, Pittsburgh, Pa)
Contraception 54:19–22, 1996   15–1

Introduction.—Intramuscularly administered methotrexate followed by intravaginal misoprostol can effectively induce abortion at 2 months' gestation or less. Now that the efficacy of this regimen is established, its clinical feasibility must be demonstrated. Women's experiences with methotrexate and misoprostol for early abortion were studied.

TABLE 4.—Main Reasons for Patients Finding Their Experience "Positive"

	% of Women With Positive Experience $n = 207$	% of Total $n = 285$
Avoid surgical procedure	29.8	21.1
More natural than surgical abortion	18.9	13.3
Liked doctor and staff	11.4	8.1
Easy to tolerate cramping/ pain	10.4	7.4
Emotionally easy	10.0	7.0
More private/personal	3.5	2.5
Study will help other women	3.5	2.5
Few side effects	3.0	2.1
Abortion earlier than with surgery	2.5	1.8
Less invasive than surgery	1.5	1.1
Free	1.5	1.1
"Took too long"*	1.0	0.7
"Didn't work"*	1.0	0.7

Note: Reasons given are those cited by more than 1 respondent. Six questionnaires were not included because of interviewer error.
*Despite citing a negative response as their "main reason," these patients described their overall experience as positive.
(Reprinted by permission of the publisher, courtesy of Creinin MD, Burke AE: Methotrexate and misoprostol for early abortion: A multicenter trial. Acceptability. *Contraception* 54:19–22. Copyright 1996 by Elsevier Science Inc.)

TABLE 5.—Main Reasons for Patients Finding Their Experience
"Negative"

	% of Women with Negative Experience $n = 20$	% of Total $n = 285$
Severe pain or cramping	30.0	2.1
Emotionally hard	25.0	1.4
Required surgical procedure	25.0	1.4
Nausea/vomiting	15.0	1.1
Severe bleeding	10.0	0.7
"Took too long"	5.0	0.3

Note: Includes only responses given by more than 1 subject.
(Reprinted by permission of the publisher, courtesy of Creinin MD, Burke AE: Methotrexate and misoprostol for early abortion: A multicenter trial. Acceptability. *Contraception* 54:19–22. Copyright 1996 by Elsevier Science Inc.)

Methods.—The analysis included 300 pregnant women participating in a large multicenter trial. All received methotrexate, 50 mg/m² IM, followed 1 week later by misoprostol, 800 µg vaginally, for early abortion. Misoprostol was repeated if the first dose did not induce abortion. The women were asked why they chose medical abortion, their past experience with surgical abortion, and their perceptions of the medical abortion experience.

Results.—Nearly half of the subjects chose medical abortion to avoid some aspect of surgical abortion. The importance of avoiding surgical abortion varied by study center and the woman's previous experience with surgical abortion. Seventy-three percent of the women reported that medical abortion was a good experience (Table 4). Twenty percent found it a neutral experience and 7% found it a bad experience (Table 5). Eighty-three percent of patients said they would choose medical abortion over surgical abortion if they had to have another abortion.

Conclusion.—Methotrexate plus misoprostol is an acceptable method of medical abortion to patients. Most patients, by far, report that the experience of medical abortion is not a negative one and that they would undergo it again if they needed another abortion. Women's reasons for choosing medical rather than surgical abortion vary by location.

Methotrexate and Misoprostol for Early Abortion: A Multicenter Trial: I. Safety and Efficacy
Creinin MD, Vittinghoff E, Keder L, et al (Univ of Pittsburgh, Pa; Univ of California, San Francisco; Women's Health Care Services, Wichita, Kan)
Contraception 53:321–327, 1996   15–2

Background.—Several studies have shown that IM injection of methotrexate, 50 mg/m², followed by misoprostol insertion induces abortion in the first 56 days of gestation. However, the safety and efficacy of this procedure have yet to be assessed at multiple sites, using a single protocol.

Methods.—This multicenter study included 300 pregnant women seeking elective abortion. Seven days after the IM injection of 50 mg/m^2 of methotrexate, the patients returned for vaginal misoprostol, 800 µg. Four 200 µg tablets were placed in the vagina through a speculum. As the speculum was removed, the tablets were pushed into the posterior fornix with a large cotton swab. Patients were permitted to get up immediately after misoprostol was administered. Vaginal ultrasonography was performed 1 and 5 days later. A surgical abortion was performed if cardiac activity was still present after the second ultrasonography. Patients returned 4 weeks later for a follow-up assessment.

Findings.—Overall, abortion occurred with no need for surgery in 87.7% of the women. The complete abortion rate was 90.6% in women with gestations of less than 49 days and 81.6% in women with gestations of 50 to 56 days (Table 2). In 65% of women, abortion occurred within 24 hours of the initial or repeat misoprostol dose. In the remaining 22.7% of women who aborted, abortion was delayed by a mean of 23.6 days. The success rate after the first misoprostol dose was greater between days 43 and 56 compared with before day 43. In almost all the women, bleeding and/or cramping began within 3.3 hours after the first misoprostol dose. Patients in whom the procedure was immediately successful had vaginal

TABLE 2.—Outcomes of Abortion With Methotrexate and Misoprostol by Gestational Age

Number	≤42 108	43–49 94	50–56 98
	Treatment success		
Abortion before misoprostol	2 1.9%	0	0
Abortion after first dose of misoprostol	47 43.5%	53 56.4%	52 53.1%
Abortion after second dose of misoprostol	22 20.4%	10 10.6%	9 9.2%
Immediate success	71 65.7%	63 67.0%	61 62.3%
Delayed success	28 25.9%	21 22.3%	19 19.5%
	Treatment failure		
Continuing pregnancy	1 0.9%	0	11 11.2%
Dropped out before day 63	1 0.9%	1 1.1%	2 2.0%
No passage by day 63	3 2.8%	3 3.2%	1 1.0%
Incomplete	4 3.7%	6 6.4%	3 3.1%
Hemorrhage	0	0	1 1.0%

(Reprinted by permission of the publisher, courtesy of Creinin MD, Vittinghoff E, Keder L, et al: Methotrexate and misoprostol for early abortion: A multicenter trial. I. Safety and Efficacy. *Contraception* 53:321–327. Copyright 1996 by Elsevier Science Inc.)

bleeding that lasted a mean of 10 days and spotting for a mean of 4 days. In women with delayed abortion, vaginal bleeding and spotting lasted a mean of 7 and 4 days, respectively. None of the women needed a transfusion. In a univariate analysis, gravidity of less than 3, lower gestational age, and lower serum β–human chorionic gonadotropin on the day of methotrexate injection significantly predicted treatment success.

Conclusion.—Methotrexate followed by misoprostol is an effective and safe alternative to surgical abortion and the use of antiprogestins and prostaglandin for medical abortion. The adverse effects of methotrexate and misoprostol administration were minimal.

▶ These 2 papers (Abstracts 15–1 and 15–2) deal with the use of 2 widely used drugs to treat a condition never formally approved by the FDA as responding to either, although methotrexate alone has been successfully used to induce abortion in pregnancies of less than 2 months duration. Clearly, there are many women who prefer a pharmacologic abortion to a surgical one, even if multiple visits are required, as well as waiting for the pregnancy to pass. The drugs are not expensive and seem to work well.

L. Lasagna, M.D.

Local Administration of Prostaglandin E₂ for Cervical Ripening and Labor Induction: The Appropriate Route and Dose

Nuutila M, Kajanoja P (Helsinki Univ)
Acta Obstet Gynecol Scand 75:135–138, 1996   15–3

Objective.—Vaginally or intracervically administered prostaglandin E_2 serves to ripen the uterus before induction of labor. The preferred route of administration has not been determined. The safety, efficacy, and dose of intravaginal and intracervical PGE_2 gel in preinduction cervical ripening in high-risk obstetric patients were compared.

Methods.—Labor was induced by amniotomy and/or oxytocin infusion in 110 women, aged 17–44 years, with high-risk pregnancies and an unripe cervix after administration of PGE_2, 1 mg intravaginally (group A, $n = 35$); 2 mg intravaginally (group B, $n = 36$); and 0.5 mg intracervically (group C, $n = 39$) a maximum of 3 times at 6-hour intervals.

Results.—Ripening time was significantly shorter in groups B (12.2 hours) and C (10.8 hours) than in group A (16.7 hours). Labor was nonsignificantly shorter in groups B (7.9 hours) and C (6.5 hours) than in group A (9.3 hours). The cesarean section rates were 28.6% in group A, 19.4% in group B, and 15.4% in group C, primarily resulting from cervical dystocia and fetal asphyxia. Labor could not be induced in 10.3% of group C, 2.9% of group B, and 2.8% of group A patients. All group C patients required 3 gel applications for cervical ripening. Neonatal outcomes were uneventful. One group B and 1 group C patient had uterine hypertonus with prolonged fetal bradycardia.

Conclusion.—Multiple intravaginal applications of 2 mg of PGE_2 gel is a safe and effective technique for ripening the cervix before induction of labor in women with high-risk pregnancies. Careful fetal monitoring during this process is important.

▶ An unripe cervix is bad news for pregnant women and their health care team because it increases the probability of a failed induction of labor and a lengthy, exhausting delivery. This study provides a basis for using prostaglandin E$_2$ intravaginally instead of intracervically, because the former route is easy and can be used by midwives.

L. Lasagna, M.D.

Fetal Cardiac Function and Ductus Arteriosus During Indomethacin and Sulindac Therapy for Threatened Preterm Labor: A Randomized Study
Räsänen J, Jouppila P (Univ of Oulu, Finland)
Am J Obstet Gynecol 173:20–25, 1995   15–4

Background.—The prostaglandin synthesis inhibitor indomethacin has long been used as a tocolytic agent for the prevention of preterm labor. This treatment may be associated with a reversible, partial constriction of the fetal ductus arteriosus. The closely related drug sulindac has been reported to be just as effective for refractory preterm labor but with fewer side effects. To study the effects of indomethacin and sulindac on fetal ductus arteriosus and fetal cardiac function in pregnancies with threatened premature labor, Doppler techniques were used.

Methods.—The randomized study included 20 pregnant patients with threatened premature labor; the fetuses were between 28 and 32 weeks' gestation. The women were assigned to receive 4 days of treatment with indomethacin or sulindac. Pulsed color Doppler ultrasound and M-mode echocardiography were performed before, during, and after treatment to evaluate fetal cardiac function and ductus arteriosus.

Results.—By 4 hours after indomethacin administration, the mean pulsatility index in fetal ductus arteriosus had decreased significantly. As treatment continued, the ventricular inner end-diastolic diameters increased and the right ventricular fractional shortening decreased. By 24 hours after the end of indomethacin treatment, the mean pulsatility index values had returned to pretreatment levels. Sulindac also decreased the mean pulsatility index in fetal ductus arteriosus, but not until 24 hours after the start of treatment. All other mean pulsatility index values were not significantly different from baseline, and all other cardiac measurements were unchanged.

Conclusions.—In pregnancies with threatened preterm labor, indomethacin treatment has a significant but reversible constrictive effect on the fetal ductus arteriosus. Secondary changes are observed as well, particularly in the right ventricle. Randomized comparison shows that sulindac has a milder and transient constrictive effect.

▶ Studying medications in preterm labor has been very difficult. Ritodrine, terbutaline, alcohol, and magnesium sulfate have been studied, with each drug's defects and deficiencies occurring later. Researchers have not produced good data supporting them. Therefore, a treatment such as a nonsteroidal anti-inflammatory agent may be a better selection. Unfortunately, the nonsteroidal agents are also used to close a patent ductus arteriosus. That would not be a good outcome in the preterm infant. However, all nonsteroidal drugs apparently do slow labor by blocking prostaglandin-induced uterine contractions. This paper may have shown, at least in a small number of patients, that sulindac has less of an effect on the patent ductus than does indomethacin.

M. Weintraub, M.D.

Decline in Cerebral Thromboembolism Among Young Women After Introduction of Low-dose Oral Contraceptives: An Incidence Study for the Period 1980–1993
Lidegaard Ø (Univ of Copenhagen)
Contraception 52:85–92, 1995   15–5

Introduction.—Oral contraceptive (OC) use has been statistically linked to the risk of cerebral thromboembolism, but it remains uncertain whether this association reflects a causal relationship or some type of selection phenomenon. The possible effects of OC use on the incidence of cerebral thromboembolic attacks (CTAs) were examined using a Danish central database.

Methods.—The database was used to identify patients with discharge diagnoses reflecting CTA in Denmark from 1980 to 1993. This information was used to determine the age-specific incidence rates (IRs) of CTA among men and women aged 15 to 44 years. Information for analysis of the possible contribution of OCs to the incidence of CTA was derived from comprehensive sales statistics covering the study period and from cross-section studies of type-specific OC use at various ages.

Results.—Cerebral thromboembolic attacks occurred in 2,522 men and 2,100 women during the period studied. In men, the IR of CTA increased exponentially with age. From 1980 to 1986, women in the 20–35-year age group had more CTAs than men of the same age. This difference became nonsignificant after 1987. From the first to the second half of the study period, the IR of CTA declined significantly by 20% for women younger than 30 years of age, whereas men of the same age group had a nonsignificant decline of 9.5%. Women older than 30 years had a nonsignificant increase of 4% from the first to the second half of the study, men had a significant increase of 11%. Further calculations assumed that OC use carried an average relative risk of CTA of 2.5 and pregnancy carried a relative risk of 4. After correction for incident cases among women, women's and men's IRs had a close covariation up to the age of 35 years. In older age groups, the IR was high in men.

Conclusions.—Young, fertile women have higher IRs of CTA than men of similar age, and this difference may be explained by the contribution of pregnancy and OC use. The IR of CTA among young women has declined since 1980, possibly because the hormonal content of OCs has decreased. There are no other known exposures to explain the described trends in CTA among young Danish men and women.

▶ It has for some time been believed that the lowering of hormonal content in OCs has resulted in fewer strokes. This nifty study supports recent studies reporting an estrogen dose-dependent association with cerebral thromboembolism. Progestogen pills do not seem to confer any increased risk.

L. Lasagna, M.D.

Differential Effects on Bone Density of Progestogen-only Methods for Contraception in Premenopausal Women
Naessen T, Olsson S-E, Gudmundson J (Univ Hosp, Uppsala, Sweden)
Contraception 52:35–39, 1995   15–6

Background.—Few investigators have studied the effects of different progestogens on bone metabolism and bone mass. Furthermore, the findings of these studies have often been contradictory. No previous randomized studies have compared the effect of different progestogens on bone mass in premenopausal women.

Methods.—To determine whether the short-term effects of standard contraceptive doses of levonorgestrel and depot-medroxyprogesterone acetate (DMPA) on bone mass and bone metabolism differ, data from a 6-month prospective clinical study were analyzed. Twenty-two premenopausal women (age range, 20–45 years) participated. The women had been randomly assigned to receive either levonorgestrel or DMPA.

Findings.—Proximal forearm bone density increased by 2.9% in women given levonorgestrel. Women given DMPA had stable values. At 6 months, the group difference was 3.4% for proximal forearm bone density and 4.1% for distal bone density. The bone density changes were consistent with the changes in biochemical indices for bone metabolism. In women using DMPA, evidence of increased bone turnover was found. Levonorgestrel users had increased bone formation with higher levels of both alkaline phosphatase and osteocalcin.

Conclusions.—Bone density is increased in levonorgestrel users and stable in DMPA users when these agents are taken in standard clinical contraceptive doses. The bone mass changes were consistent with changes in bone metabolism indices.

▶ The lesson here is simple: contraceptive progestogens are not identical in their effects on bone density. Because some women may take such birth control methods for decades, these differences may have considerable impact on fracture risks later in life.

L. Lasagna, M.D.

Case-Control Study of Oral Contraceptive Use and Risk of Breast Cancer
Rosenberg L, Palmer JR, Rao RS, Zauber AG, Strom BL, Warshauer ME, Harlap S, Shapiro S (Boston Univ, Brookline, Mass; Mem Sloan-Kettering Cancer Ctr, New York; Univ of Pennsylvania, Philadelphia; et al)
Am J Epidemiol 143:25–37, 1996   15–7

Background.—Several reports on the relationship between oral contraceptive (OC) use and breast cancer have been published. Based on data from a multipurpose hospital-based surveillance system initiated 20 years ago, this relationship has been found to be nonexistent or weakly positive among older women. However, an increased risk of breast cancer among younger women using OCs has been reported. The association between OC use and breast cancer in white women aged 25–59 years was investigated.

Methods.—Data were collected between 1977 and 1992 in a case–control surveillance system in hospitals in Boston, New York, and Philadelphia. Data on 3,540 patients with breast cancer were compared with data on 4,488 patients with nonmalignant nongynecologic conditions unassociated with OC use.

Findings.—Comparing women using OCs for at least 1 year with those using them for less than 1 year, the multivariate relative risk estimates were 1.7 in women aged 25–34, 0.9 in women aged 35–44, and 1.2 in women aged 45–59. The relative risk estimates were greatest for prolonged use among women aged 25–34 years, but this trend was not significant. Also, duration of use was associated with recency of use; their effects could not be distinguished. The relative risk estimate declined with increasing duration of use among women aged 35–44. Among women aged 45–59, some relative risk estimates were increased but not in any consistent pattern.

Conclusions.—These findings provide more evidence of an association between OC use and an increased risk of breast cancer among women younger than 35 years. This association was strongest for women who had used OCs the longest, but the duration of use trend was not statistically significant.

▶ Drs. Shapiro and Strom are among our most talented pharmacoepidemiologists. This paper tackles an important problem, but it represents not a final answer but another contribution to a complex area in which risks are tricky to identify beyond peradventure of doubt and in which age and duration of contraceptive use seem to make simple conclusions and advice almost impossible.

Meanwhile, there's no room for agnostics. Either a woman uses oral contraceptives or not. Not using them is not a delay of judgment but a judgment that their risk–benefit equation is less favorable than the alternatives.

L. Lasagna, M.D.

Effect of Physician Gender on the Prescription of Estrogen Replacement Therapy

Seto TB, Taira DA, Davis RB, et al (Brockton/West Roxbury Veterans Affairs Med Ctr, West Roxbury, Mass; Harvard School of Public Health, Boston; Beth Israel Hosp, Boston)
J Gen Intern Med 11:197–203, 1996   15–8

Background.—Although there is considerable evidence of the benefits of postmenopausal estrogen replacement therapy (ERT), only 3% to 15% of eligible women receive it. This may be partially related to uncertainty regarding its risks. However, research has also suggested that physician-specific factors may influence the use of ERT. The effect of physician gender on the use of ERT was evaluated in a case-control study.

Methods.—Seventy-two women older than age 50 years receiving new prescriptions for ERT during an 18-month period were identified from a computer-based patient medication profile. Each was matched for age and time of visit with 2 controls who were not receiving ERT. The charts of both cases and controls were reviewed. All of the patients were interviewed by telephone to determine whether they had selected their primary care physician and the factors contributing to their decision. They were asked about their interest in ERT and preventive testing and whether the physician or the patient had initiated discussion regarding ERT.

Results.—Female physicians cared for 63% of the case patients and 38% of the control patients. Estrogen replacement therapy was used by 45% of the patients cared for by a female physician and 23% of the patients cared for by a male physician. Compared with the control patients, the case patients were significantly more likely to have received Papanicolaou smears, mammograms, breast examinations, and fecal occult blood testing. Patients were still significantly more likely to use ERT if they had a female physician, after controlling for the performance of these preventive health measures. Case patients were also more likely to have selected their primary care physician, had a hysterectomy, be interested in ERT, and be concerned about perimenopausal symptoms. After controlling for all of these potential confounders, patients with female physicians were still 11.4 times more likely to be using ERT than patients with male physicians.

Conclusion.—There are gender-related differences in the likelihood of physicians to prescribe ERT that are not explained by patient preferences. Women cared for by female physicians are significantly more likely to be prescribed ERT than are women cared for by male physicians. Further study is needed to determine the reasons for these gender-related differences.

▶ I hope this was not intended as a male doctor–bashing article. However, the YEAR BOOK OF DRUG THERAPY and many journal articles have pointed out that physicians, in general, should be checking on a woman's desire to have ERT. Obviously, there was a large standard error associated with this study given that the odds ratio was 11.4, but the 95% confidence interval was 1.1 to 113.6. It still means that the male physicians had not yet gotten it.

M. Weintraub, M.D.

Prevalence of Menopausal Symptoms Among Women With a History of Breast Cancer and Attitudes Toward Estrogen Replacement Therapy
Couzi RJ, Helzlsouer KJ, Fetting JH (Johns Hopkins Med Insts, Baltimore, Md)
J Clin Oncol 13:2737–2744, 1995   15–9

Background.—Whether women with a history of breast cancer should be given estrogen replacement therapy (ERT) for menopausal symptoms has been much debated. To determine the prevalence and severity of vasomotor, gynecologic, and other symptoms in women with a history of in situ or invasive locoregional breast cancer and the impact of these symptoms on quality of life, a survey was conducted. These women's attitudes toward ERT and the factors affecting their willingness to take estrogen were elicited.

Methods.—Three hundred twenty women, aged 40 to 65 years, were mailed a questionnaire. All study participants had received a diagnosis of in situ or invasive locoregional breast cancer between 1988 and 1992. The response rate was 77%.

Findings.—One hundred ninety of the 222 respondents were postmenopausal. Sixty-five percent of these women had hot flashes; 44%, night sweats; 48%, vaginal dryness; 26%, dyspareunia; 44%, sleep problems; and 44%, feelings of depression. The frequency of sleep disturbances and feelings of depression increased with worsening vasomotor symptoms. Forty-one percent of the menopausal women thought that they had a physical or emotional problem associated with menopause since their diagnosis of breast cancer. Half of these women said they needed treatment. Overall, 31% of the postmenopausal women said they would consider ERT. Women reporting a problem associated with menopause were more likely to consider ERT than women without such problems, those proportions being 42% and 22%. The percentage willing to take estrogen increased with the increasing severity of symptoms, especially symptoms of depression and sleep disturbances. Awareness that ERT reduces the risks of heart disease and osteoporosis was uncorrelated with an increased willingness to take it. However, women who believed that ERT increases the risks of recurrent breast and uterine cancer were less willing to consider this treatment.

Conclusions.—Vasomotor symptoms significantly affect the quality of life of postmenopausal women who have had breast cancer. The safest, most effective methods for alleviating these symptoms need to be established.

▶ Although not every postmenopausal woman suffers from hot flashes, many do, and for some it is not merely a matter of mild transient feelings of warmth, but severe disabling waves of heat, with drenching sweats and insomnia. The first 2 years after menopause are the worst, usually, but a significant number of women suffer symptoms for 6 to 10 years, and a few for over a decade. By contrast, urogenital complaints tend to get worse with increasing age.

Chemotherapy for breast cancer may induce ovarian failure, and the anti-estrogen tamoxifen can cause hot flashes. This article provides valuable insight into the perceptions and attitudes toward health and of ERT for women with a history of breast cancer. The topic of vasomotor symptoms in such patients deserves additional study.

L. Lasagna, M.D.

Superior Compliance and Efficacy of Continuous Combined Oral Estro-gen-Progestogen Replacement Therapy in Postmenopausal Women
Dören M, Reuther G, Minne HW, et al (Westfälische Wilhelms-Universität, Münster, Germany; Ruprecht-Karls-Universität, Münster, Germany)
Am J Obstet Gynecol 173:1446–1451, 1995   15–10

Background.—Estrogen replacement therapy is not widely accepted. Regular withdrawal bleeding is thought to be the major reason for this. Compliance, relief of climacteric symptoms, and effects on lumbar bone mineral density were compared in patients given a sequential estrogen-progestogen, continuous combined replacement treatment, or placebo.

Methods.—Patients in group 1 were given 2 mg of estradiol valerate daily and 5 mg of medroxyprogesterone acetate daily for 12 days a month sequentially to induce withdrawal bleeding. Patients in group 2 received 2 mg of estradiol, 1 mg of estriol, and 1 mg of norethisterone acetate daily continuously to maintain amenorrhea. Group 3 consisted of control patients.

Findings.—In group 1, compliance at 1 year was 66% and 49% at 2 years, compared with 93% for 1-year compliance and 73% for 2-year compliance in group 2. The 2 groups showed similar improvement in climacteric symptoms. The main reason for quitting therapy was uterine bleeding, cited by 24% of the patients in group 1 and 3% of the patients in group 2. Bone mineral density improved at 1 and 2 years in group 2 only, compared with baseline values. No significant changes in bone mineral density occurred in groups 1 or 3. Age at menopause was unassociated with compliance.

Conclusions.—Women in whom postmenopausal amenorrhea was maintained complied better with estrogen replacement therapy than women receiving the sequential regimen. The continuous combined and sequential hormone therapies were similar in their relief of climacteric symptoms, but the former was more effective in protecting against decreased lumbar bone mineral density.

▶ There are good reasons for postmenopausal women to take estrogen, but withdrawal bleeding has disenchanted many women who do not regret that their periods have stopped.

This study suggests that continuous combined estrogen replacement therapy is more acceptable to women than a sequential estrogen-progestogen regimen and is superior with regard to prevention of bone loss.

L. Lasagna, M.D.

Effects of Continuous Combined Hormone-replacement Therapy on Lipid Levels in Hypercholesterolemic Postmenopausal Women
Denke MA (Univ of Texas, Dallas; Veteran's Affairs Med Ctr, Dallas)
Am J Med 99:29–35, 1995   15–11

Background.—In postmenopausal women, estrogen lowers low-density lipoprotein (LDL)-cholesterol levels while increasing high-density lipoprotein-(HDL) cholesterol levels. However, the addition of progestogens—especially the androgenic progestogens—can lessen these effects. Because medroxyprogesterone is only weakly androgenic, its use in combination with estrogens may have less of a negative effect on lipids. The lipid-lowering effects of continuous combined hormone replacement therapy (HRT) were assessed in postmenopausal women with hypercholesterolemia.

Methods.—Thirty-two postmenopausal women with LDL cholesterol levels of greater than 130 mg/dL and fasting triglyceride levels of less than 250 mg/dL were studied. Half of the women had undergone hysterectomy. All of the women were asked to follow a standardized diet high in saturated fat for 1 month, then to follow the fat-modified Step-One diet, which supplies 30% of calories from fat, 10% saturated fat, and less than 300 mg of dietary cholesterol per day. After 3 months on this diet, the patients took daily placebo tablets for 3 months. They then started 3 months of supplementation with conjugated estrogens, 0.625 mg/day, plus medroxyprogesterone, 2.5 mg/day.

Results.—Compliance with the Step-One diet was good. This diet reduced total cholesterol level by 11 mg/dL and LDL cholesterol level by 8 mg/dL. With HRT, further reductions of 17 mg/dL for total cholesterol level and 23 mg/dL for LDL cholesterol level occurred. This form of HRT also resulted in significant increases in HDL and very low density cholesterol levels and in triglyceride levels.

The distribution of LDL values showed a further shift to the left with continuous combined HRT vs. diet alone. The LDL value was greater than 190 mg/dL in 10 women during the high-saturated-fat diet, compared with only 1 woman during the Step-One diet plus HRT. The number of women with LDL values greater than 160 mg/dL was 26 (high-saturated-fat diet) vs. 10 (Step-One diet plus HRT). Two women had HDL cholesterol values of less than 35 mg/dL during the placebo period, compared to none during the HRT period. Eleven of 16 women with an intact uterus reported bleeding during HRT; only 5 of them reported frank bleeding.

Conclusions.—Continuous combined HRT—consisting of conjugated estrogens plus medroxyprogesterone—yields a significant reduction in

LDL cholesterol level and a mild increase in HDL cholesterol levels. The latter effect is not as great as that achieved with estrogen therapy alone. This HRT regimen may be useful in postmenopausal women with hyper-cholesterolemia who have not undergone hysterectomy.

▶ Chalk up another plus for combined HRT for postmenopausal women!

L. Lasagna, M.D.

Postmenopausal Hormone Use and Risk of Large-bowel Cancer
Newcomb PA, Storer BE (Univ of Wisconsin, Madison)
J Natl Cancer Inst 87:1067–1071, 1995   15–12

Background.—The production of secondary bile acids is thought to promote colon carcinogenesis. Because progestins and exogenous estrogens may reduce the production of these acids, women receiving hormone replacement therapy (HRT) might lower their risk of large-bowel cancer. Clear evidence for such an effect is lacking, however, and a case-control study was conducted to investigate the potentially important relationship between HRT and cancer risk.

Methods.—Patients considered for the study were all Wisconsin women with a new diagnosis of cancer of the colon or rectum who were younger than 75 years at diagnosis and had been reported to a statewide cancer registry from 1990 through 1991. The final case group included 694 menopausal women, 480 with a diagnosis of colon cancer and 214 with a diagnosis of rectal cancer. Controls were 1,622 women randomly selected from a list of licensed drivers and a roster of Medicare beneficiaries in Wisconsin. Telephone interviews were conducted to obtain information on medical history, postmenopausal HRT use, and family history.

Results.—The risk of developing colon cancer was about 30% lower among women who reported ever using HRT, compared with women who never used HRT. Recent use only, not former use, was associated with reduced risk. Risk reduction was similar for estrogen-only users and for women who took estrogen and progestin. Hormone use, whether at any time or recently, had no effect on the risk of rectal cancer. There was a trend for an inverse association between decreasing time since last use of HRT and the risk for colon cancer, but not for rectal cancer. The inverse association between HRT and cancer risk appeared to be strongest among women at lower absolute risk of disease, particularly among those with leaner body mass.

Conclusions.—A significant reduction in colon cancer incidence was found among postmenopausal women who used HRT. The reduction was about 30% for ever use and 46% for recent use. No association was observed between HRT and rectal cancer. Because adenocarcinoma of the large bowel is among the most common cancers in Western populations, the finding of a reduced risk for women taking postmenopausal hormones may have important public health implications.

▶ Wow! Hold on to your epidemiologic thinking caps. If this paper had turned out the other way, as the authors originally thought, it would have made the front page of the *New York Times*. However, it showed a clear-cut decrease in the relative risk for colon cancer and a nonsignificant relative risk for rectal cancer. Ah well, off the pages of the local newspaper and onto the pages of the *Journal of the National Cancer Institute.*

M. Weintraub, M.D.

16 Pain

Variation in the Placebo Effect in Randomised Controlled Trials of Analgesics: All Is as Blind as It Seems
McQuay H, Carroll D, Moore A (Univ of Oxford, England)
Pain 64:331–335, 1995   16–1

Background.—The placebo response has often been misunderstood to involve both a fixed fraction of the population and a fixed extent of reaction. However, data have shown a varied proportion of the population to be affected across studies and an effect that can vary systematically with the efficacy of the active agent. These findings have brought into question the possibility of both selection bias and observer bias in randomized, double-blind, placebo-controlled trials. The variations in placebo responses were examined in 5 randomized, double-blind, parallel-group trials of analgesic agents to examine this possibility.

Methods.—Individual patient data from 5 placebo-controlled, double-blind, randomized trials of analgesic agents were analyzed. Each of the trials used 3 scales to determine pain intensity and 2 scales to determine pain relief. The relationship between pain relief and time was calculated for each patient and was compared against the maximum possible pain relief in relation to time.

Results.—Of the 525 patients in the 5 trials, 130 received placebo. These patients experienced 0% to 100% of the maximum possible pain relief, whereas the patients who received active agents experienced 0% to 97% of the maximum possible pain relief (Fig 1). When the patients in the placebo groups who had less than 50% of the maximum possible pain relief were compared with those with more than 50% of the maximum possible pain relief, they differed only in age, with no differences in sex, height, weight, initial pain intensity, or mood. The mean percent of maximum possible pain relief varied from 11% to 29% in the placebo study arms and from 12% to 49% in the active study arms. There was a significant relationship between the mean values in the placebo and the active study arms of each study, with the mean placebo results averaging 54% of the mean active results. However, there was no significant relationship between the median active and placebo responses; the median placebo response averaged less than 10% of the median active response.

Conclusions.—The use of inappropriate statistical methods has led to the recognition of a constant relationship between active analgesic and

Percentage

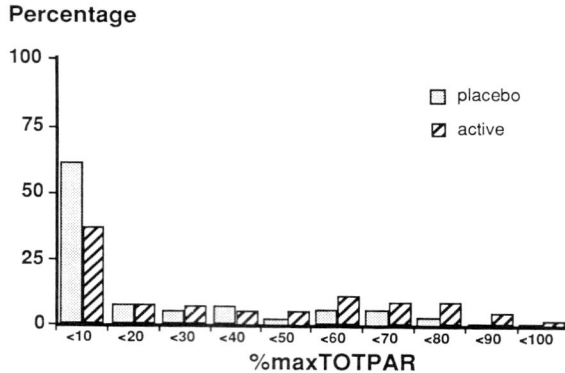

FIGURE 1.—Distribution of percentage of maximum possible pain relief (*%maxTOTPAR*) scores for the 130 patients given placebo and for the 395 patients given active drugs. (Reprinted from McQuay H, Carroll D, Moore A: Variation in the placebo effect in randomised controlled trials of analgesics: All is as blind as it seems. *Pain* 64:331–335, 1995, with kind permission of Elsevier Science-NL, Sara Burgerhartstraat 25, 1055 KV Amsterdam, The Netherlands.)

placebo response. Median responses, and not mean responses, should be used to evaluate the efficacy of analgesic agents in clinical trials.

▶ If the placebo beats the active drug or comes close to doing so, there won't be a meaningful or statistically significant difference. The most common result in 395 patients taking active drug and 130 taking placebo was less than 10% of maximum! Of the active drug, the variation in these cases was from 12% to 49% of the maximal score. The authors recommend several changes in reportage for analgesic trials. They suggest looking at median values. I'm more interested in achieving a meaningful goal, no matter how it's measured. We also should look very carefully at the individual patient responses to achieve a clinically significant goal.

M. Weintraub, M.D.

Age as a Risk Factor for Inadequate Emergency Department Analgesia
Jones JS, Johnson K, McNinch M (Michigan State Univ, Grand Rapids)
Am J Emerg Med 14:157–160, 1996   16–2

Introduction.—Recent studies suggest that many patients who come to the emergency department (ED) do not receive adequate analgesia. This problem appears to be most common among elderly patients, in whom pain may be ignored or inadequately treated. A retrospective analysis examined whether elderly trauma patients were less likely than younger patients to receive ED analgesia.

Methods.—The records of a community hospital and tertiary care facility were reviewed for an 18-month period (August 1992–January 1994) to identify adult patients with an ED discharge diagnosis of isolated long-bone fracture. Excluded were cases of multiple trauma and patients who denied pain on admission. Data recorded included patient demographics, ED treatment, and final disposition. Analgesic use was classified as low or high dose, narcotic or nonnarcotic, and oral or parenteral.

Results.—Eligibility requirements were met by 231 patients, 109 of whom were older than 70 (mean age, 80.6 years). Most (88%) elderly patients had fallen and sustained a fracture of the femur; falls accounted for 31% and motor vehicle accidents accounted for 57% of fractures in younger patients. The elderly were more likely than the nonelderly to receive no analgesic (34% vs. 20%) and to have analgesic administration delayed. Narcotics were given to 98% of the nonelderly vs. 89% of the elderly, and high dose analgesics were given to 44% of the nonelderly vs. 19% of the elderly. Advanced age was the strongest predictor of no analgesic in multiple logistic regression analysis.

Conclusion.—Among ED patients with isolated long-bone extremity fractures, younger patients were more likely to receive a narcotic for pain. The nonelderly also received the analgesic within a shorter period of time and at a higher equivalent dose. Elderly patients may underreport symptoms, and physicians may be concerned with the adverse side effects of analgesics in older patients with underlying medical conditions.

▶ I like the term *oligoanalgesia* but dislike its clinical manifestations. The elderly are more sensitive than younger people to opiates, but they don't deserve to be undertreated. (Many nonelderly are also undertreated, I admit.)

L. Lasagna, M.D.

Age Is the Best Predictor of Postoperative Morphine Requirements
Macintyre PE, Jarvis DA (Univ of Adelaide, Australia; Royal Adelaide Hosp, Australia)
Pain 64:357–364, 1995   16–3

Background.—Traditionally, the opioid dose prescribed for postoperative pain relief has been based on the patient's weight. Although dose reductions are often considered in elderly patients, age-related dose changes are generally not considered in younger patients. The factors that best predict the amount of morphine used in the first 24 hours after surgery were determined.

Methods.—The medical records of 1,010 patients younger than 70 years were reviewed. All had been prescribed morphine in a patient-controlled analgesia (PCA) system after major surgery. Variables studied were patient age, sex, weight, operative site, verbal numeric pain score, and a nausea/vomiting score. The effects of intraoperative and recovery room doses of opioid were analyzed in a subgroup of 78 patients.

Findings.—Interpatient variability in PCA morphine doses was great, with differences as high as tenfold in each age group. However, the best predictor of PCA morphine requirement in the first 24 hours postoperatively was the patient's age. For patients older than 20 years, these requirements could be estimated by the following formula: *Mean first 24-hour morphine requirement (mg) = 100 − age* (Fig 1).

Conclusions.—Previous studies have reported a correlation between patient age and the amount of opioid needed. In this study, the association was quantified, providing a guideline for opioid dosing. Prescriptions for

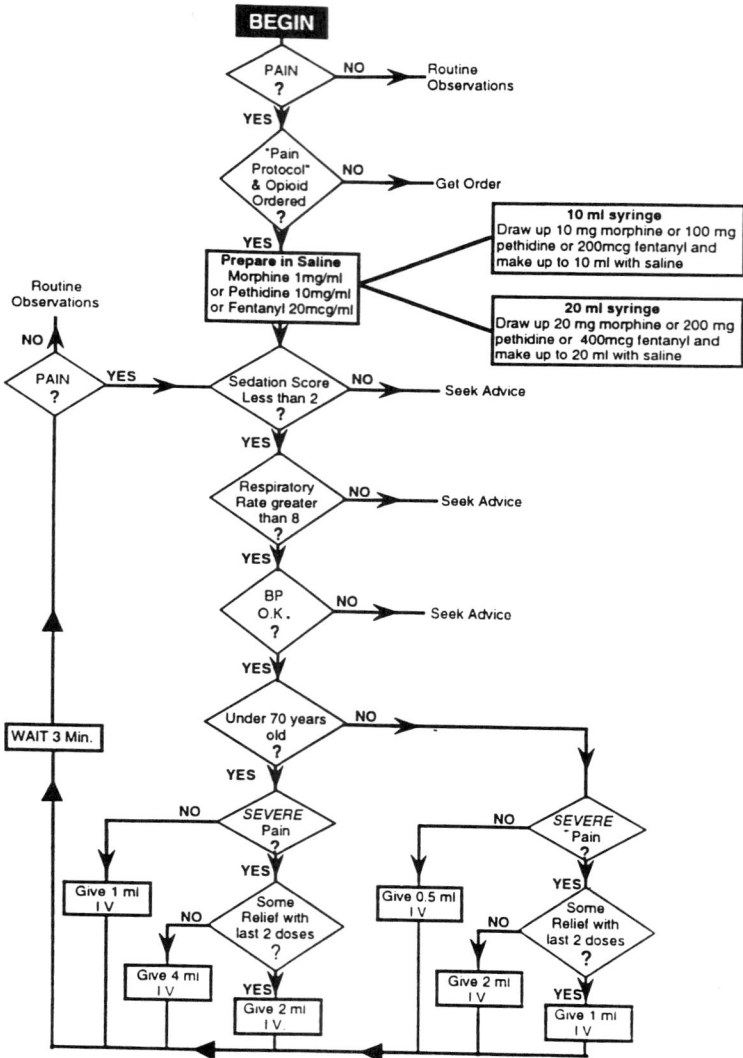

FIGURE 1.—Acute Pain Service 'Recovery Room Intravenous Pain Protocol.' (Reproduced with permission of the Acute Pain Service). (Courtesy of Macintyre PE, Jarvis DA: Age is the best predictor of postoperative morphine requirements. *Pain* 64:357–364. Copyright 1995, with kind permission of Elsevier Science-NL, Sara Burgerhartstraat 25, 1055 KV Amsterdam, The Netherlands.)

conventional analgesic regimens should include a dose range centered on values from the formula above to allow for the wide variation among patients in each age group. Although initial morphine dose should be determined by patient age and not weight, subsequent doses must be titrated based on effect.

▶ The authors' recommendations are very sensible—be aware of the general relationship (an inverse one) between age and postoperative morphine requirements but be flexible enough to titrate according to the adequacy or inadequacy of pain relief.

L. Lasagna, M.D.

Ethnic Differences in Analgesic Consumption for Postoperative Pain
Ng B, Dimsdale JE, Shragg GP, et al (Univ of California San Diego, La Jolla)
Psychosom Med 58:125–129, 1996   16–4

Introduction.—Although many reports have examined the relation between ethnicity and pain, it is difficult to draw any general conclusions. One recent study suggested that Hispanic patients were less likely to receive pain medication in the emergency department than non-Hispanic whites. Differences in analgesic usage by ethnicity were compared for patients undergoing the same painful procedure.

Methods.—The retrospective study included 250 consecutive hospitalized patients undergoing open reduction and internal fixation of a limb fracture. One hundred and fourteen patients were classified as white, 100 as Hispanic, and 36 as black. The 3 groups were compared in terms of analgesic consumption during the postoperative period, measured in morphine equivalents.

Results.—The mean analgesic dosage was 22 mg/day for whites, 16 mg/day for blacks, and 13 mg/day for Hispanics. The difference remained significant even after controlling for demographic and clinical variables such as age, sex, insurance status, and number of diagnoses. There were no ethnic differences in the use of acetaminophen or nonsteroidal anti-inflammatory drugs.

Conclusions.—Analgesic usage for postoperative pain varies by ethnicity, being highest for whites and lowest for Hispanics. The source of these differences is unknown: it could be related to differences in the patients' pain behavior or in the caregivers' perceptions and treatment of them. Ethnic differences in patient-controlled analgesia might be a fruitful area for further investigation.

▶ One of the problems with this study is that we do not know for sure whether there was a bias on the part of the house officers in giving the pain medication to the different racial groups. As the authors point out, ethnicity is a "slippery" concept to define. In this case, however, it would have been easier to classify the patients by race. For example, one does not know whether in the white population the patients were all of Scandinavian or all of Southern European background.

M. Weintraub, M.D.

Improving Analgesic Prescribing in a General Teaching Hospital
McQuillan R, Finlay I, Branch C, et al (Holme Tower Marie Curie Centre, South Glamorgan, Wales; Univ Hosp of Wales, Cardiff)
J Pain Symptom Manage 11:172–180, 1996   16–5

Objective.—In 1 teaching hospital, patients with cancer or HIV disease had poorly controlled pain because of inaccurate diagnosis of the cause of the pain and inappropriate analgesia. Changes implemented to improve patient care were reviewed. Guidelines for physicians and nurses and pain control information for patients were presented.

Methods.—In interviews, 178 patients with cancer or HIV were asked to record their pain on a 4-point scale. Their drugs were recorded. Patients reported pain (40%), nausea, constipation, and mouth soreness. The results were reported and a palliative care service was instituted, which included an acute pain service that developed guidelines, educated staff, had treatment discussions, and convened quarterly meetings with physicians. The survey was repeated 1 year later and 146 patients were interviewed.

Results.—From 1991 to 1993, the use of nonsteroidal anti-inflammatory drugs increased from 6.2% to 13.7% ($P = 0.022$), subcutaneous diamorphine infusions increased from 5.6% to 14.4% ($P = 0.005$), and inappropriate opioid use decreased from 7.3% to 0.7% ($P = 0.004$). Meperidine use (6%) was unchanged. Patients who were interviewed a second time reported a decrease in "worse" scores from 22% in 1991 to 15% to 1993. Of the 53% of staff members who returned their questionnaires, 64% thought the guidelines were useful or very useful, 10% used them frequently or very frequently, and 26% were aware of nurses' guidelines. The palliative medicine registrar was rated helpful by 90% and prompt in responding to referrals by 88%.

Conclusion.—Guidelines and education has improved pain control in hospitalized patients. Continuing education is necessary to sustain this improvement.

▶ These folks deserve credit for doing something constructive about a common problem—inadequate analgesic prescribing. They developed some good guidelines (see the appendixes in the original article), didactic teaching, and "a rapidly responsive clinical advisory service." They wisely conclude that "...ongoing education will be required to maintain this trend to improve patient care." Amen.

L. Lasagna, M.D.

Acute Pain Management: Programs in U.S. Hospitals and Experiences and Attitudes Among U.S. Adults

Warfield CA, Kahn CH (Beth Israel Hosp, Boston; Harvard Med School, Boston)
Anesthesiology 83:1090–1094, 1995   16–6

Introduction.—Inadequate management of acute postoperative pain increases patient discomfort, prolongs recovery, and increases health care costs. The current state of pain management in U.S. community and teaching hospitals is unknown. Two surveys were performed to evaluate the status of pain management in American hospitals and the attitudes of American adults toward postoperative pain management.

Methods.—One hundred teaching hospitals, 100 community hospitals with fewer than 200 beds, and 100 community hospitals with more than 200 beds were surveyed by telephone about their current pain management programs and their plans for future programs. In addition, adults from 500 American households were asked about their attitudes toward, and experiences with, postoperative pain and pain management.

Results.—An acute postoperative pain management program was in place at 42% of the hospitals, and another 13% planned to institute such a program. Almost all the programs offered patient-controlled analgesia, consultation, direct patient management, continuous nerve block techniques, and intraspinal opioids. The most frequent characteristics of these programs included written guidelines, quality assurance measures, on-call personnel, and standards for postoperative pain management.

In the household survey, more than three fourths of adults believed that some pain is necessary after surgery. For 57% of patients who had undergone surgery, postoperative pain was their main fear before surgery. Postoperative pain was reported by 77% of individuals, and 80% of these respondents had moderate-to-extreme pain. More than three fourths had postoperative pain even after receiving their first dose of medication. About half received counseling about postoperative pain, and nearly all believed it was acceptable to complain about postoperative pain.

Discussion.—These surveys document growing professional and public awareness of the importance of postoperative pain management. Formal pain management programs are becoming more common at U.S. hospitals, and pain management is becoming more aggressive. Still, further public and professional education is required to make the problem of postoperative pain less frequent and less severe.

▶ Acute and chronic pain tend to be managed poorly, in large part because of stupidity on the part of physicians and nurses. The opiates, for example, are often given less often and in lower doses than are needed postoperatively because of unfounded fears on the part of medical personnel about the likelihood that patients will have severe respiratory depression or become addicts.

Patients awaiting surgery are rightfully apprehensive about how much pain they will have postoperatively, but their fears could be allayed by talking to them before surgery about what will happen *and* dosing them properly postoperatively. Indeed, our group at Rochester studied this in 1983.[1] Doses "q4h" inevitably lead to poor pain management. If an injection hasn't relieved pain within the first hour, it's not likely to work over the next 3 hours.

L. Lasagna, M.D.

Reference

1. Weis OF, Sriwatanakul K, Weintraub M, Lasagna L: Reduction of anxiety and postoperative analgesic requirements by audiovisual instruction: *Lancet* 8:43–44, 1983.

Intramuscular Ketorolac Versus Oral Ibuprofen in Acute Musculoskeletal Pain
Turturro MA, Paris PM, Seaberg DC (Mercy Hosp, Pittsburgh, Pa; Univ of Pittsburgh, Pa)
Ann Emerg Med 26:117–120, 1995   16–7

Background.—Ketorolac tromethamine, the only parenteral nonsteroidal anti-inflammatory drug (NSAID) available in the United States, may be as effective as other NSAIDs given orally and rectally in relieving postoperative pain. The analgesic efficacy of intramuscular ketorolac was compared with that of oral ibuprofen in patients seeking care in an emergency department for acute musculoskeletal pain.

Methods.—Eighty-two patients, aged 18–70 years, were enrolled in the randomized, prospective, double-blind study. All reported mild-to-moderate acute musculoskeletal pain caused by trauma. Forty-two patients were given 60 mg of ketorolac intramuscularly and a placebo pill. The remaining 40 patients were given 800 mg of ibuprofen and a saline intramuscular injection. Pain was assessed on a visual analogue scale at baseline, at 15-minute intervals for 1.5 hours, and again at 2 hours.

Findings.—Average pain scores improved in both groups during the course of the study. Between-group differences were nonsignificant at all intervals studied. The numbers of patients in the 2 groups dropping out of the study because of insufficient pain relief were also comparable. The prevalence of side effects did not differ significantly between groups.

Conclusions.—Although ketorolac tromethamine is a useful NSAID for patients with acute pain syndromes in whom oral NSAID administration is not possible or practical, ketorolac does not appear to have any other advantages over less costly oral NSAIDs. Because the administration of ketorolac is painful and its cost is so high, its routine use for minor-to-moderate acute musculoskeletal pain is unjustified.

▶ These 2 NSAIDS appeared similar in the doses used, although the pain score averages were a bit better with ibuprofen. If you have a patient who can take oral medication, ibuprofen is at least as good and a *lot* cheaper than parenteral ketorolac.

L. Lasagna, M.D.

Recovery and Complications After Tonsillectomy in Children: A Comparison of Ketorolac and Morphine
Gunter JB, Varughese AM, Harrington JF, et al (Univ of Cincinnati, Ohio)
Anesth Analg 81:1136–1141, 1995   16–8

Hypothesis.—The analgesic equivalence of ketorolac and morphine suggested that the former agent, if administered after tonsillectomy, might hasten recovery and discharge while decreasing vomiting, hopefully without increasing the risk of posttonsillectomy bleeding.

Study Plan.—In a prospective, randomized, double-blind study, 96 children undergoing tonsillectomy received either 0.1 mg of morphine per kg or 1 mg of ketorolac per kg intravenously after the procedure. Recovery was monitored while the patients were hospitalized, and their parents were contacted 24 hours and 2 weeks after tonsillectomy.

Results.—Ketorolac was given to 49 patients after tonsillectomy and morphine to 47. About one third of patients in each group received supplemental morphine in the postanesthesia care unit. There were no significant differences in times to awakening, recovery, or readiness for discharge. Four patients in each group were admitted to the hospital. The ketorolac-treated patients vomited less than those given morphine. Two patients given ketorolac and 1 given morphine required a second operation to control bleeding. Major bleeding in the first 24 hours was more prevalent in the ketorolac group, but there was no subsequent increase in major bleeding after this time.

Conclusions.—Ketorolac increases the risk of bleeding even when given after tonsillectomy. Although it does limit vomiting compared with morphine, ketorolac does not hasten recovery or eliminate unplanned hospital admissions, and its use probably is contraindicated in this setting.

▶ Tonsillectomy, although usually not a serious surgical procedure, can at times lead to significant complications. Opioids can control postoperative pain in such patients but may cause somnolence, respiratory depression, and nausea.

Ketorolac, a nonsteroidal anti-inflammatory drug (NSAID), can provide analgesia equal to that achieved with morphine with less of the adverse effects described here. The drawbacks are that ketorolac depresses platelet function and increases bleeding time, and the incidence of clinically significant bleeding in this study led its authors to conclude that, overall, the risk-benefit ratio does not justify use of the NSAID either before or after adenotonsillectomy.

L. Lasagna, M.D.

Analgesic Efficacy and Safety of Tramadol Enantiomers in Comparison With the Racemate: A Randomised, Double-Blind Study With Gynaecological Patients Using Intravenous Patient-controlled Analgesia

Grond S, Meuser T, Zech D, et al (Univ of Cologne, Germany; Grünenthal GmbH, Stolberg, Germany)
Pain 62:313–320, 1995   16–9

Purpose.—Tramadol (T) is an opioid analgesic that chemically is a racemic mixture of 50% (+) and 50% (−) enantiomers. Studies in animal models revealed that T enantiomers exert their analgesic effects via different modes of action and that the (+) T enantiomer is the more potent one. This randomized, double-blind, phase-II trial was done to assess the analgesic efficacy and safety of the 2 T enantiomers compared with the T racemate.

Patients.—Of 98 patients with severe or maximum postoperative pain after major gynecologic operations under opioid-free halothane anesthesia, 33 were randomized to (+) T analgesia, 33 to (±) T, and 32 to (−) T. After acceptable pain relief was obtained after an IV loading dose of up to 200 mg of the study medication, patients were connected to a patient-controlled analgesia (PCA) device and observed for 24 hours. Patients who dropped out of the study were rated as nonresponders.

Results.—Four patients (12%) in the (+) T group, 5 (15.2) in the (±) T group, and 17 (53%) in the (−) T group dropped out because of inefficacy. Twenty-two patients (67%) from the (+) T group, 16 (48%) from the (±) T group, and 12 (38%) from the (−) T group were responders, defined as those experiencing a decrease of pain intensity on a 5-point scale from severe or maximum pain to mild or no pain within the first hour after the loading dose. Fifty-five patients had 149 episodes of nonserious adverse events, and most episodes occurred in the (+) T group. Twenty-seven patients (82%) in the (+) T group, 25 (76%) in the (±) T group, and 13 (41%) in the (−) T group expressed satisfaction with the pain relief obtained when interviewed.

Conclusions.—The racemate of T is clinically superior to either T enantiomer alone for the treatment of severe postoperative pain because its efficacy is similar to that of (+) T but with fewer side effects.

▶ For years, a few people have been trying to get others to investigate the possibility of interesting differences between a racemate and its component enantiomers. The present study beautifully exemplifies what the enantiomer enthusiasts are talking about.

In animal studies, both enantiomers showed antinociceptive effects, but these were achieved by different modes of action—one behaved like a typical opioid and inhibited serotonin uptake, whereas the other did not behave this way and inhibited noradrenaline reuptake.

In the clinic, the "opioid" enantiomer was clearly superior to the other enantiomer and to the racemate, regardless of whether one was dealing with satisfaction or premature termination of the study because of inefficacy. The price paid for this superior efficacy was an increased incidence of nausea and vomiting, but without a further exploration of dose-response, it is impossible to say whether the superior enantiomer, at lower doses, might still be superior but with equivalent side effects. Fascinating.

L. Lasagna, M.D.

Does Patient-Controlled Analgesia Achieve Better Control of Pain and Fewer Adverse Effects Than Intramuscular Analgesia?: A Prospective Randomized Trial
Nitschke LF, Schlösser CT, Berg RL, et al (Marshfield Clinic, Wis)
Arch Surg 131:417–423, 1996   16–10

Background.—Providing adequate postoperative pain relief while minimizing adverse effects can be frustrating. Three analgesic regimens were compared in a group of patients who underwent colon resection.

Methods.—The prospective, randomized study included 31 patients given patient-controlled morphine sulfate analgesia (PCA), 31 given IM morphine, and 28 given IM ketorolac tromethamine. Patients rated pain on numerical and visual analogue scales in the first 5 postoperative days.

Findings.—Adverse effects were reported by only 2 patients, both receiving PCA. Neither needed to be switched to another group, however. Significantly more patients receiving IM ketorolac needed alternative analgesics than patients in the morphine groups. The patients receiving ketorolac also had a significantly shorter duration of ileus than the patients in either morphine group, and significantly lower pain scores and less postoperative confusion, although missing data complicate the interpretation of these latter findings. Patients given ketorolac had significantly shorter hospital stays than patients given morphine. The 2 morphine groups did not differ significantly in length of stay.

Conclusions.—Ketorolac appears to be superior to IM or PCA morphine for the control of pain, to lessen postoperative confusion, and to minimize length of stay and ileus duration. However, 18% of the patients given ketorolac needed additional analgesia. Also, patients strongly preferred PCA. Most patients should probably receive PCA narcotics for postoperative pain. The addition of ketorolac, however, may decrease narcotic dose and resultant adverse effects. Patients who are especially vulnerable to adverse effects should primarily receive ketorolac.

▶ Patient-controlled analgesia is not perfect (what is?), but it works remarkably well for most patients.

L. Lasagna, M.D.

Morphine Overdose From Patient-controlled Analgesia Pumps

Kwan A (United Christian Hosp, Hong Kong)
Anaesth Intensive Care 24:254–256, 1996   16–11

Introduction.—The use of patient-controlled analgesia (PCA), using a programmable syringe pump to manage acute pain, has increased. This technique reduces staff workload and is associated with high patient satisfaction. Both the technique and the devices have been shown to be extremely safe. However, 2 cases of morphine overdose caused by PCA malfunction were reported.

> *Case 1.*—Man, 30, was given a morphine solution (1 mg/mL) via PCA, programmed for a bolus of 1 mg with a 10-minute lockout time and a 4-hour maximum of 15 mg, after emergency repair of a perforated peptic ulcer. The PCA device was placed on top of the patient's locker. The patient was stable 2 hours after surgery, and the PCA device had 40 mL of morphine left. Two hours later, there was only 30 mL left in the PCA syringe, although the patient was still stable, pain-free, and awake. The nurse found that the syringe was being continually emptied slowly, an action that could not be stopped. Within 5 minutes, 25 mg of morphine was administered, at which time the tubing was disconnected. The patient remained stable but drowsy. He was observed closely and required no treatment to counteract the overdose. He remained pain-free until the fourth postoperative day. Inspection of the PCA device revealed that no alarms had occurred, and the program recorded only 4 total demands and 2 good demands.
>
> *Case 2.*—Man, 72, underwent drainage of a psoas abscess. He was given PCA-delivered morphine at a concentration of 1.0 mg/mL. The device was programmed to deliver a 1-mg bolus with a 10-minute lockout time and a 4-hour limit of 12 mg. The PCA pump was placed on top of the patient's locker. When the patient complained of pain, the nurse encouraged him to make a demand. When he did, the plunger detached from the plunger clamp and completely emptied the syringe, resulting in the delivery of 30 mg of morphine within 1 minute. The patient required IV naloxone and supplementary oxygen. He remained drowsy for 20 hours and pain-free for another day. The PCA pump showed 6 recorded demands, with 3 good demands, and no record of the additional 37 mg delivered.

Discussion.—Although PCA devices are generally safe, problems can occur. Syphoning can occur when the PCA pumps are placed above the level of the patients and no antisyphon valve is used. In addition, unintentional delivery may occur if the plunger breaks away from the plunger clamp.

► In the 15 years since PCA was first described, very few cases of opioid overdoses have been reported. (Additional ones must exist because under-reporting of adverse events is a perennial problem, but the problem seemingly occurs rarely.) When troubles occur, they may be explained by pump failure, incorrect programming, or faulty drug dilution. If the glass syringe is disengaged from the drive mechanism, syphoning of the contents can occur.

L. Lasagna, M.D.

Oral Methadone for Managing Chronic Nonmalignant Pain
Gardner-Nix JS (Scarborough Gen Hosp, Ont, Canada)
J Pain Symptom Manage 11:321–328, 1996   16–12

Objective.—Five patients treated with oral methadone for chronic non-malignant pain unresponsive to other oral or parenteral opioids were described.

> *Case 1.*—Woman, 60, with multiple sclerosis was treated with methadone for radiating back pain of 10 years' duration unrelieved by hydrocodone. With oral methadone, 225 mg 3 times per day, her pain rating subsided to 2 on a scale of 0 to 10. Her methadone treatment costs Can$103.75 per month compared with Can$3,631.16 for hydromorphone given with a subcutaneous pump. Sedation effects improved after a few weeks.
> *Case 2.*—Woman, 36, with unremitting back pain of 10 years' duration unrelieved by surgery received hydromorphone, 56 mg 6 times daily. Her pain rating was 7 on a scale of 0-10. With methadone, 300 mg in the morning and 500 mg at night, and with 32 mg of hydromorphone every 4 hours for breakthrough pain, her pain rating improved to 4. The monthly treatment cost for methadone is Can$133 as compared with Can$931.39 for oral hydromorphone.
> *Case 3.*—Woman, 47, with back pain since her teens, worsening after a traffic accident, was treated unsuccessfully with intravenous hydromorphone infusion at 8 mg/hr plus 8 mg/hr as needed for breakthrough pain. With methadone, 350 mg every 12 hours, as well as 16 mg of oral hydromorphone every 4 hours for break-through pain, her pain rating was 2. Her monthly methadone cost is Can$133 compared with Can$3,204 for hydromorphone.
> *Case 4.*—Man, 56, with radiating left loin pain exacerbated by passing kidney stones, despite using 12–16 tablets of acetamino-phen-oxycodone per day, was given 300 mg of methadone every 8 hours, with 5 oxycodone tablets daily as needed. He had insomnia, a decrease in appetite, weight loss, and a bitter taste. He was given trazodone for insomnia but impotence occurred. Methadone was discontinued. He was given a fentanyl patch, 150 µg/hr with 50 mg

of morphine every 4 hours as needed for breakthrough pain. His weight loss and impotence resolved and his pain rating was 2. His monthly cost for methadone was Can$202.16, for oxycodone Can$349.14, and for fentanyl Can$454.84.

Case 5.—Man, 43, with radiating left loin pain exacerbated when passing kidney stones did not have pain relief with meperidine or morphine injections, a transcutaneous electrical nerve stimulator, or 20–25 tablets of oxycodone-acetaminophen daily. He had sedation at methadone dosages of 125 mg every 12 hours, and a fentanyl patch, 100 µg/hr failed to control his pain. His pain was controlled with long-acting hydrocodone, 96 mg every 12 hours, and 24 mg of hydromorphone every 4 hours for breakthrough pain. He is less sedated. The monthly cost for his oxycodone was Can$349.14 as compared with Can$887.04 for fentanyl and Can$83.00 for methadone. Monthly hydromorphone costs are Can$1,059.84.

Conclusion.—Oral methadone is a cost-effective alternative to other opioids for management of chronic nonmalignant pain in certain patients.

▶ Oral morphine is often effective in patients with chronic pain but doesn't always provide adequate pain relief and sometimes produces intolerable side effects. In some of these latter cases, oral methadone can be effective, convenient to take, and cost-effective.

L. Lasagna, M.D.

NMDA Receptor Blockade in Chronic Neuropathic Pain: A Comparison of Ketamine and Magnesium Chloride
Felsby S, Nielsen J, Arendt-Nielsen L, et al (Aarhus Univ, Denmark; Aalborg Univ, Denmark)
Pain 64:283–291, 1995   16–13

Background.—The clinical characteristics of neuropathic pain conditions have much in common, regardless of different causes and localization, suggesting a possible common pathophysiology. The spinal hyperexcitability observed in neuropathic pain may be related to excitatory amino acids acting at N-methyl-D-aspartate (NMDA) receptor sites. Two drugs that block the NMDA channel in different ways—ketamine and magnesium chloride—were studied for their effects on chronic neuropathic pain.

Methods.—The double-blind, placebo-controlled study included 10 patients with peripheral neuropathic pain. Ketamine was given by a 10-minute bolus infusion of 0.84 µmol/kg = 0.2 mg/kg, followed by a continuous infusion of 1.3 µmol/kg/hr = 0.3 mg/kg/hr. Magnesium was given by a 10-minute bolus infusion of 0.16 mmol/kg, followed by a continuous infusion of 0.16 mmol/kg/hr. Pain was assessed by various methods, including visual analog scale, area of touch-evoked allodynia, and detection and pain thresholds to mechanical and thermal stimuli.

Results.—With ketamine, spontaneous pain was reduced by 57% and the area of allodynia by 33%. These reductions were significant. In contrast, the 29% reduction in pain and the 18% reduction in allodynia achieved by magnesium chloride was not significant. With ketamine, the reduction in pain was significantly correlated with the reduction in area of touch-evoked allodynia. Neither treatment affected thresholds of pain or detection in response to mechanical or thermal stimuli.

Conclusions.—The ongoing pain and allodynia observed in patients with neuropathic pain appear to be interrelated phenomena. Both may be mediated by the same mechanism, which may involve an NMDA receptor. In the current study, some patients responded to ketamine but not magnesium, whereas others responded to magnesium but not ketamine.

▶ Neuropathic pain responds poorly to nonsteroidal anti-inflammatory drugs and opiates. It frequently responds to tricyclic antidepressants, particularly the "old-fashioned" representatives of the class, which do not include the specific serotonin reuptake inhibitors. In any case, we are still searching for therapies for neuropathic pain that are useful in the paroxysms of shooting pain, the burning or lightning-like pain, and the hyperalgesia that some patients feel. This study may allow us to think about a mechanism of the neuropathic pain and its relation to the NMDA receptor.

M. Weintraub, M.D.

The Analgesic Response to Intravenous Lidocaine in the Treatment of Neuropathic Pain
Ferrante FM, Paggioli J, Cherukuri S, et al (Brigham and Women's Hosp, Boston; Harvard Med School, Boston)
Anesth Analg 82:91–97, 1996   16–14

Background.—Intravenous lidocaine has long been used to provide analgesia in patients with neuropathic pain of different causes. However, basic pharmacologic relations, such as dose-response curves, have not been elucidated fully. Concentration-effect and dose-response relations for the clinical administration of IV lidocaine in patients with neuropathic pain of varying etiologies were determined.

Methods.—Thirteen patients received IV lidocaine, 500 mg, at a rate of 8.35 mg/min over 60 minutes. Every 10 minutes during that time, visual analog pain scores and venous blood samples were obtained. Serum samples also were taken for determining serum and serum water lidocaine levels at the onset of analgesia and when pain was relieved completely.

Findings.—The dose-response relation showed large increases in pain relief for concomitant minimal increases in dosage. The ED_{50} and ED_{90} differed by 44.5 mg of lidocaine. The concentration-effect also was steep. Pain scores abruptly declined over a range of 0.62 µg/mL of lidocaine. The free concentration of lidocaine was not better correlated with analgesia onset or complete analgesia than the serum concentration of lidocaine.

Thus, the mechanism of analgesia to IV lidocaine may not be based on a conventional concentration-effect relation.

Conclusions.—In patients with neuropathic pain, large increases in analgesic response appear to be attained with very minimal dosage increases in IV lidocaine. The analgesic response to IV lidocaine is best described as a precipitous "break in pain" over a narrow dosage and concentration range.

▶ The traditional dose-response curve for analgesics tends to be relatively flat. Thus, in clinical trials, it is very hard to distinguish different doses of analgesics, even when they are separated by a factor of 2 or 3. Nonsteroidal anti-inflammatory drugs frequently have such a dose-response relation. Apparently, that is not true for lidocaine, which has a remarkably steep dose-response curve, according to this abstract. Certainly, the study has to be repeated with a placebo, but it is very interesting and exciting. It seems that lidocaine-induced analgesia developed in many of the patients as if a switch had been turned on at a particular concentration of lidocaine. It appears that the lidocaine concentration between 2.5 and 3 µg/mL of whole blood was the critical concentration.

M. Weintraub, M.D.

Opioid-induced Muscle Activity: Implications for Managing Chronic Pain
Sylvester RK, Levitt R, Steen PD (North Dakota State Univ, Fargo; Univ of North Dakota, Grand Forks)
Ann Pharmacother 29:1118–1121, 1995   16–15

Introduction.—Involuntary muscle contractions are now recognized as an adverse effect of opioid therapy. However, opioid-related muscle hyperactivity remains a little-recognized problem of unknown mechanism. Management options for a case of opioid-induced involuntary muscle hyperactivity were studied.

> *Case Report.*—Man, 71, with primary mucinous adenocarcinoma of the lung, was referred for radiation therapy of a spinal metastatic lesion. The patient, who was ventilator dependent, had metastasis-related pain. His transdermal fentanyl therapy was titrated to 200 µg/hr, and he began receiving increasing doses of orally administered morphine solution for breakthrough pain. Two days later, continuous morphine infusion was begun. The patient's responsiveness declined and involuntary muscle hyperactivity began; the hyperactivity appeared to represent breakthrough pain. By this time, the patient was unable to communicate. Over a 7-day period, his morphine infusion rate increased from 22 to 717 mg/hr, with no change in muscle hyperactivity. A consulting pharmacist suggested that the muscle hyperactivity could be an adverse effect

of opioid therapy, and recommended decreasing the patient's morphine infusion while monitoring for changes in muscle hyperactivity and level of consciousness. The family decided to withdraw the patient's ventilator support before this or another intervention could be implemented.

Discussion.—The possibility of opioid toxicity must be remembered when muscle hyperactivity develops in an unresponsive patient receiving chronic opioid therapy. Assuming that the involuntary muscle movements simply indicate breakthrough pain may lead to unnecessary escalation of opioid doses. In this situation, the opioid dose should be reduced by 20% to 30% per day until the muscle hyperactivity resolves or the patient can communicate again. Alternatively, clonazepam, 0.5 mg 3 times a day, can be tried, with incremental doses of 0.5–1.0 mg every 3 days to achieve the desired response.

▶ The first reports of opioid-induced involuntary muscle activity incriminated meperidine and fentanyl. These movements have included tremors, twitches, myoclonus, and tonic-clonic seizures. Since then, morphine, hydromorphone, and heroin have been added to the list. The mechanism is unknown.

If such activity occurs during general anesthesia, one can give a neuromuscular blocker, with or without thiopental, and quickly stop the muscular manifestations. In conscious patients, the therapeutic options are nowhere as clear. Benzodiazepines (and especially clonazepam) seem to help.

L. Lasagna, M.D.

Opioid Therapy for Chronic Nonmalignant Pain: A Review of the Critical Issues
Portenoy RK (Mem Sloan-Kettering Cancer Ctr, New York)
J Pain Symptom Manage 11:203–217, 1996   16–16

Objective.—Physicians avoid prescribing opioids for chronic nonmalignant pain because of exaggerated fears of addiction, side effects, tolerance, and impaired psychosocial functioning for the patient and potential regulatory sanctions for themselves. Favorable experiences with opioid-treated patients call these fears into question and argue for a reevaluation of prescribing practices.

Discussion.—Reviews of 9 published surveys of opioid therapy for treatment of chronic nonmalignant pain were summarized. Contrasting results from other reports emphasize the variability of patient responses. Critical issues to consider in patient populations likely to realize sustained pain relief from opioid drugs include therapeutic efficacy, adverse effects, and dependence/addiction/abuse. Therapeutic efficacy is evaluated in terms of the balance between analgesia and side effects, length of response, and effect on functional outcome. Adverse effects are measured in terms of organ toxicity and side effects. Physical dependence resulting in withdrawal effects, addiction or risk of addiction leading to aberrant behavior, and abuse resulting in overmedication are major areas of concern. Guidelines for the management of opioid therapy, based on clinical experience, were proposed and included recommendations for opioid use only after other types of analgesia have failed, informed consent, dosing regimens, patient involvement in care, a maximum of 1 month between patient visits and prescriptions initially, specific assessments, and appropriate documentation. The guidelines also provided a list of contraindications for opioid treatment, a list of behaviors that may indicate addiction/dependence/abuse, and suggestions on when hospitalization may be appropriate.

Conclusion.—Current experience with treatment of chronic nonmalignant pain with opioids does not support the fears many physicians have about such prescribing. Long-term controlled trials are needed to validate clinical experience.

▶ Opioid therapy for chronic nonmalignant pain is often avoided because of exaggerated worries on the part of physicians about addiction, tolerance, side effects, and psychosocial functioning. This article pleads for a less fearful approach wedded to the safe assumption that no 2 patients are alike.

L. Lasagna, M.D.

Randomized Evaluation of Controlled-Release Codeine and Placebo in Chronic Cancer Pain
Dhaliwal HS, Sloan P, Arkinstall WW, et al (Ontario Cancer Treatment and Research Found, Thunder Bay, Canada; Univ of Kentucky, Lexington; Kelowna Gen Hosp, BC, Canada et al)
J Pain Symptom Manage 10:612–623, 1995   16–17

Objective.—Codeine is commonly combined with analgesics for treating mild to moderate pain. There are few data on the use of codeine on its own for the management of chronic cancer pain. Controlled-release (CR) codeine was assessed for efficacy and safety in the treatment of chronic cancer pain.

Methods.—The randomized, double-blind, crossover study included 35 patients with chronic cancer pain. The patients received 7 days of treatment with CR codeine and 7 days of treatment with placebo in double-blind fashion. Pain intensity was assessed on a visual analog scale and a 5-point categorical scale. The need for acetaminophen-plus-codeine as "rescue" medication also was recorded.

Results.—All pain scores were significantly lower with CR codeine than with placebo. In addition, the patients used about half as much rescue medication while using CR codeine compared with placebo. Patients and investigators alike expressed a preference for CR codeine over placebo.

Conclusions.—Controlled-release codeine is an effective therapy for chronic cancer pain. It is a flexible and convenient treatment with a

12-hour duration of action, which permits uninterrupted sleep and improves compliance. It also has the potential to reduce dependence on caregivers, improve quality of life, and increase control over pain management.

▶ I used to think that codeine alone was not very effective. It was, of course, used as an adjunct to various other drugs, but my feeling was that in amounts necessary to achieve pain control, it caused pretty bad constipation and had a ceiling effect. In addition, it is not as good as other drugs, particularly the anti-inflammatory agents, in bone pain. However, this study makes us reevaluate the use of codeine. One weakness of this study is that the dose-response data are unclear because all the doses were merged together. Investigators often have trouble separating doses of analgesics from one another. Even a doubling of dose may not be easily distinguished. Still and all, we have to reevaluate codeine treatment in cancer pain.

M. Weintraub, M.D.

Patient-controlled Analgesia With Nitrous Oxide in Cancer Pain
Keating HJ III, Kundrat M (Veterans Affairs Med Ctr, Des Moines, Iowa; Univ of Iowa, Iowa City)
J Pain Symptom Manage 11:126–130, 1996   16–18

Background.—Patients with cancer often have inadequate pain relief and/or breakthrough pain with movement. Nitrous oxide has been suggested as an approach to prompt control of breakthrough pain. However, there have been concerns about its environmental safety. The efficacy and environmental safety of an improved patient-controlled delivery system for nitrous oxide were studied.

Methods.—Six patients with uncontrolled pain related to advanced cancer were studied. In a room with an exhaust fan enabling 12 room air exchanges per hour, the patients were instructed in the use of a bedside, patient-controlled inhalation system delivering nitrous oxide and oxygen at a 50%/50% concentration, which patients received by inspiring through a plastic mouthpiece with a 1-way valve. Pain was rated subjectively and objectively, and a quality-of-life questionnaire was administered before and 15 minutes after use of the system. Nitrous oxide detection badges were worn by the nursing staff and kept at the patients' bedsides.

Results.—The patients required a mean of 10.3 inhalations (range, 1–16) to relieve pain. The treatments were well tolerated and usually described as pleasant. The few negative reactions included lightheadedness, dry mouth, nausea, headache, anxiety, and a cold feeling. The monitoring badges recorded nitrous oxide levels of less than 2 ppm, a level well below safe environmental requirements. Pain was significantly improved, by both subjective and objective ratings, with pain relief lasting 30 minutes to 2 hours. There were significant reported improvements in stress and life satisfaction by the patients.

Conclusions.—Nitrous oxide can be safely delivered with a patient-controlled device, with minimal environmental exposure. This technique produces significant improvements in controlling cancer-related pain and in quality of life. Further study is warranted.

▶ The analgesic properties of nitrous oxide have been known for 2 centuries, and in the mid-nineteenth century Horace Wells, a dentist, noticed at a stage show that 1 of the participants, while under the influence of nitrous oxide, injured himself but seemingly felt no pain. The next day Wells had one of his own teeth painlessly extracted by a colleague while breathing the gas.

This study is a follow-up to a 1983 report by Fosburg and Crone[1] on the usefulness of nitrous oxide in treating refractory pain in the terminally ill. Improved delivery systems have been developed to allay concerns about the environmental safety of nitrous oxide.

L. Lasagna, M.D.

Reference

1. Fosburg MT, Crone RK: Nitrous oxide for refactory pain in the terminally ill. *JAMA* 250:511–513, 1983.

Aspirin or Acetaminophen? A Comparison From Data Collected by the Spanish Drug Monitoring System
Carvajal A, Prieto JR, Requejo AA, et al (Univ of Valladolid, Spain)
J Clin Epidemiol 49:255–261, 1996   16–19

Background.—Aspirin and acetaminophen are the most commonly prescribed and used self-medications. They have been shown to have comparable efficacy for some indications. However, they may have differing toxicity profiles. The characteristics of adverse reactions to the 2 drugs were compared.

Methods.—All records of adverse reactions to aspirin or acetaminophen occurring between 1982 and 1991 were obtained from the database of the Spanish Drug Monitoring System and reviewed.

Results.—There were 423 reports of adverse reactions related to aspirin use and 147 reports related to acetaminophen use. The mean patient age was significantly older in the aspirin group than in the acetaminophen group. There were no significant gender differences. The rate of adverse reactions to acetaminophen remained stable across patient age groups, whereas the rate of aspirin-related adverse reactions increased with age. Reaction severity was significantly associated with exposure time and cumulative dose and was significantly greater with aspirin than with acetaminophen overall. Severity also increased with age. Hepatic reactions were related to aspirin use in 2 patients and to acetaminophen use in 4 patients. Renal damage occurred in 2 aspirin users and no acetaminophen users. Congenital malformations were attributed to aspirin use in 25 patients (3%) and to acetaminophen use in 16 patients (7%). There were 8 fatal adverse reactions in the aspirin group, including 5 gastrointestinal tract reactions and 3 cases of blood dyscrasias. Of the 5 fatal acetaminophen reactions, 3 were blood dyscrasias and 2 were fetal deaths.

Conclusions.—Aspirin-related adverse reactions appear to be more severe than acetaminophen-related adverse reactions. The 2 drugs had similar proportions of death, malformation, and renal damage, whereas hematologic and hepatic effects were more common with acetaminophen use.

▶ Spain has had, since 1982, a collaborative network for reporting and assessing adverse drug reactions. This report deals with 2 old and widely used antipyretic analgesics. They both work and both can produce side effects, but their pharmacologic profiles differ with regard to details of both harm and benefit.

Aspirin clearly poses a greater risk of gastrointestinal bleeding, whereas acetaminophen use (at least at high doses) carries with it the risk of liver damage.

L. Lasagna, M.D.

Chronic Use of Symptomatic Headache Medications
Von Korff M, Galer BS, Stang P (Group Health Cooperative of Puget Sound, Seattle; Univ of Washington, Seattle; Applied Health Care Research, Glaxo, Research Triangle Park, NC)
Pain 62:179–186, 1995   16–20

Background.—Headache patients commonly use symptomatic headache medications, including acetaminophen, aspirin, opioids, non-steroidal anti-inflammatory medications, muscle relaxants, and ergotomine tartrate. However, frequent use of these medications may increase the likelihood of chronic headache. The prevalence of chronic use of symptomatic headache medications and the predictors of chronic use were investigated among primary care patients with headache.

Methods.—A total of 662 patients complaining of headache during a 1-year period were interviewed at 3–6 weeks, 1 year, and 2 years after their primary care visit. During the interview, data were collected on medication use patterns within the previous month, headache diagnosis, pain, depressive symptoms, and the use of pain-focused coping strategies. Chronic/frequent users were defined as patients who reported (during at least 2 of the interviews) the use of a medication at least 14 days during the previous month.

Results.—Chronic/frequent use of a class of symptomatic headache medication was reported by 21% of the patients, and 2.6% were classified as chronic/frequent polypharmacy users. Chronic/frequent use was twice as common with over-the-counter medications as with prescription medications. In multivariate analysis, chronic/frequent use was significantly associated with increasing age and the number of headache days.

Conclusions.—There is a high prevalence of chronic/frequent use of symptomatic headache medications among primary care patients with headache. Older patients and those with persistent headache may be at particular risk. Primary care physicians should elicit information about long-term patterns of medication use in their patients with headache and counsel these patients about the risks of frequent and long-term use of headache medications. Prophylactic and psychological approaches to headache management should be emphasized.

▶ Headaches are all too common, and some are caused by drugs by mechanisms that are not all that clear. Chronic headache sufferers do, of course, take drugs to relieve their pain, so it's not easy to decide in a given patient whether chronic medication is a cause of headache or a response to the headaches.

L. Lasagna, M.D.

Ketoprofen, Paracetamol and Placebo in the Treatment of Episodic Tension-Type Headache

Dahlöf CGH, Jacobs LD (Gothenburg Migraine Clinic, Sweden; Rhône-Poulenc Rorer GMBH, Köln, Germany)
Cephalalgia 16:117–123, 1996   16–21

Background.—The most common headache type is the episodic tension-type headache. The occasional use of analgesics is an important complementary therapy for such headaches. The efficacy and tolerability of a single oral dose of ketoprofen 25 mg were compared with those of single doses of ketoprofen 2 × 25 mg, paracetamol 500 mg and 1,000 mg, and placebo in patients with episodic tension-type headache.

Methods.—Twenty-seven women and 13 men, aged 19 to 56 years, were included in the double-blind, randomized, placebo-controlled trial. In each of 30 patients, 5 attacks of episodic tension-type headache were treated with a single dose of each medication. The minimum interval between attacks was 72 hours. Reductions in headache pain intensity from baseline to 2 hours after intake were assessed on a 100-mm visual analog scale.

Findings.—Ketoprofen 50 mg was significantly better than placebo and paracetamol in decreasing headache pain intensity. Neither paracetamol dose differed significantly from placebo. There were few adverse effects, usually mild or moderate in severity. Such events did not differ among treatments.

Conclusions.—Ketoprofen 50 mg appears to be an effective analgesic in the treatment of moderate or severe episodic tension-type headache. Its tolerability seems to be satisfactory compared with that of placebo and paracetamol.

▶ In a conference held at the Food and Drug Administration, the consensus of the group of visiting experts was that, although many pains could be included under the rubric of "aches and pains," 2 types of pain would be necessary to tease out because of either a specificity or a difficulty in studying them. The first was menstrual cramps, which were felt to be specifically related to prostaglandin synthesis, and the second was headache. To a certain extent, this was because of the difficulty of studying headache populations, of characterizing them, and of encompassing different types of headache. Even in this study published in *Cephalalgia,* one could question the diagnostic criteria used for episodic tension-type headache. For example, the headaches could be occurring with migraine headaches. They had to have a history of at least 1 year, although many people with sudden onset or recent onset of headache would require a workup, in my opinion. This study was done as a Latin Square, which is very sensitive to drop-outs, and, in fact, 10 patients dropped out of the study. They did find that ketoprofen was an effective drug and that the others, including 1,000 mg of acetaminophen, were not distinguishable from placebo. Perhaps the study worked out in the end.

M. Weintraub, M.D.

ACE Inhibitors for Prophylaxis of Migraine Headaches
Bender WI (Spokane Headache Clinic, Wash)
Headache 35:470–471, 1995

16–22

Introduction.—For individuals with headache frequency that impedes their daily life, migraine headache prophylaxis with daily medication is helpful. Current available agents have several side effects, including fatigue, drowsiness, dry mouth, impotence, and weight gain. For migraine prophylaxis, a good response was obtained with angiotensin-converting enzyme (ACE) inhibitors.

Methods.—Seventeen patients (age range, 18–59 years) with moderate-to-severe migraine headaches occurring at least twice a month were given an ACE inhibitor for prophylaxis. Most were given enalapril; some were given lisinopril. The mean daily dose was 16.4 mg (range, 10–25 mg).

Results.—Treatment lasted 3 months to 3 years. Ten patients reported marked improvement, 6 had moderate improvement, and 1 had slight improvement. Cough was the main side effect; it was intolerable in 3 patients.

Conclusions.—The presence of sustained benefit and the lack of side effects should prompt further investigation of the use of ACE inhibitors as migraine prophylaxis, even though their mechanism of action is unknown. Doses of the ACE inhibitors were considerably higher than those usually used for treating hypertension. A high degree of satisfaction with their quality of life was noted by patients who continued to receive this treatment.

▶ This is another example of serendipity (a term coined by the 18th century English novelist Horace Walpole, after 3 princes of Serendip, the ancient name for then Ceylon, now Sri Lanka, who were constantly stumbling upon truths for which they were not searching). One lady reported that migraines ceased when she went on an antihypertensive medication, enalapril.

This was an open study, with doses of ACE inhibitors higher than those usually employed to lower blood pressure. Impressive results!

L. Lasagna, M.D.

The Efficacy and Safety of Subcutaneous Sumatriptan in the Acute Treatment of Menstrual Migraine

Facchinetti F, for the Sumatriptan Menstrual Migraine Study Group (Istituto di Clinica Ostetrica e Ginecologica, Modena, Italy; Constantiaberg Medi-Clinic, Capetown, South Africa; Lääkärikeskus Meditori, Turku, Finland; et al) *Obstet Gynecol* 86:911–916, 1995   16–23

Introduction.—Menstrual migraine may affect anywhere from 7% to 30% of the total population of patients who have migraines. Among the many approaches to treatment of menstrual migraine is sumatriptan, a serotonin agonist at the vascular receptor subtype. Retrospective and open-label studies have suggested that subcutaneously administered sumatriptan is an effective treatment for menstrual migraine. Sumatriptan's efficacy and safety in the acute treatment of menstrual migraine were evaluated in a double-blind, placebo-controlled trial.

Methods.—The study included outpatients with menstrual migraine at 40 centers in 6 countries. On enrollment, the patients were given a syringe containing either sumatriptan 6 mg or placebo and instructed to inject the medication as the first treatment for their next 2 attacks of menstrual migraine. The medications were administered with an autoinjector device. Two hundred sixty patients were randomized; 179 injected either sumatriptan or placebo to treat at least 1 attack. The study definition of headache relief was reduction of a severe or moderately severe headache to a mild headache, or complete resolution of the headache.

Results.—No significant difference in efficacy was found between the first and second attacks. Two hours after treatment, patients receiving sumatriptan reported headache relief in 73% of first attacks and 81% of second attacks. In contrast, relief was reported after placebo treatment in only 31% of first attacks and 29% of second attacks. In both groups, headache recurred within 24 hours after treatment of the first attack in more than 50% of patients. Sumatriptan was fairly well tolerated. The adverse events—including dizziness or vertigo, nausea or vomiting, and paresthesia—were similar to those previously reported.

Conclusions.—Subcutaneously administered sumatriptan appears to be an effective and well-tolerated treatment for menstrual migraine. Although sumatriptan does have some adverse effects, most are short-lived and resolve on their own. Patients at risk for coronary artery disease should be carefully evaluated before receiving subcutaneously administered sumatriptan.

▶ Menstrual migraine is a fairly common type of migraine. It obviously responds to sumatriptan.

L. Lasagna, M.D.

Preemptive Oral Treatment With Sumatriptan During a Cluster Period
Monstad I, Krabbe A, Micieli G, et al (Hedmark Sentralsykehus, Elverum, Norway; Rigshospitalet, Copenhagen; Clinica Neuropatologica, Policlinico, Pavia, Italy; et al)
Headache 35:607–613, 1995   16–24

Introduction.—Characterized by recurrent unilateral attacks of headache of great intensity and brief duration (30 to 120 minutes), cluster headache often is accompanied by local signs and symptoms of autonomic dysfunction. In the acute treatment of cluster headache, a single 6-mg subcutaneous injection of sumatriptan has been shown to be effective in 2 previous placebo-controlled studies. Some patients, however, have more than 1 attack per day, and the recommended number of sumatriptan injections is 2 in a 24-hour period. For these patients, it would be better if the number of attacks could be reduced or prevented. The effectiveness of oral treatment with 100 mg of sumatriptan 3 times a day for 7 days in aborting the cluster period or reducing the number of attacks was evaluated in a placebo-controlled study.

Methods.—The effect of a 1-week period of preemptive treatment with oral sumatriptan was studied on 169 patients in this multinational, multicenter, randomized, double-blind, placebo-controlled study. The frequency and severity of the cluster headaches were measured during this period, as were the safety and tolerability of the drug. The patients were randomly assigned to receive 100 mg of sumatriptan 3 times a day or a placebo.

Results.—There was not a significant reduction in the number or severity of cluster headache attacks among the patients who received sumatriptan. During the treatment period, oral sumatriptan was not associated with an altered or increased adverse event profile. There was a 50% reduction in the number of attacks in 22% of the patients who received the placebo. This 50% reduction also was achieved by 23% of the patients who took sumatriptan.

Conclusion.—Preemptive oral treatment with sumatriptan is ineffective in reducing or preventing cluster headache attacks.

▶ A friend of mine used to say that no one did large clinical trials unless the outcome was known beforehand. This trial, of course, was a money-saving activity and ensured that the investigators would all be doing good work toward their promotion or attainment of tenure. Unfortunately, this multinational, multicenter, randomized, double-blind, placebo-controlled trial in 169 patients did not work out that way. If anything, the placebo group did somewhat better than the sumatriptan group, at least in the last 4 days of the observation week. In all other parameters, the 2 groups were identical. In fact, the means were identical and even looked "cooked" or "dry-labeled."

M. Weintraub, M.D.

Oral Acyclovir Therapy Accelerates Pain Resolution in Patients With Herpes Zoster: A Meta-analysis of Placebo-controlled Trials
Wood MJ, Kay R, Dworkin RH, et al (Birmingham Heartlands Hosp, England; S-Cubed, Sheffield, England; Columbia Univ, New York; et al)
Clin Infect Dis 22:341–347, 1996   16–25

Background.—The pain associated with herpes zoster is the primary reason that patients desire medical care. Four placebo-controlled, randomized, double-blind trials of 800 mg of oral acyclovir given 5 times daily for 7 to 10 days for the treatment of herpes zoster have been completed. A meta-analysis of these studies was conducted to assess the effects of acyclovir on zoster-associated pain.

Study Design.—A total of 691 patients were involved in the 4 studies. The analysis was performed on an intent-to-treat basis. The pain end points were complete cessation of pain, cessation of moderate to severe pain, cessation of postherpetic neuralgia, and the first pain-free period. The numbers of patients with postherpetic neuralgia at 3 and 6 months also were determined.

Results.—Greater age and more severe pain at presentation were associated with more and prolonged pain. Acyclovir increased pain resolution at all pain end points. The benefit of acyclovir was greatest in patients older than 50 years of age. Fewer patients treated with acyclovir had postherpetic neuralgia at 3 and 6 months than those treated with placebo.

Conclusions.—This meta-analysis demonstrated that acyclovir was effective in the treatment of zoster-associated pain, especially in the higher-risk group of older patients with herpes zoster.

▶ This was a "good" meta-analysis because it supported my own analysis of the literature and refuted the one study with negative results. Using freedom from pain as the outcome criterion also was very good. In fact, although we frequently can help patients feel better when we cannot cure them, it is better to know that we can treat people and completely eradicate their pain.

M. Weintraub, M.D.

Hemodialysis-Related Pruritus: A Double-blind, Placebo-controlled, Crossover Study of Capsaicin 0.025% Cream

Tarng D-C, Cho Y-L, Liu H-N, et al (Veterans Gen Hosp-Taipei, Taiwan; Natl Yang-Ming Univ, Taipei, Taiwan)
Nephron 72:617–622, 1996   16–26

Background.—Between 37% and 86% of all patients receiving maintenance hemodialysis experience pruritus, which has a major effect on their quality of life. Although many causes of this complication have been identified, the underlying mechanisms are not well understood, and the many treatments proposed for it remain controversial. The local application of capsaicin depletes the peripheral neurons of substance P, a neuropeptide implicated in pain mediation and some itch sensations. The safety and efficacy of capsaicin 0.025% cream in treating hemodialysis-related pruritus was evaluated in a double-blind, placebo-controlled, crossover study.

Methods.—Nineteen patients receiving hemodialysis with idiopathic, moderate to severe pruritus were enrolled and 17 completed the trial. Capsaicin or placebo base cream was applied to localized areas of pruritus 4 times a day. Pruritus severity and adverse treatment effects were recorded weekly.

Findings.—Fourteen of the 17 study completers reported marked relief. Five had complete remission of pruritus during capsaicin use. Capsaicin was significantly more effective than placebo. A prolonged antipruritic effect was observed 8 weeks after treatment. There were no serious adverse effects or significant changes in serum albumin, calcium, phosphorus, alkaline phosphatase, or intact parathyroid hormone levels during capsaicin or placebo use.

Conclusions.—In some patients receiving maintenance hemodialysis, idiopathic pruritus may be transmitted by substance P from the peripheral sensory neurons to the CNS. Topical capsaicin markedly improves pruritus in such patients.

Clinical and Urodynamic Effects of Intravesical Capsaicin Treatment in Patients With Chronic Traumatic Spinal Detrusor Hyperreflexia

Geirsson G, Fall M, Sullivan L (Reykjavik City Hosp, Iceland; Univ Hosp, Göteborg, Sweden)
J Urol 154:1825–1829, 1995   16–27

Background.—Intravesical capsaicin has been recommended as a way to reduce detrusor hyperreflexia in patients with incontinence from various spinal cord diseases. Hypothetically, capsaicin could block afferent signals from the bladder mechanoreceptors in patients with chronic spinal lesions, reducing hyperreflexia. It also may block the afferent signals from the bladder cooling reflex. The efficacy of capsaicin in reducing bladder hyperreflexia in patients with chronic traumatic spinal detrusor hyperreflexia was investigated.

Methods and Findings.—Ten men with traumatic chronic spinal lesions were included in the study. Capsaicin solution, 2 mM, dissolved in 30% alcohol was instilled into the bladder and left in place for 30 minutes. Improvement in bladder function, expressed as an increase in cystometric capacity or a reduction in maximal detrusor pressure, was documented in all but 1 patient. Treatment effects persisted for 2 to 7 months. The ice water test was negative in half the patients immediately after capsaicin administration.

Conclusions.—Capsaicin treatment was beneficial in these patients with chronic traumatic spinal detrusor hyperreflexia. Its positive effects may be explained by the blocking of C fiber afferents. The optimal dosage and treatment interval have yet to be established. The ice water test may be used to monitor the ideal dosage.

Double-blind, Placebo-controlled Study of the Application of Capsaicin Cream in Chronic Distal Painful Polyneuropathy
Low PA, Opfer-Gehrking TL, Dyck PJ, et al (Mayo Found, Rochester, Minn)
Pain 62:163–168, 1995   16–28

Background.—Capsaicin (CAPS) has been reported to show a weak beneficial effect in the treatment of painful diabetic neuropathy. It is an alkaloid that depletes tissues of substance P (SP) and reduces neurogenic plasma extravasation, the flare response, and chemically induced pain. The efficacy of topical CAPS in the treatment of chronic distal painful polyneuropathy was evaluated in a double-blind, placebo-controlled, randomized study.

Study Design.—The 2 study limbs were assigned to CAPS, in a 0.075% cream, or placebo (PLAC) applied 4 times a day for 8 consecutive weeks. The first tube contained the active PLAC, methyl nicotinate. In the final 4-week, single-blind, washout phase, PLAC was administered bilaterally. The following scales were used to assess efficacy: investigator global; patient global; visual analog (VAS) of pain severity; VAS of pain relief; activities of daily living; and allodynia. Safety was assessed using a neurologic disability scale, nerve conduction studies, computer-assisted sensory examination for vibration and thermal cooling and warming, quantitative sudomotor axon reflex test (QSART), and quantitative flare response.

Patients.—Forty patients with bilateral symmetric chronic painful neuropathy of the lower extremities were enrolled, and 39 completed the 12-week study. All had neuropathic pain of long duration (median, 56 months) and moderate, relatively nonselective impairment of large- and small-fiber function. Half the patients had idiopathic distal small-fiber neuropathy and only 7 had diabetes.

Results.—The efficacy indices did not differ significantly between the CAPS and PLAC sides at 4 and 8 weeks of treatment, with no loss of benefit during the final 4-week washout phase. A few indices favored the PLAC at early time points (1–4 weeks), presumably because of the hyperalgesia and intensification of burning pain that was common on the CAPS side. The percentages of patients who reported improvement with CAPS and PLAC, respectively, were 51.4 and 53.8 at 4 weeks, 56.4 and 64.1 at 8 weeks, and 59.0 and 66.7 at 12 weeks. All the safety indices showed no differences between sides.

Conclusion.—In patients with chronic distal painful neuropathy, the large percentage of limbs that improve may reflect a pronounced PLAC response. There is no evidence of a change in neurogenic flare response, which is largely caused by SP; in quantitative sensory tests of small-fiber function using thermal cooling and thermal warming; or in postganglionic sudomotor function measured using QSART to suggest that the effects of CAPS sufficiently deplete SP when applied to intact skin.

▶ In the first of these 3 papers (Abstracts 16–26 through 16–28), the capsaicin was effective in ameliorating the itching of patients undergoing hemodialysis. Unfortunately, itching tends to worsen during and immediately after dialysis. The investigators chose to apply the therapy to a specific area, such as the anterior or posterior aspect of the legs, arms, or trunk. I believe that this is a good way to treat itching because attacking one of the worst spots seems to make the itching become milder all over. Unfortunately, the effects of capsaicin make it very difficult to carry out a crossover study, as was done in the abstracted paper.

In the second study, the capsaicin was put directly into the bladders of men with spinal cord lesions. Again, this very interesting study should be corroborated with a placebo-controlled trial.

The last study was a double-blind, placebo-controlled parallel group study, which should overcome the design defects of both the previous studies. However, this was not a positive study. The authors go to great lengths to search for possibilities, as they should, for why the study was not positive. It appears we still have quite a ways to go in understanding capsaicin and helping it work in many diseases.

M. Weintraub, M.D.

Analgesics and Cancers of the Renal Pelvis and Ureter
Linet MS, Chow W-H, McLaughlin JK, et al (Natl Cancer Inst, Bethesda, Md; Internatl Epidemiology Inst, Rockville, Md; Univ of Southern Calif, Los Angeles; et al)
Int J Cancer 62:15–18, 1995   16–29

Background.—Although renal pelvis and ureter (RPU) cancers are relatively rare, their incidence has been increasing in the United States. An increased risk of these cancers has been associated with cigarette smoking and analgesic use. The carcinogenic risks of analgesic agents were further investigated in a large, population-based, case-control study.

Methods.—The study was conducted in 3 regions of the United States. Five hundred two patients with RPU cancers and 496 control patients were interviewed between 1983 and 1986.

Findings.—None of the nonprescription nor prescription analgesics evaluated were associated with an increased risk of RPU cancer. Regular users of phenacetin, acetaminophen, and aspirin did not have a significantly increased risk. In addition, increased risk was not correlated with cumulative lifetime intake or duration of regular use of these drugs alone or combined. A slight increase in risk was noted among long-term acetaminophen users. Patients reporting the highest cumulative doses, the longest duration of phenacetin use, or both did not have an increased risk.

Conclusions.—Neither phenacetin nor aspirin was found to be associated with a significantly increased risk of RPU cancer. The nonsignificant excess risk observed among long-term acetaminophen users suggests the need for continued surveillance of the long-term effects of this analgesic agent.

▶ This study contradicts several earlier studies that found trouble from phenacetin (rarely ever used alone). This may simply reflect the past removal of this analgesic from most analgesic combinations. I do not know what to make of the data on acetaminophen, because overall the drug's troubles have generally involved the liver and not the genitourinary tract.

L. Lasagna, M.D.

17 Psychiatric Disorders

Long-term, Nightly Benzodiazepine Treatment of Injurious Parasomnias and Other Disorders of Disrupted Nocturnal Sleep in 170 Adults
Schenck CH, Mahowald MW (Univ of Minnesota, Minneapolis; Hennepin County Med Ctr, Minneapolis)
Am J Med 100:333–337, 1996   17–1

Introduction.—Studies of benzodiazepine treatment have reported a low risk of inappropriate use, psychological dependence, and physiologic tolerance. However, there is little information on these risks with long-term treatment with benzodiazepines. To examine the efficacy, dose stability, adverse effects, and abuse potential with benzodiazepines, a 12-year experience with these agents in a large number of patients with chronic severe sleep disorders was reviewed.

Methods.—Over 12 years, 170 adults with long-term sleep disorders were treated by 1 physician. The specific sleep disorder diagnoses included injurious sleepwalking and sleep terrors (in 69 patients), rapid-eye-movement sleep behavior disorder (in 52), chronic severe insomnia (in 25), and restless legs syndrome/periodic limb movement disorder (in 24). All were treated with benzodiazepines (most commonly clonazepam) nightly for at least 6 months.

Results.—Complete or nearly complete control of the sleep disorders was achieved by 86% of the patients. After 6 months, the benzodiazepine dose was the same or lower than the starting dose in 71% of the patients. Drug discontinuation or dose reduction generally did not produce withdrawal symptoms. Adverse effects, including mild morning sedation, subjective memory dysfunction, and alopecia, occurred in 15.9%. Thirteen patients required dose reduction or substitution of another benzodiazepine. Relapses of alcohol- or substance-abuse disorders occurred in 4 patients, and 3 other patients occasionally took excessive doses.

Conclusions.—Benzodiazepines are highly effective in the long-term treatment of disruptive sleep disorders, with dose stability, safety, and a low risk of abuse. A history of alcohol or substance abuse need not be automatically considered a contraindication for benzodiazepine treatment.

The findings in the patients with chronic insomnia, however, cannot be generalized to the treatment of typical insomnia.

▶ Sleep gurus tend to decry the chronic use of hypnotic drugs, fearful that these drugs will lose effectiveness and cause addiction. This has always seemed to me a philosophy of despair for the millions of patients with chronic insomnia. This study is welcome news: long-term benzodiazepine use was effective and safe. Bravo!

L. Lasagna, M.D.

Effects of Triazolam on Sleep, Daytime Sleepiness, and Morning Stiffness in Patients With Rheumatoid Arthritis

Walsh JK, Muehlbach MJ, Lauter SA, et al (St Luke's Hosp, Chesterfield, Mo)

J Rheumatol 23:245–252, 1996   17–2

Background.—Patients with rheumatoid arthritis (RA) frequently complain of disordered sleep and undue fatigue during the day. As many as two thirds of patients are affected, and a number of them try hypnotic medications. Usually musculoskeletal pain and stiffness is blamed, but appropriate treatment does not necessarily improve sleep, and some anti-inflammatory drugs may themselves disrupt sleep.

Objective.—A polysomnographic study was planned in 15 patients with definite or classic RA to compare the effects of the benzodiazepine hypnotic triazolam and placebo on insomnia and daytime sleepiness.

Methods.—Using a double-blind crossover design, triazolam or placebo was given 30 minutes before retiring on 7 consecutive nights. The initial dose was 0.25 mg for patients aged 30–59 years and half that for older patients. The dose was doubled after the second night if the clinical response was inadequate. The last 2 nights of each week were spent in the sleep laboratory. Daytime sleepiness and the severity of arthritic symptoms were estimated using visual analog scales.

Results.—Total sleep time was significantly greater during triazolam therapy, chiefly because of increased stage 2 sleep. Slow-wave sleep was significantly less during triazolam therapy, whereas rapid eye movement latency was longer. Twelve of the 15 patients were less sleepy during the day when given triazolam. Morning stiffness lasted longer during placebo treatment, but there were no other significant differences in arthritic activity.

Conclusion.—The judicious use of a short-acting hypnotic agent may provide better sleep and decrease morning stiffness in patients with RA.

▶ Insomnia, from whatever cause, exacts a considerable toll in productivity, car accidents, and other undesirable consequences. The present study shows the benefits of effective hypnotic therapy in patients with RA during the short term but leaves unanswered what the effects of chronic hypnotic intake would be. Would triazolam taken repeatedly for many months (or years) lose its effectiveness or lead to physical dependence? Because RA is almost invariably a chronic illness, poor sleep is going to be a challenge for lots longer than a week. I was fascinated by the mysterious (or at least unexplained) decrease in morning stiffness.

L. Lasagna, M.D.

Continuing Clozapine Despite Neutropenia
Wesson ML, Finnegan DM, Clark PI (Clatterbridge Hosp, Bebington, Wirral, England)
Br J Psychiatry 168:217–220, 1996   17–3

Background.—Clozapine treatment carries approximately a 3% cumulative risk of neutropenia and almost a 1% cumulative risk of agranulocytosis. Patients receiving clozapine are monitored to ensure their safety. In some cases, a strict policy of stopping clozapine because of neutropenia may unnecessarily deny patients the chance to benefit from this treatment, especially if the neutropenia is not related to clozapine. A patient who continued to benefit from clozapine treatment despite unrelated neutropenia is reported.

> *Case Report.*—Man, 40, began taking clozapine for chronic schizophrenia, with dramatic improvement in his behavior. Two years later, he was found to have a right testicular swelling that was suspected of being malignant. He initially refused treatment but ultimately underwent orchidectomy and cytotoxic chemotherapy for testicular teratoma with pulmonary metastases. With the agreement of the Clozaril Patient Monitoring Service, it was decided that the patient should continue taking clozapine despite the hematopoietic suppression caused by his chemotherapy. The rationale was that stopping the drug would lead to worsening of the patient's behavior and thus prevent him from receiving chemotherapy. The patient was treated under close supervision on the oncology ward, with daily monitoring of his blood counts. After 4 courses of chemotherapy, the patient's metastases resolved, and his predicted 5-year survival was 85%.

Discussion.—A patient in whom clozapine treatment was continued despite non–clozapine-related neutropenia is described. The patient and everyone involved in his or her treatment must give consent in exceptional cases of this type. The situation would be different for a patient designated as an exceptional case for psychiatric reasons only—for safety, such a patient should not be allowed to restart clozapine after a "red alert."

▶ Clozapine causes agranulocytosis in approximately 1% of patients taking it, but 3 times that number develop neutropenia. This case suggests that neutropenia due to other causes need not be an absolute contraindication to the use of clozapine in patients with refractory schizophrenia.

L. Lasagna, M.D.

Antidepressant Use in the Elderly: Association With Demographic Characteristics, Health-related Factors, and Health Care Utilization
Brown SL, Salive ME, Guralnik JM, et al (Natl Inst on Aging, Bethesda, Md; Universita Cattolica, Rome; Ctrs for Disease Control, Atlanta, Ga; et al)
J Clin Epidemiol 48:445–453, 1995   17–4

Background.—Depression occurs in up to 45% of hospitalized elderly persons, and more than 10% of elderly persons living in the community may have been reported to have significant depressive symptoms. The characteristics of antidepressant use and its correlates were investigated.

Methods and Findings.—Data were obtained on a total of 13,074 persons in the 4 Established Populations for Epidemiologic Study of the Elderly (EPESE) communities. Antidepressants were significantly more likely to be prescribed for women than for men. African Americans were significantly less likely than whites to take antidepressant medication. The health-related measures associated with antidepressant use were poor self-perceived health, polypharmacy, disability in activities of daily living, and a history of stroke. Each variable pertaining to health care utilization (number of physician visits, overnight hospitalization in the preceding year, and use of a regular physician) was correlated with antidepressant use in at least 2 of the communities. A multivariate regression model indicated that higher antidepressant use was significantly correlated with female gender, race, poor self-perceived health, and a greater number of contacts with physicians in the past year.

Conclusion.—This analysis indicated that antidepressant use among the elderly was associated with demographic factors, health-related variables, and health care utilization. The differences found in treatment by race were striking and merit additional research.

Antidepressants and the Elderly: Double-blind Trials 1987-1992
Anstey K, Brodaty H (Univ of Queensland, Australia; Prince Henry Hosp, Little Bay, Australia)
Int J Geriatr Psychiatry 10:265–279, 1995   17–5

Background.—Although the empirical evidence from antidepressant trials in elderly patients has been reviewed, the studies included were performed between 1964 and 1986. Since that time, several new drugs with the promise of fewer adverse effects have been introduced. The new data were reviewed to determine whether particular antidepressants were superior in the treatment of depression in elderly persons.

Methods and Findings.—The review included all double-blind studies of antidepressants reported between 1987 and 1992 and involving subjects aged 55 years or older with a primary diagnosis of major or clinical depression. The annual rate of trials conducted since 1987 was higher than that during the period between 1964 and 1986. About 27% of the patients initially enrolled withdrew before the trials were completed. Study completers had a general decrease of about 55% in scores on the Hamilton Rating Scale for Depression. The agents studied did not vary in efficacy. Although the newer antidepressants (especially the selective serotonin reuptake inhibitors) seemed to have fewer side effects, methodologic shortcomings limited the interpretation of the findings.

Conclusion.—Currently, the efficacies of the major antidepressants do not differ from one another in elderly patients. Thus, detailed information on the adverse effects associated with an antidepressant, the symptoms for which it is of most value, and the reasons for withdrawal would be most useful to clinicians. Future studies would benefit from more standardized methodology and reporting of results.

▶ I always have trouble separating out poorer self-perceived health, greater contact with physicians, and more significant health problems as a cause or a result of antidepressant use, particularly in the elderly. This paper (Abstract 17–4) relates to another one in this edition of the YEAR BOOK as hip fracture was significantly associated with antidepressant use in 2 of the 4 communities. Although underutilization of antidepressants does occur, we still have to worry about adverse effects, such as hip fractures.

The second paper (Abstract 17–5) reviews data from the 5-year period 1987 to 1992 and critiques the types of studies and their manner of being carried out. The authors believe that the studies were underpowered. Also, the study populations did not include people who were very old, people in institutions, and physically frail people as well. In any case, the trials in the elderly, although they at least exist and have supplied very important kinds of information, could be better.

M. Weintraub, M.D.

Dosing of Antidepressants: The Unknown Art
Jerling M (Karolinska Inst, Huddinge, Sweden)
J Clin Psychopharmacol 15:435–439, 1995   17–6

Objective.—It can be difficult to determine the right dose of a tricyclic antidepressant (TCA) because of treatment failure, individual kinetic variability, and other reasons. Plasma therapeutic concentration ranges have been suggested for the TCAs amitriptyline (AT) and nortriptyline (NT). The principles followed by physicians in the dosing of AT and NT were studied; a comparison of the concentrations achieved with the suggested therapeutic ranges and the effects of therapeutic drug monitoring (TDM) was included.

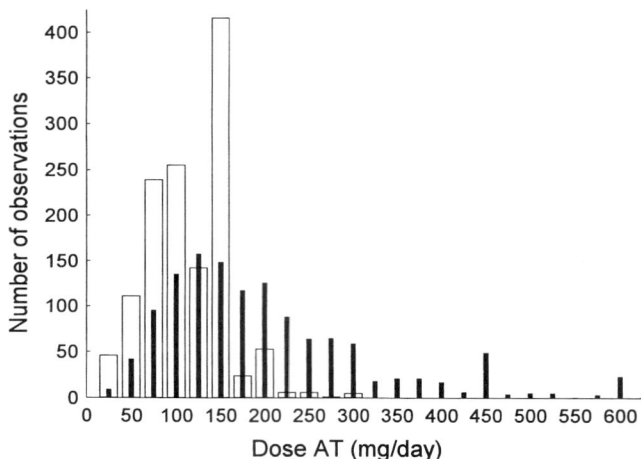

FIGURE 4.—Prescribed doses (*open bars*) and the doses calculated to give a concentration of amitriptyline (*AT*) plus nortriptyline in plasma of 150 ng/mL (*filled bars*) in a therapeutic drug-monitoring study of patients treated with AT. (Courtesy of Jerling M: Dosing of antidepressants: The unknown art. *J Clin Psychopharmacol* 15(6):435–439, 1995.)

Methods.—Data from a hospital TDM laboratory on 2,393 observations in 1,606 patients taking AT or NT were analyzed. Factors related to the prescribed doses and the measured antidepressant concentrations were evaluated by linear multiple regression.

Results.—Older patients received significantly smaller doses of both AT and NT, although age does not have any major impact on the kinetics of

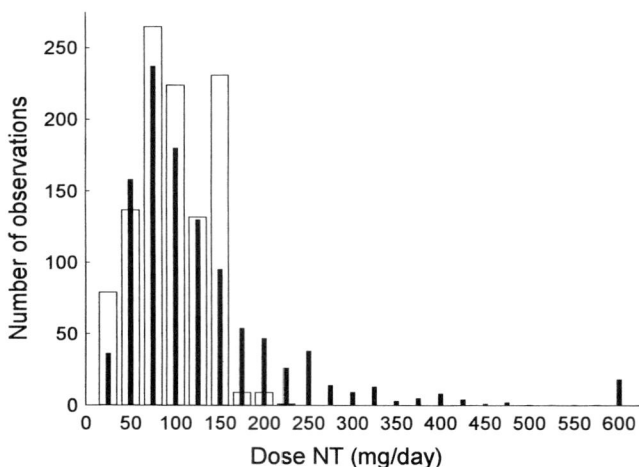

FIGURE 5.—Prescribed doses (*open bars*) and the doses calculated to give a concentration of nortriptyline (*NT*) in plasma of 100 ng/mL (*filled bars*) in a therapeutic drug-monitoring study of patients treated with NT. (Courtesy of Jerling M: Dosing of antidepressants: The unknown art. *J Clin Psychopharmacol* 15(6):435–439, 1995.)

these drugs. When interactions with other drugs occurred, they were not managed by adjusting the dose of the antidepressant. The effects of drugs that inhibited the effects of the cytochrome P450 enzyme CYP2D6 were not considered, and inpatients and outpatients had similar dose-adjusted concentrations. In patients taking AT for whom more than 1 concentration analysis was available, TDM increased the proportion of concentrations within the suggested therapeutic range. However, this was not the case for patients taking NT. With both drugs, there was a tendency to give low doses (Figs 4 and 5).

Conclusion.—This TDM study shows large kinetic variability for TCAs in the population, which must be managed by individualized dosing. However, as currently practiced, this individualization is often based on incorrect principles. The role of TDM in identifying kinetic outliers who need higher or lower than usual doses is particularly important at the start of treatment.

▶ The author is correct to criticize inept prescribing of antidepressants in terms of dosage. However, he should be more accepting of the possibility that physicians prescribe lower doses for older patients *not* because they believe there to be age-dependent differences in their pharmacokinetics, but because of a belief that there may be age-dependent differences in pharmacodynamics, with resultant greater predisposition in the elderly to adverse effects.

L. Lasagna, M.D.

Outcomes of "Inadequate" Antidepressant Treatment
Simon GE, Lin EHB, Katon W, et al (Univ of Washington, Seattle)
J Gen Intern Med 10:663–670, 1995   17–7

Background.—Antidepressant treatment in primary care may often be inadequate. Depressed patients in primary care frequently receive low doses of antidepressants or stop medication before its benefits are apparent. The outcomes of patients given low levels of antidepressants in primary care were investigated.

Methods.—Twenty primary care physicians prescribed antidepressants to 88 patients. Thirty-nine percent received imipramine; 23%, desipramine; 11%, fluoxetine; 11%, nortriptyline; and 16%, other antidepressants. Fifty-six percent of the patients received at least 30 days of antidepressant therapy at the recommended dosages. Treatment classified as adequate consisted of mean daily doses of 141 mg (expressed as imipramine-equivalent doses), and that considered inadequate, 56 mg.

Findings.—The likelihood of receiving adequate drug therapy was unassociated with patient age, gender, medical comorbidity, and the severity of depression at baseline. After 4 months, all patients had marked clinical improvement. Patients receiving low-intensity treatment were less likely to respond clinically than patients receiving adequate pharmacotherapy.

However, at 4 months the between-group differences in scores on the Symptom Checklist depression scale and the proportion of patients with continuing major depression were not significant. These findings were replicated in another 157 patients.

Conclusions.—Although the improvement rates among patients receiving recommended dosages of drug therapy were somewhat higher than among those receiving inadequate dosages, the latter group also had good short-term outcomes. Efforts to improve pharmacotherapy for depressed patients in primary care should focus on the subgroup who do not respond to initial treatment.

▶ It's hard to criticize a physician who prescribes "low" doses of an antidepressant for patients who respond to such doses. But criticism *is* deserved if failure to respond to such low doses is not followed by an escalation of dose. The latter often is done by medical center physicians to whom "failures" are referred, with good outcomes.

L. Lasagna, M.D.

Treatment Discontinuation With Selective Serotonin Reuptake Inhibitors Compared With Tricyclic Antidepressants: A Meta-analysis
Anderson IM, Tomenson BM (Univ of Manchester, England)
BMJ 310:1433–1438, 1995   17–8

Introduction.—Per tablet, the first-generation tricyclic antidepressants (TCAs) are less expensive than the newer selective serotonin reuptake inhibitors. However, the TCAs may actually be less expensive if there are problems with compliance and treatment failure. Previous research was analyzed to compare the treatment discontinuation rates of selective serotonin reuptake inhibitors vs. TCAs.

Methods.—The meta-analysis included 62 randomized, controlled trials comprising 6,029 patients with major unipolar depression. The studies compared 1 of 5 selective serotonin reuptake inhibitors against a TCA. The 2 types of drugs were compared for their rates of treatment discontinuation, including cases caused by side effects and treatment failure.

Results.—The selective serotonin reuptake inhibitors had an overall discontinuation rate 10% lower than that of the TCAs. The dropout rate related to side effects was 25% lower with the newer drugs, whereas no significant difference was noted in dropout rate related to treatment failure. The various selective serotonin reuptake inhibitors analyzed had similar dropout rates.

Conclusion.—In terms of overall dropout rate, the selective serotonin reuptake inhibitors appear to be better tolerated than the TCAs. This difference is explained by the smaller number of dropouts related to side effects. However, the difference is fairly small and may, therefore, be clinically irrelevant; the compliance advantage of selective serotonin reuptake inhibitors should not be overestimated in analyses of cost effectiveness.

▶ As the authors point out, it is important to see not only how often different drugs for the same indication are discontinued because of side effects, but also how large the differences are, how clinically relevant they are, and how much they cost.

L. Lasagna, M.D.

Falls Among Older People: Relationship to Medication Use and Ortho-static Hypotension
Liu BA, Topper AK, Reeves RA, et al (Univ of Toronto)
J Am Geriatr Soc 43:1141–1145, 1995   17–9

Background.—Falling has significant consequences for the health and independence of older people. Medication use and orthostatic hypotension are 2 factors that have been widely proposed as risk factors for falls among the elderly. The significance of these 2 factors was examined prospectively among healthy, independent older people.

Methods.—One hundred older residents of self-care residential facilities who could stand unaided were studied. Prescription medications were documented at baseline. Blood pressure measurements were obtained after 5 minutes of supine rest, immediately upon standing, and after 5 minutes of standing. Orthostatic symptoms were determined by direct inquiry. Falls were monitored for 1 year by weekly report.

Results.—At least 1 fall was reported by 61% of the subjects, with 39% falling at least twice. Antidepressant use was significantly associated with an increased risk of falling. However, no other classes of medication were associated with falling. There were no differences in the prevalence of either orthostatic hypotension or orthostatic symptoms between fallers, recurrent fallers, and nonfallers. Antidepressant use was not significantly associated with orthostatic hypotension.

Conclusion.—Antidepressants were the only class of medications associated with falling. In contrast to some other studies, the risk of falling was not related to the use of either diuretics or sedative-hynotics. Also in contrast to other reports, orthostatic hypotension and orthostatic symptoms were unrelated to the risk of falling.

▶ Some epidemiologists say that unless the risk ratio is 2 or greater, the result of a study is not really significant, even if the *P* value is < 0.05. We really do not know why elderly people fall, although we have suspected that medications play a role. However, even long-acting benzodiazepines have not been uniformly shown to cause falls in various studies. Still, falls are so dangerous because of their almost inevitable, often irreversible, negative cycle. We have to be careful and attack every cause that we can find. That is why, even though a risk ratio of 1.6, as found in this particular study, is not very high, we should still pay attention to antidepressants and long-acting benzodiazepines. We should even be paying attention to medications that cause postural hypotension. With the aging of the population (the mean age in this particular study was 83 years), falls will be an increasingly important topic. We do know that classes in exercise training can help elderly people avoid falls, and we should be recommending them for all our elderly patients.

M. Weintraub, M.D.

Serotonin Syndrome: A Potentially Fatal Complication of Antidepressant Therapy
Corkeron MA (Sir Charles Gairdner Hosp, Perth, Australia)
Med J Aust 163:481–482, 1995   17–10

Background.—Serotonin syndrome is a potentially fatal complication of drugs that have a serotonergic effect on the CNS. This syndrome is not widely recognized. Serotonin syndrome in a patient taking monoamine oxidase inhibitors and selective serotonin reuptake inhibitors was studied.

Case Report.—Man, 39, sought medical care for a 3-hour history of tremor, sweating, and agitation. He had taken his first dose of the selective serotonin reuptake inhibitor sertraline 12 hours before seeking treatment. Chronic therapy with the monoamine oxidase inhibitor tranylcypromine was stopped 36 hours before the sertraline dose. On initial assessment, this patient was drowsy and restless, with marked tremor, global hypertonia, and hyperreflexia. Increased salivation and bowel sounds were noted. The patient's condition deteriorated markedly during the next half hour. He became increasingly confused and had gross hypertonia and myoclonus, fixed midsize pupils, increasing tachycardia, a rapid temperature increase to 38.8°C, profuse sweating, and skin flushing. Serotonin syndrome caused by interaction between tranylcypromine and sertraline was diagnosed provisionally, and ventilation with paralysis and sedation was instituted. The patient's condition improved progressively thereafter.

Conclusions.—Patients with serotonin syndrome may die of rhabdomyolysis, disseminated intravascular coagulation, respiratory distress syndrome, or cardiovascular collapse. The diagnosis of serotonin syndrome is made when the patient has at least 3 of the following: altered mental state, agitation, myoclonus, hyperreflexia, diaphoresis, tremor, shivering, diarrhea, incoordination, and fever; has had agents with serotonergic properties recently prescribed or increased in dose; and has had other causes or the use of neuroleptic agents excluded.

▶ This author suggests that this potentially fatal complication of antidepressant therapy is most likely to occur in patients on either monoamine oxidase inhibitors or selective serotonin reuptake inhibitors. Prescribing physicians need to know the presenting features. Ideally, the patient should also know what to look for and to report promptly to the doctor. (One should try to inform without producing an exaggerated anxiety, which may be tough to do!)

The syndrome is not the same as the tyramine-related hypertensive crisis or the neuroleptic malignant syndrome.

L. Lasagna, M.D.

Renal Function On and Off Lithium in Patients Treated With Lithium for 15 Years or More: A Controlled, Prospective Lithium-Withdrawal Study
Bendz H, Sjödin I, Aurell M (Univ Hosp, Lund, Sweden; Univ Hosp, Linköping, Sweden; Univ of Göteborg, Sweden)
Nephrol Dial Transplant 11:457–460, 1996   17–11

Background.—Studies of the reversibility of lithium effects of renal function have yielded conflicting results. The magnitude and reversibility of reduced renal function in patients on long-term lithium treatment were further investigated.

Methods.—Thirteen patients who had taken lithium for 15–24 years were included in the study. The patients were studied at 5 and 9 weeks after lithium was discontinued. A control group of age- and sex-matched psychiatric patients not taking lithium was studied for comparison.

Findings.—After lithium was stopped, the glomerular filtration rate (GFR) improved from 69 to 74 mL/min/1.73 m^2 body surface area, which did not differ significantly from control values. Only 2 of the previous lithium users had decreased GFR, compared with none of the control subjects. There was no improvement in maximal urinary concentration capacity, which was 637 mOsm/kg H_2O in the lithium patients and 856 mOsm/kg H_2O in the control subjects. Two lithium users had isothenuria.

Conclusions.—Patients who receive lithium often have irreversible, clinically important decreases in maximum urinary concentration capacity. This condition can progress to nephrogenic diabetes insipidus. In most lithium users, GFR is well preserved.

▶ The withdrawal study is a powerful technique for the assessment of drug effects. Of course, it's better if done with substitution of a placebo, but it can be very valuable to help understand whether people need a therapy or, as in this case, whether renal function will return to normal when the drug is stopped. This particular study was done as a comparison, not of certain individuals with others who remained on lithium, but of all patients removed from lithium and a matched control group of psychiatric patients. Patients in this study could not concentrate their urine even after withdrawal from lithium.

The thyroid effects of lithium are also well described. I wonder how many patients had an increased thyroid gland size and what happened to the gland after discontinuation of lithium. In any case, this was a valuable assessment of the effects of lithium during withdrawal.

M. Weintraub, M.D.

Pharmacologic Therapies in Dementia
Fleming KC, Evans JM (Mayo Clinic Rochester, Minn)
Mayo Clin Proc 70:1116–1123, 1995   17–12

Introduction.—It may be difficult, in a given case, to decide whether dementia-related behaviors require intervention or should merely be observed and tolerated. Possible approaches include psychosocial intervention, assessment of concurrent medical disorders, and training caregivers in behavioral management. Drugs may often help but are best used in conjunction with nonpharmacologic measures.

Impaired Cognition.—Acetylcholinesterase inhibitors counter cognitive symptoms in a few patients with mild-to-moderate Alzheimer's disease (AD). Ergoloid mesylates have proved ineffective for this purpose. Some have recommended a trial of psychostimulants such as methylphenidate, but improved cognitive function has not been documented in patients with dementia. Chelation treatment—popular for a time—is no longer in favor. Aspirin has been proposed in late-onset AD because of the presence of vascular risk factors.

Psychiatric and Behavioral Disorders.—Demented patients may have substantial symptoms of depression and anxiety. Patients who are agitated, uncooperative, or hallucinatory have occasionally responded to neuroleptic therapy. If a neuroleptic drug is tried, a shorter-acting agent such as haloperidol is preferred. Benzodiazepines have not been established as effective in the setting of dementia, and they may themselves impair cognition, produce sedation, and increase the risk of falling. Antidepressant therapy is appropriate when major depression supervenes in a patient with dementia. Patients with AD who are resistant to neuroleptic therapy reportedly have become less hostile and more cooperative when given carbamazepine. β-Blockers have been used to control aggression in patients with traumatic brain injury, but they have not been systematically evaluated in patients with dementia-related behavioral problems.

▶ The demented elderly are a growing problem as our civilization "grays," but the drugs available to slow down cognitive decline are pretty poor. For the lonely folks in nursing homes, drugs are a staff cop-out and no substitute for human attention.

L. Lasagna, M.D.

Resolved: Autistic Children Should Have a Trial of Naltrexone
Campbell M (New York Univ)
J Am Acad Child Adolesc Psychiatry 35:246–247, 1996   17–13

Objective.—There is evidence that treatment with the opiate antagonist naltrexone can reduce hyperactivity, and possibly self-injurious behavior, in children with autism. However, there have been no placebo-controlled studies demonstrating naltrexone's ability to reduce a range of severely maladaptive behaviors in a clinically meaningful way. The research supporting the use of naltrexone treatment for children with autism is reviewed.

Naltrexone in Autism.—Naltrexone treatment for children with autism is of interest because of the possible role of the endogenous opioid system in the development of autism and self-injurious behavior and because of the need for psychoactive agents not associated with tardive dyskinesia. The author's research group assigned 41 hospitalized children with autism to receive naltrexone or placebo. The naltrexone dose was 1 mg/kg/day, given in a single morning dosage for 3 weeks. Naltrexone was associated with significant reductions in hyperactivity and "hyperactivity factor," with a significant increase in hypoactivity and a trend toward lower restlessness. There were no significant changes in weight or laboratory parameters, and side effects were rare and transient. The findings need confirmation in larger, double-blind, placebo-controlled studies.

The author's study did not show a significant reduction in self-injurious behavior with naltrexone, although there was some rebound of self-injurious behavior after the end of naltrexone treatment. Naltrexone-related reductions in self-injurious behavior may have been related to the baseline level of such behavior.

Recommendations.—The available evidence suggests that naltrexone may be helpful in a subgroup of children with autism. Its effectiveness and safety should be further examined in patients with prominent symptoms of hyperactivity, self-injurious behavior, or both. Pending further studies, naltrexone should be used only in children with autism who do not respond to haloperidol or another standard neuroleptic drug.

▶ Pharmacotherapy has made only minor contributions to the management of children with autism, so one can appreciate Dr. Campbell's unwillingness to dismiss the possibility that naltrexone might be helpful for a subset of these children.

L. Lasagna, M.D.

Pharmacotherapy of Adult Attention Deficit/Hyperactivity Disorder: A Review

Wilens TE, Biederman J, Spencer TJ, et al (Massachusetts Gen Hosp, Boston; Harvard Med School, Boston)

J Clin Psychopharmacol 15:270–279, 1995   17–14

Background.—The persistence of attention deficit/hyperactivity disorder (ADHD) into adulthood is an increasingly recognized disorder. The use of pharmacotherapy for adults with this disorder is not as well established as its use in children and adolescents. The efficacy and dosing parameters of various agents used in the treatment of adult ADHD were reviewed.

The Use of Pharmacotherapy in Adult ADHD.—Seven studies of psychostimulants in a total of 193 subjects and 10 studies of nonstimulant medications in a total of 167 subjects were identified. The latter group of studies included antidepressants, antihypertensives, and amino acids. Most double-blind studies were of psychostimulants, and most open studies were of the nonstimulant agents, generally antidepressants. Diagnostic criteria, dosing parameters, and response rates varied markedly among the studies. The aggregate controlled studies demonstrated that the stimulants had a clinically and statistically significant effect on the decrease of ADHD symptoms. Open studies of the nonserotonergic antidepressants showed a moderate anti-ADHD effect.

Conclusions.—The current literature appears to support the use of robust doses of stimulants and antidepressants for adult ADHD. Additional controlled studies with strict diagnostic criteria and outcome methodology are needed to better delineate the pharmacotherapeutic options in this patient population.

▶ The average reader of this review should take away a couple of points: that adult ADHD exists and it's not even so rare, and that there are a whole host of adequate treatments for the signs and symptoms of this syndrome. In addition to the symptoms that really do define the syndrome (impulsive behavior, hyperactivity, and inattention or distractibility), there are common adult symptoms, such as poor concentration ability, that lead to marked inattention, easy distractibility, day dreaming and forgetfulness (although not of names in those of us who are older than 50 years of age), and a frequent shift in activities. Of course, as the syndrome gets away from these core and main symptoms, it begins to describe almost everybody who is an adult.

I believe that adult deficit disorder happens after head injuries, strokes, and CNS infectious diseases, although without any data, I hasten to add, in a number of people who had attention deficit disorder as children. The article found that stimulants did work and that in open trials antidepressants of the nonserotonergic type were helpful as well. What's needed now is a repeat of these studies in large groups of patients who have the very well-documented core symptoms and main ancillary symptoms.

M. Weintraub, M.D.

The Acute Management of Aggressive Behaviour in Hospitalized Children and Adolescents

Measham TJ (McGill Univ, Montreal)
Can J Psychiatry 40:330–336, 1995   17–15

Background.—Health care professionals must manage acutely aggressive behaviors among children and adolescents in various hospital settings. The efficacies of different practices were assessed and research needs determined.

Review.—The available literature on management techniques used in child psychiatric wards was reviewed. Pharmacotherapy, psychotherapy, seclusion, restraint, and the use of *pro re nata* medications were described in the literature. Some aspects of aggression in child psychiatric settings have been associated with caregiver and setting characteristics. Diphenhydramine was found to be ineffective. Time-out procedures were the only management strategies found to be effective. There are currently no studies comparing different management strategies. Restrictive management strategies were found to be most successful in milieus enriched enough so that children prefer to remain in them. Restrictive management strategies should be used only when there is an open discussion of patients and staff interactional styles and when these methods are reviewed regularly.

Conclusions.—Little evidence exists for the long-term efficacy of most strategies used to manage acutely aggressive behaviors. More research is needed before safer and more effective management techniques can be established.

▶ This important problem has not been adequately studied in the past. This thoughtful paper deserves to be read in full, because there are no neat "bottom lines."

L. Lasagna, M.D.

A Long-term, Double-blind, Placebo-controlled Crossover Trial of the Efficacy of Fluoxetine for Trichotillomania

Streichenwein SM, Thornby JI (Baylor College of Medicine, Houston)
Am J Psychiatry 152:1192–1196, 1995   17–16

Background.—There is no generally recognized treatment for trichotillomania. However, trichotillomania has recently been linked to the spectrum of obsessive-compulsive disorders that can be effectively treated with new drugs such as clomipramine and selective serotonin reuptake inhibitors. Trials of serotonin reuptake inhibitors have had mixed results in patients with trichotillomania. The efficacy of long-term treatment with high-dose fluoxetine in patients with trichotillomania was examined with a double-blind, placebo-controlled, crossover study.

Methods.—Sixteen patients with trichotillomania without psychiatric comorbidity completed a 31-week trial that included an initial 2-week placebo washout phase, a 12-week treatment with either fluoxetine or placebo, a 5-week washout period, and a 12-week treatment phase with the alternate substance. The patients underwent a physical examination at the beginning and end of the trial. Laboratory tests were performed at baseline, week 6, week 17, and at the end of the trial. Depression was evaluated at weeks 1, 6, 12, 18, 23, and 29. The patients were asked to place all hairs pulled into an envelope each day.

Results.—The patients had a history of hair-pulling behavior that ranged from 2 to 40 years (mean, 19 years). Most patients had comorbid disorders, particularly anxiety disorders. There were no significant improvements in any of the studied variables during treatment, compared with placebo. The physical examinations and laboratory tests were all normal. Adverse effects were experienced during both treatment phases and included nightmares, insomnia, dizziness, irritability, anxiety, and gastrointestinal and genitourinary symptoms.

Conclusions.—Fluoxetine treatment, even at high doses, does not improve symptoms in patients with trichotillomania. This suggests that trichotillomania is different from other obsessive-compulsive disorders in that serotonin may not be the primary dysfunctional neurotransmitter.

▶ The theoretical background for this particular study was quite good. Fluoxetine is effective in obsessive-compulsive disorder. Trichotillomania is, in a sense, more than an impulse control disorder as defined in the *Diagnostic and Statistical Manual of Mental Disorders,* ed 4, but it has a flavor of an obsessive-compulsive disorder. Individuals note an increasing tension immediately before they act out and pull out their hair, or when they attempt to avoid that particular behavior. They also feel a sense of relief when pulling out the hair. Well, this is one of those negative studies that got published. Fluoxetine was ineffective in halting hair pulling behavior in this crossover study. I guess we're stuck with clomipramine in the treatment of trichotillomania.

M. Weintraub, M.D.

18 Pulmonary Disorders

Iodinated Glycerol Has No Effect on Pulmonary Function, Symptom Score, or Sputum Properties in Patients With Stable Chronic Bronchitis
Rubin BK, Ramirez O, Ohar JA (St Louis Univ, Mo)
Chest 109:348–352, 1996   18–1

Introduction.—A previous study showed that treatment with iodinated glycerol (IG) improved subjective well-being for patients with chronic bronchitis. However, this study did not provide objective data on pulmonary function or sputum clearance. The effects of IG therapy on quality of life, pulmonary function, and sputum properties were studied in patients with chronic bronchitis.

Methods.—The randomized, placebo-controlled trial included 26 adult patients with stable chronic bronchitis. The patients received 16 weeks each of treatment with placebo and with IG, 60 mg qid. Spirometry and plethysmography were performed to assess pulmonary function, and patient questionnaires were given to assess symptoms. The physical, transport, and surface properties of sputum also were assessed.

Results.—Treatment with IG did not produce significant improvement in pulmonary function, clinical scores, or sputum properties. The global symptom score was improved with both treatments compared with baseline, but there was no significant difference between the treatments. Changes occurring in the global symptom score during treatment were positively correlated with changes in sputum spinnability.

Conclusions.—Treatment with IG does not significantly improve pulmonary function, well-being, or sputum properties in patients with chronic bronchitis. This treatment may produce a small increase in sputum hydration, but the change has no significant effect on sputum viscoelasticity or transportability.

▶ This paper gave a good test of IG over 16 weeks compared with placebo in a double-blind, randomized, placebo-controlled, crossover study. Iodinated glycerol had no major beneficial effect.

M. Weintraub, M.D.

The Benefits and Risks of Over-the-Counter Availability of Nicotine Polacrilex ("Nicotine Gum")

Oster G, Delea TE, Huse DM, et al (Policy Analysis Inc, Brookline, Mass; Med Research Internatl Inc, Burlington, Mass; Harvard School of Public Health, Boston; et al)
Med Care 34:389–402, 1996
18–2

Background.—Because nicotine is highly addictive, smoking cessation attempts have a low rate of success. However, smoking cessation can be facilitated with nicotine-replacement therapy. It has been suggested that nicotine gum be offered over the counter (OTC). However, there may be some risks. Smokers may use nicotine gum and ignore more effective methods of quitting, thus reducing the chance of success, or may delay smoking cessation by using the gum to cope with temporary periods of nicotine abstinence, such as during the work day. The risks and benefits of making nicotine gum available OTC were analyzed with a model for predicting smoking behavior among adult smokers in the United States.

Methods.—Data on the current population of adult smokers were obtained from national data sources. The population was stratified by sex, age, and smoking intensity. The annual occurrences of continued smoking, abstinence, or death were predicted for a 10-year period in 4 scenarios for smoking cessation. It was assumed that light and heavy smokers would remain abstinent for 1 year at rates of 5% and 3.4%, respectively, with smoking cessation without assistance; 10% and 6.8% with prescription nicotine replacement therapy; 20% and 13.6% with formal smoking cessation programs; and 7.5% and 5.1% with OTC nicotine gum. Sensitivity analyses were performed by varying the assumed quit rates with OTC nicotine gum.

Results.—Using the assumed quit rates of the original model, a 10-year period would result in abstinence in 7.5 million smokers if nicotine gum were available by prescription only and in approximately 8 million smokers if nicotine were available OTC. Sensitivity analyses showed that the number of current smokers who would be abstinent at 10 years would vary considerably, depending on the efficacy of OTC nicotine gum, but would remain substantial regardless of the quit rate.

Conclusion.—The effect of OTC availability of nicotine gum on future smoking behavior is sensitive to a number of variables, including the decision to quit, the methods used, and the effectiveness of the nicotine gum. It would, nevertheless, expand the options for smokers wanting to quit and might increase the rate of abstinence among current smokers, conferring substantial public health benefits.

▶ As in all studies that use models, this one is very much dependent on the numbers of people who will buy nicotine gum OTC. Nicotine patches are also now available OTC, and I will bet that this has really influenced the purchase of nicotine gum. Still and all, this is an important discussion of the smoking cessation methods and their value.

M. Weintraub, M.D.

Safety of Nicotine Polacrilex Gum Used by 3,094 Participants in the Lung Health Study

Murray RP, for the Lung Health Study Research Group (Univ of Manitoba, Winnipeg, Canada; Univ of Alabama, Birmingham; Univ of Minnesota, Minneapolis)
Chest 109:438–445, 1996   18–3

Objective.—Nicotine polacrilex (NP) chewing gum is an effective aid for smoking cessation when used properly. A few studies that included relatively few patients followed up for brief periods of time have reported predominantly minor side effects of NP use. None have examined the safety of NP in larger samples for an extended period. Cardiovascular and other side effects of NP were studied as part of a large smoking cessation trial.

Methods.—The analysis included data on 3,094 participants in the Lung Health Study who used NP chewing gum during the first year of the study. All were adult smokers with evidence of early chronic obstructive pulmonary disease. They were followed up annually for hospitalizations and every 4 months for side effects of NP use.

Results.—Throughout the 5-year study, there was no relationship between cardiovascular hospitalization and death rate and the use of NP, the dose of NP, or the concomitant use of NP and cigarettes. Although approximately one fourth of NP users experienced side effects of some type, most of these effects were minor and transient. At least 5% of users experienced side effects when they stopped using NP, including headache, indigestion, oral irritation or ulcers, and nausea. Using NP and smoking cigarettes at the same time did not appear to increase the risk of side effects. Intensive instruction and monitoring of NP use as part of the study protocol appeared to reduce the occurrence of side effects, such as dizziness, headaches, and throat irritation.

Conclusions.—Using NP as an aid for smoking cessation does not appear to increase the risk of adverse cardiovascular events or any other serious side effects. It may be best to provide careful instruction in and monitoring of NP use to maximize the effectiveness and minimize the side effects of NP.

▶ This study predicted a number of things, none of which was a great surprise. Being a current smoker, being male, being older, and having elevated diastolic blood pressure were factors that predicted fatal and nonfatal cardiovascular events among 3,332 special intervention participants. One of the interesting points in this paper is that there was no evidence of simultaneous smoking and use of nicotine-containing chewing gum. In addition, the nicotine levels of people who use the gum were typically one third of those found in cigarette smokers. The gum is available now over-the-counter. Thus, it is likely that fewer patients will be receiving intensive smoking cessation training. Still, if patients plan their cessation attempt appropriately, decide on a "quit" date, and pay attention to the written materials that come with the package as well as the tapes, they may have equal or more success than other people who have received the gum under prescription. The company is supplying "Smoke-Enders" or other program numbers to call, paid for by the manufacturer. Even if just a few people stop smoking and many continue to use the gum beyond the usual time of cessation, it still is beneficial to the patients. It is a nonharmful, clean way of satisfying their nicotine addiction.

M. Weintraub, M.D.

Inhalation of Antibiotics in Cystic Fibrosis
Touw DJ, Brimicombe RW, Hodson ME, et al (Free Univ Hosp, Amsterdam; Leyenburg Hosp, 's-Gravenhage, The Netherlands; Royal Brompton Hosp, London)
Eur Respir J 8:1594–1604, 1995   18–4

Background.—Antipseudomonal antibiotics are commonly used in aerosol form in patients with cystic fibrosis. However, their influence on lung function, infection, and quality of life has not been clearly documented.

Methods and Findings.—Studies of antibiotic inhalation treatment in patients with cystic fibrosis published between 1965 and the present were reviewed. The use of nebulizers with limited ability to produce particles in the respirable range reportedly compromises effective aerosol delivery. Twelve studies on maintenance therapy have been published. In 4 uncontrolled investigations of antibiotic aerosol maintenance in stable patients, the number of patients needing hospitalization was reduced. Six of 8 placebo-controlled trials showed that treated patients had significantly improved lung function. Four studies demonstrated a reduction in the number of patients hospitalized. Some studies showed that nebulized placebo solution negatively affects outcome, probably because the choice of osmolarity was improper. In studies of antibiotic aerosols used as an adjunct to IV treatment in patients with an acute exacerbation, antibiotic administered in aerosol form failed to enhance the effects of IV antibiotic. However, sputum colony counts were lower in these studies. Studies of toxicity to date have shown no renal toxicity or ototoxicity.

Conclusions.—Aerosol maintenance therapy with an appropriate antibiotic at a sufficient dose appears to be beneficial for patients with cystic fibrosis and chronic *Pseudomonas aeruginosa* infection. It may improve lung function and decrease the number of hospitalizations resulting from acute exacerbations.

Long-term investigations of toxicity using higher doses are still needed. Although the introduction or selection of resistant bacteria is relatively rare, it is still of concern.

▶ All too many patients with cystic fibrosis find their lungs colonized by pathogenic bacteria, most often *Haemophilus influenzae* and *Staphylococcus aureus* at first, but later *Pseudomonas aeruginosa*. Aerosols with appropriate concentrations of the right antibiotic should be used as maintenance therapy in many patients with cystic fibrosis who are chronically infected with *Pseudomonas aeruginosa.*

L. Lasagna, M.D.

Dornase Alfa: A New Option in the Management of Cystic Fibrosis
Witt DM, Anderson L (Kaiser Permanente of Colorado, Westminster; Multum Information Services, Inc, Denver)
Pharmacotherapy 16:40–48, 1996   18–5

Background.—Recombinant human dornase alfa (DNase I), a mucolytic that selectively digests extracellular DNA and decreases the viscosity of purulent sputum, is the first new therapy developed specifically for cystic fibrosis (CF) in nearly 3 decades. It was approved by the Food and Drug Administration in 1993 for use in conjunction with standard treatments in selected patients with CF. Features of this agent and its use were discussed.

Dornase Alfa in the Management of CF.—Objectively, clinical trials have shown that DNase I modestly improves pulmonary function compared with placebo and slightly reduces the number of respiratory exacerbations, which necessitates parenteral antibiotics. Subjectively, patients may report substantial improvement. In phase III trials, patients given DNase I have been noted to have slightly shorter hospital stays than those given placebo. Such trials have also shown that DNase I reduces the risk of infectious exacerbations regardless of the initial effects on pulmonary function. Aerosolized DNase I preparations are safe and generally well tolerated. The most common side effects are voice alterations and sore throat. Dornase alfa should be used only as an adjunct to traditional CF treatments. To sustain its therapeutic effect, DNase I must be administered on a continuous daily basis.

Long-term studies of the effects of DNase I on morbidity and mortality are still needed to define its role in patients with CF. Further research is also needed to determine the best time to begin such therapy and to determine its safety in children younger than 5 years. In addition, studies are needed to prospectively identify patients most likely to benefit from DNase I.

Dornase alfa is very expensive, which necessitates careful monitoring of clinical response to identify patients who will benefit from the treatment. Variables to be monitored include severity of dyspnea, cough frequency, sputum production, fatigue, appetite, sleep patterns, exercise tolerance, ease of sputum expectoration, and sputum clearance. Spirometry may be useful in the identification of treatment responders. However, because DNase I has been reported to have positive subjective effects, the decision to continue treatment should not be based only on the results of pulmonary function tests.

Conclusions.—Dornase alfa has been shown to be safe, to modestly improve lung function, and to decrease the number of respiratory exacerbations that necessitate parenteral antibiotics in patients with CF. However, this agent is very costly and should always be given in conjunction with standard CF treatments such as antibiotics, chest physiotherapy, and pancreatic enzyme supplementation.

▶ The life span of people born with CF has increased from a median of 3 years to a median of 30 years as a result of aggressive treatment with antibiotics, bronchial drainage, and pancreatic enzyme supplementation, but their lives are still all too short.

Dornase alfa is an imaginative approach because it selectively digests extracellular DNA and, thus, reduces the viscosity of purulent sputum. It seems safe enough, and provides some benefits to some patients, but it is expensive and is in no way a substitute for the aforementioned aggressive therapy.

L. Lasagna, M.D.

Liposomal Prostaglandin E₁ in Acute Respiratory Distress Syndrome: A Placebo-controlled, Randomized, Double-blind, Multicenter Clinical Trial
Abraham E, Park YC, Covington P, et al (Univ of Colorado, Denver; Liposome Company, Princeton, NJ; Pharmaceutical Product Development, Morrisville, NC; et al)
Crit Care Med 24:10–15, 1996   18–6

Background.—The mortality rate of patients with acute respiratory distress syndrome (ARDS) remains high. Prostaglandin E_1 (PGE_1) produces vasodilation, downregulates inflammatory responses, and blocks platelet aggregation. The safety and efficacy of liposomal PGE_1 (TLC C-53) were evaluated in a randomized, prospective, multicenter, double-blind, placebo-controlled phase II clinical trial.

Methods.—The study group consisted of 25 patients with ARDS, who were prospectively randomized to be infused for 60 minutes every 6 hours over 7 days with either drug or placebo. The starting dosage was 0.15 µg/kg/hr, which was increased every 12 hours until intolerance developed, invasive monitoring was halted, or the maximum dosage of 3.6 µg/kg/hr was reached. Patients received aggressive care throughout the study period. The outcome measurements were PaO_2/FIO_2, dynamic pulmonary compliance, ventilator dependence on day 8, and 28-day mortality.

Results.—On day 8, all 8 patients in the placebo group required mechanical ventilation, whereas 8 of the 17 patients in the treatment group were no longer on the ventilator. PaO_2/FIO_2 improved more in the treatment group, and this reached significance on day 3. Lung compliance increased significantly more in the treatment group than in the placebo group by day 8. The 28-day mortality rate was 6% in the treatment group and 25% in the placebo group, but this difference did not reach significance because of the small sample size. Drug-related adverse events were reported in 82% of the treatment group, but half of these were localized infusion site irritations. TLC C-53 was well tolerated hemodynamically.

Conclusions.—In a small group of patients with ARDS, the liposomal prostaglandin E_1, TLC C-53, was associated with improved oxygenation, increased lung compliance, and decreased ventilator dependency compared to placebo. The trend in mortality rates with this drug was favorable, but did not reach significance because of the small sample size. Larger clinical studies will be required to confirm the beneficial effects of TLC C-53 in the treatment of patients with ARDS.

▶ One of the problems with smaller studies, even if they are multicentered in 8 centers, is that they often do not produce very convincing results. Unfortunately, the 28-day mortality was not statistically significant in this study. The question we have to ask ourselves is, based on these data, would we be able to use liposomal PGE_1? Further studies will have to be done, but only because this particular study was not large enough. Finally, would we be worried about the ethics of doing another study with PGE_1?

M. Weintraub, M.D.

Aspirin *Versus* Indomethacin Treatment of Patent Ductus Arteriosus in Preterm Infants With Respiratory Distress Syndrome
Van Overmeire B, Brus F, Van Acker KJ, et al (Univ Hosp Antwerp, Belgium; Univ Hosp, Groningen, The Netherlands)
Pediatr Res 38:886–891, 1995   18–7

Background.—Treatment of patent ductus arteriosus (PDA) is indicated in neonates with respiratory distress syndrome (RDS), to avert potentially serious pulmonary, hemodynamic, renal, and gastrointestinal effects of left-to-right shunting of blood. A comparison was made of the effectiveness of, and the incidence of side effects from, treatment of PDA with indomethacin and with aspirin.

Methods.—Seventy-five neonates met the criteria of gestational age younger than 34 weeks, RDS requiring assisted ventilation or continuous positive airway pressure, and a postnatal age between 24 and 96 hours. Each patient underwent initial echocardiographic-Doppler evaluation to demonstrate the presence and severity of the PDA. If the PDA did not rapidly improve over another 24 hours, the neonates were randomly assigned to receive either 0.2 mg of indomethacin per kilogram IV every 12 hours for 3 doses, or 15 mg of aspirin per kilogram IV every 6 hours for 4 doses. Another echocardiogram was performed 24 hours after the last dose. Any neonate whose PDA failed to close then received a course of indomethacin.

Results.—Of the 75 neonates, 38 received indomethacin and 37 received aspirin. The rate of successful PDA closure was significantly higher for indomethacin (92%) than for aspirin (43%). After successful closure, no PDA reopened. Urine output for the 72 hours after starting treatment was significantly lower in the neonates receiving indomethacin, but it remained above 1 mL of urine per kilogram per hour, and the decrease was transient. The 2 groups did not differ significantly with regard to treatment intensity for RDS, development of bronchopulmonary dysplasia, or development of side effects of therapy. Logistic regression analysis showed that PDA closure correlated positively with use of indomethacin and with younger gestational age.

Conclusions.—Indomethacin is significantly more effective than aspirin in closing PDA in premature neonates with RDS. The decrease in urine output experienced with indomethacin is transient.

▶ Patent ductus arteriosus is quite common in preterm infants, but the duct may close spontaneously in the first few days after delivery. Indomethacin has long been known to achieve nonsurgical closure, but its administration is not invariably successful.

In this elegant trial, aspirin was clearly inferior to indomethacin, although the latter treatment did temporarily decrease urine flow. (Oliguria, anuria, and transient renal failure have been seen fairly frequently after indomethacin.)

I agree with the authors that there is little incentive to study aspirin further in this situation. It seems unlikely that bigger doses would achieve the needed inhibition of cyclooxygenase.

L. Lasagna, M.D.

19 Rheumatic and Arthritic Diseases

A Cost Effectiveness Analysis of Cyclosporine in Rheumatoid Arthritis
Anis AH, Tugwell PX, Wells GA, et al (St Paul's Hosp, Vancouver, BC, Canada; Univ of British Columbia, Canada; Univ of Ottawa, Canada)
J Rheumatol 23:609–616, 1996   19–1

Background.—Rheumatoid arthritis (RA) is a progressive disease that is both complicated and expensive to treat over the long term. Five recent clinical trials determined that cyclosporine (CyA) is a safe and effective second-line treatment for patients with RA. A meta-analysis of these 5 studies that included a cost-effectiveness analysis was performed. The cost study is presented in this report.

Study Design.—Data from 5 randomized, controlled, blinded parallel group clinical trials were selected for the meta-analysis. Three of the trials were placebo controlled and the other 2 trials had D-penicillamine (D-Pen) and azathioprine (Aza) as active treatment comparisons. An incremental economic analysis was performed from a societal perspective and from the perspective of the Ontario Ministry of Health.

Results.—The treatment of patients with RA using CyA produced at least a 25% reduction in tender joint count in 35% of the patients, compared to 17% of the patients treated with placebo. There was no difference between the results with CyA and those with the other 2 drugs. From the perspective of the Ontario Ministry of Health, the annual incremental cost of using CyA to achieve this improvement was $1,473 higher than with Aza and $1,618 higher than with D-Pen. From a societal perspective, the annual incremental cost of CyA was $2,886 higher than with Aza and $3,731 higher than with D-Pen.

Conclusions.—Because CyA is significantly more expensive than other effective second-line treatments for patients with severe RA, it would be beneficial to investigate which patients would benefit most from this therapy. Society must decide whether this drug provides good value for the cost of treatment of patients with severe RA.

▶ This study clearly damaged the thought of giving CA compared to almost any other therapy or, in fact, even placebo on a cost-effectiveness basis. The real judgment will have to be made by society in choosing to pay for the scarce resources in patients with RA who have tried, and failed to respond to, all the other therapies.

M. Weintraub, M.D.

Comparison of Intramuscular Gold and Sulphasalazine in the Treatment of Early Rheumatoid Arthritis: A One Year Prospective Study
Peltomaa R, Paimela L, Helve T, et al (Kivelä Hosp, Helsinki; Helsinki Univ)
Scand J Rheumatol 24:330–335, 1995   19–2

Introduction.—Erosive changes of rheumatoid arthritis (RA) may occur during the first few years of the disease; hence, early treatment with disease-modifying antirheumatic drugs (DMARDs) is indicated for prevention of irreversible joint destruction. Recent studies have suggested sulfasalazine as the drug of choice over gold compounds for early treatment of RA. However, these 2 forms of therapy have not been previously compared based on early radiologic progression of disease. The efficacies of sulfasalazine and IM gold as the first DMARD given were compared with respect to both clinical and radiologic findings in patients with recent-onset RA.

Methods.—Prospectively studied were 128 patients with newly diagnosed (within 1 year of first symptoms) RA. The first 70 consecutive patients received standard adjusted therapy with IM gold (sodium aurothiomalate). The subsequent 58 consecutive patients were treated with sulfasalazine (0.5 g daily, increasing by 0.5 g weekly to a maintenance dose of 2 g daily in most patients). Clinical and laboratory variables of disease were assessed at 3-month intervals; radiography of the hands, wrists, and feet was performed initially and at the conclusion of the study. Clinical characteristics were comparable between the 2 patient groups. A few patients in each group concurrently received low-dose systemic steroid therapy.

Results.—Forty percent of patients receiving gold therapy and 48% of patients receiving sulfasalazine were withdrawn from the study during the 1 year of follow-up, primarily because of adverse reactions. None of the drug complications were life threatening. Women were more likely to discontinue treatment than were men. Clinical and laboratory parameters improved in both groups; difference in improvement between groups was not significant. Clinical improvement was most prominent in the first 3 months, but radiologic features showed clear progression of disease in both groups. After 1 year, improvement in the erythrocyte sedimentation rate, the C-reactive protein level, the Ritchie articular index, the duration of morning stiffness, and the visual-analogue scale of pain was significant in both groups. Grip strength did not improve significantly in either group.

Discussion.—Both treatments show a beneficial effect on clinical disease activity that is greatest during the first 3 months. Radiologic progression of disease occurred regardless in all but 30% of patients receiving sulfasalazine and in all but 19% of patients receiving gold. Antirheumatic treatment should be started as soon in the disease process as possible; combination therapy might be an option for some patients.

Chronic Sulfasalazine Therapy in the Treatment of Delayed Pressure Urticaria and Angioedema

Engler RJM, Squire E, Benson P (Walter Reed Army Med Ctr, Washington, DC; Uniformed Services Univ, Bethesda, Md)
Ann Allergy Asthma Immunol 74:155–159, 1995   19–3

Background.—Workers who must stand for prolonged periods using their hands forcefully can be seriously disabled by delayed pressure urticaria/angioedema, which causes painful, chronic swelling of the hands and feet and systemic malaise and flu-like symptoms. Patients with severe disease usually do not respond to antihistamines and nonsteroidal anti-inflammatory drugs. Corticosteroids are often needed to control symptoms. The efficacy of sulfasalazine in 2 patients with refractory delayed pressure urticaria was reported.

Patients and Outcomes.—The patients were 2 men, aged 39 and 50. Both had disabling pressure urticaria and angioedema. All other treatment options (except corticosteroids) had failed. The first patient needed more than 30 mg of prednisone daily for more than 6 months to continue working. Sulfasalazine up to 4 g/day was well tolerated by both patients. There were no adverse reactions, and symptoms were resolved completely. The symptoms of the first patient remained well controlled 1 year after initiation of therapy, but 2 g or more per day was needed. The second patient had excellent symptom control 6 months after beginning treatment but was lost to follow-up.

Conclusions.—Sulfasalazine in doses used for inflammatory bowel disease is apparently an effective alternative treatment for delayed pressure urticaria and angioedema in patients whose symptoms are not controlled adequately by traditional treatment. This agent may be corticosteroid sparing.

▶ One drug doesn't have only one effect, as illustrated by these two papers (Abstracts 19–2 and 19–3). In the first, sulfasalazine (SAS) was put up against an effective treatment, IM gold, and it did pretty well in early rheumatoid arthritis. Actually, the investigators of this study were quite brave in so treating rheumatoid arthritis of less than one year's duration. Unfortunately, many patients, 40% of the gold patients and 48% of the SAS patients, withdrew either because of adverse effects or lack of efficacy. Some of the patients who were in the study probably could have been taken off the medication and it would have been seen to have worked just as well. Neither gold nor SAS patients had a stop in their development of erosions, according to the x-ray Larsen scores. Gold gives variable responses on the development of erosions and SAS, in general, does not prevent the erosions.

The radiologic status was stable in only 30% of the patients on SAS and only 19% of gold-treated patients. The investigators showed that early treatment with DMARDs, or disease modifying antirheumatic drugs (a misnomer if there ever was one), should be started soon after the diagnosis.

In another use of SAS, a small number (2) of open-labeled studies showed some value in treating pressure urticaria. Sulfasalazine has also been used in scleroderma and dermatitis herpetiformis. Sulfasalazine may be steroid sparing in this case.

M. Weintraub, M.D.

Survival and Drug Discontinuation Analyses in a Large Cohort of Methotrexate Treated Rheumatoid Arthritis Patients
Alarcón GS, Tracy IC, Strand GM, et al (Univ of Alabama, Birmingham)
Ann Rheum Dis 54:708–712, 1995   19–4

Background.—Methotrexate is now considered a standard option in the treatment of rheumatoid arthritis (RA). In a previous cohort study of patients with RA given methotrexate treatment, the probability of continuing methotrexate at 5 years was about 50%. The reasons for discontinuing the drug, overall survival, and causes of death in this cohort were reported.

Methods.—One hundred fifty-two patients with RA began methotrexate treatment between 1981 and 1986. The patients underwent annual follow-up assessment.

Findings.—The probability of continuing methotrexate at 10 years (among the first subjects to enter the cohort) was 30%. The most common reason for discontinuing therapy was toxicity (and its severity). The cumulative probabilities of survival for women and men were 85% and 45%, respectively. The number of deaths from infection were greater than expected. However, the number of deaths from cancer and cardiovascular diseases were in the expected range.

Conclusion.—In this cohort, the most common reason for discontinuing methotrexate treatment was toxicity. Survival was comparable to that reported in other cohorts with RA. However, methotrexate may have been an associated factor in deaths from infection.

▶ The rate of continuation of most patients receiving disease-modifying antirheumatic drugs is really quite low. Part of this is the result of lack of efficacy, but most of the patients drop out from inability to tolerate the medications because of adverse effects. Methotrexate has become the most used disease-modifying antirheumatic in patients with RA. Although most people who left the cohort of methotrexate-treated patients did so because of adverse drug reactions, including death, hopefully, the more recent patients are doing better because of the use of folic acid, lower doses, and, perhaps, even better patient selection. This paper should be of interest to not only rheumatologists, but to physicians treating patients with RA in general practice settings.

M. Weintraub, M.D.

Pancytopenia Related Eosinophilia in Rheumatoid Arthritis: A Specific Methotrexate Phenomenon?

Bruyn GAW, Velthuysen E, Joosten P, et al (Medisch Centrum Leeuwarden, The Netherlands)
J Rheumatol 22:1373–1376, 1995   19–5

Introduction.—Low-dose oral methotrexate (MTX) therapy is an effective means of treating rheumatoid arthritis (RA), but drug-related pancytopenia is described in approximately 3% of patients. Four patients with RA in whom pancytopenia developed while they were receiving low doses of MTX also were noted to have striking eosinophilia in both the peripheral blood and bone marrow.

Clinical Findings.—The patients were 2 men and 2 women whose average age was 65 years; they had had RA for 9 years on average. Pancytopenia developed while the patients were receiving 7.5 mg or, in 1 case, 15 mg of MTX each week. These patients had a number of risk factors for pancytopenia, including renal dysfunction, hypoalbuminemia, a low folate level, the use of multiple drugs, and nonsteroidal anti-inflammatory drug treatment. The pancytopenia was associated with relative eosinophilia ranging from 22% to 56%. No eruptions were noted, and the patients had no history of parasitic infection and no clinical evidence of malignant disease. Eosinophils peaked earlier than did neutrophils. Three of the 4 patients showed eosinophilia after receiving folinic acid. The eosinophilia persisted for 11 days on average.

Discussion.—Eosinophilia has not been described in patients with RA in whom neutropenia develops in relation to other drugs, suggesting a specific effect of MTX on myelopoiesis. Studies are needed to determine whether folinic acid releases endogenous myeloid growth factors or other cytokines in patients receiving low doses of MTX.

▶ Relative eosinophilia in the presence of pancytopenia must be a rare bird, although pancytopenia per se in patients treated with MTX for RA is well known.

L. Lasagna, M.D.

How Low Can You Go? Use of Very Low Dosage of Gold in Patients With Mucocutaneous Reactions

Klinkhoff AV, Teufel A (Univ of British Columbia, Vancouver)
J Rheumatol 22:1657–1659, 1995   19–6

Background.—Intramuscular gold treatment is often used as a second-line agent in the treatment of rheumatoid arthritis. Some patients are sensitive to both the benefits and adverse effects of this therapy. The use of very low dose gold in patients with mucocutaneous reactions was studied.

Methods and Findings.—Eleven women and 2 men with rheumatoid arthritis effectively treated at maintenance doses of IM gold were identified by record review. Eleven patients were seropositive, and 2 had Felty's syndrome. Mucocutaneous side effects developed in these patients within 20 weeks of treatment initiation, when their disease had greatly improved. Adverse effects recurred with sequential dosage adjustments. Doses exceeding 10 mg were not tolerable. These side effects were managed by temporarily stopping gold treatment. When the side effects resolved, IM gold therapy was resumed at about a 50% dosage reduction, which was decreased by a further 50% when adverse effects recurred.

Final maintenance dosages were 3 mg per week in 3 patients; 10 mg every 3 weeks in 2; 10 mg every 4 weeks in 2; 5 mg per week in 2; and, in 1 patient each, 2 mg every 4 weeks, 2 mg every week, 5 mg every month, and 10 mg every 6 weeks. All patients improved at these very low dosages. Six patients are currently in complete remission. The average duration of treatment was 5.5 years.

Conclusions.—The most effective, least toxic dosage for IM gold treatment is unknown. Patients who are sensitive to the effects of IM gold can have good long-term outcomes at very low doses.

▶ It is important to remember that treating all patients the same inevitably means that some patients will be suboptimally treated. "Fine-tuning," not homogenization, of treatment should always be the goal.

This study documents just such an individualized approach by these Canadians. Congratulations!

L. Lasagna, M.D.

20 Skin Diseases

Treatment of Hemangiomas of Infants With High Doses of Prednisone
Sadan N, Wolach B (Meir Gen Hosp, Kfar Saba, Israel; Tel-Aviv Univ, Israel)
J Pediatr 128:141–146, 1996   20–1

Purpose.—Hemangiomas in infants grow slowly and gradually resolve spontaneously, so treatment is usually unnecessary. However, some hemangiomas should be treated when they are interfering with important functions, endangering delicate structures, or causing a cosmetic problem. The use of high-dose prednisone therapy for the treatment of hemangiomas in infants was studied.

Patients.—Sixty infants with hemangiomas were treated with prednisone during a 24-year period; 45 of the patients were girls. In most cases, treatment was started between 1 week and 3 months of age. The initial dosage of oral prednisone was 3 mg/kg/day in 4 divided doses at the beginning of the study. In the latter part, this was increased to 5 mg/kg/day in 4 divided doses. Treatment was tapered after 2 weeks and discontinued after 6–8 weeks in most patients. Most patients received 1 or 2 courses of therapy. The hemangiomas were monitored for involution and regrowth.

Results.—Sixty-eight percent of patients had a rapid and excellent response, 25% had a good response, and treatment failed in 7%. All 20 patients with hemangiomas of the eye showed a reduction in the size of the lesion within 24 hours after the start of treatment (Fig 3). Patients receiving prednisone, 5 mg/kg/day, were more likely to have an excellent response. Although moon facies, behavioral changes, and other side effects were noted, they resolved after the end of prednisone therapy.

Conclusions.—High-dose oral prednisone therapy is very effective in infants with hemangiomas. An initial dose of 5 mg/kg/day works best, and treatment should continue for no less than 6 weeks. In severe cases, treatment may exceed 12 weeks.

▶ Although the natural history of hemangiomas is benign, self-curing and therefore responds well to compassionate neglect, some of the lesions can interfere with function (e.g., feeding, vision, voiding, or hearing) or are so cosmetically disturbing that treatment is indicated.

Corticosteroids have been used to treat this condition for at least 3 decades, with variable results. These authors seem to have had a very favorable experience over a 24-year period. Because these are big doses of

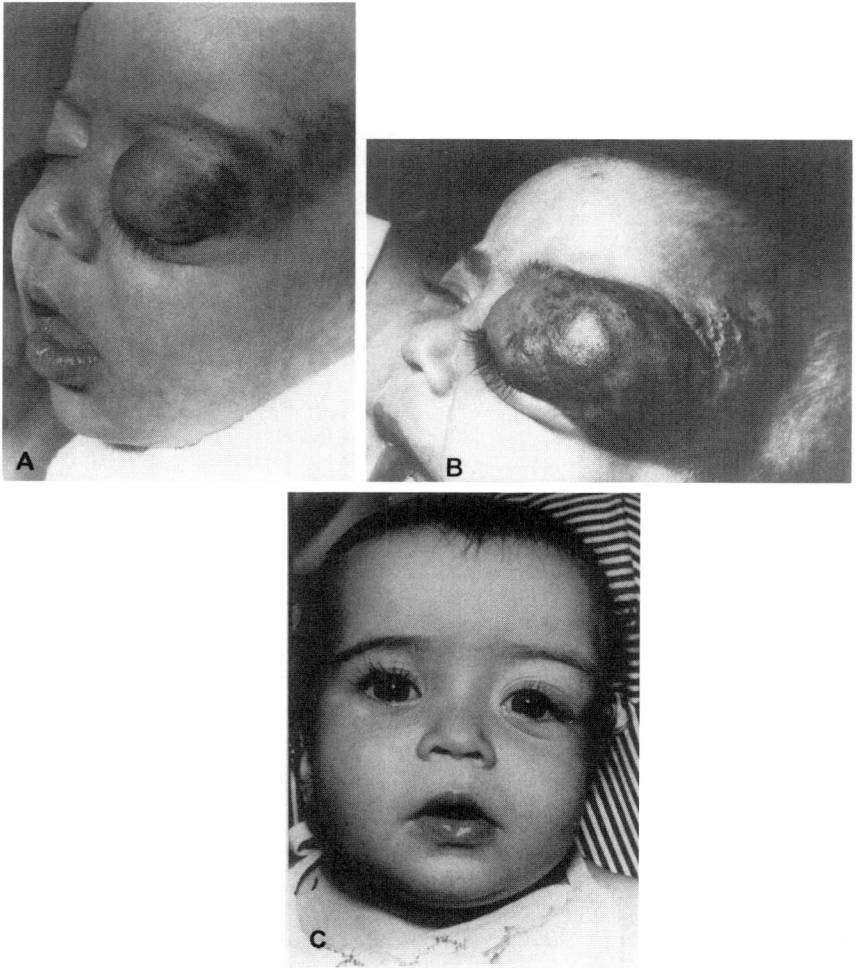

FIGURE 3.—A 3-week-old girl. A, hemangioma of left eye caused complete occlusion and considerable proptosis. Rapid regression of tumor occurred shortly after initiation of treatment. The dose of prednisone was tapered after 2 weeks of therapy from 5 to 4 mg/kg/day. B, swift regrowth of tumor occurred and the tumor reached a huge size. The dose of prednisone was increased to 5mg/kg/day for 1 month; then gradual tapering was instituted. Treatment continued for 12 weeks. C, 2 months after completion of treatment, the results were rated as excellent. (Courtesy of Sadan N, Wolach B: Treatment of hemangiomas of infants with high doses of prednisone. *J Pediatr* 128:141–146, 1996.)

corticosteroid given for weeks or months, there are side effects (moon facies, osteoporosis, and behavioral changes), but these side effects resolve when therapy is stopped.

L. Lasagna, M.D.

Duration of Remission During Maintenance Cyclosporine Therapy for Psoriasis: Relationship to Maintenance Dose and Degree of Improvement During Initial Therapy
Ellis CN, Fradin MS, Hamilton TA, et al (Univ of Michigan, Ann Arbor; Affairs Med Ctr, Ann Arbor, Mich)
Arch Dermatol 131:791–795, 1995   20–2

Background.—Cyclosporine is effective in treating severe psoriasis. However, this agent can be associated with toxic effects, depending on dose and length of treatment, especially affecting the kidneys. The efficacy of maintenance cyclosporine treatment at lesser doses in patients initially responding to such therapy was investigated.

Methods.—Sixty-one patients with clearing or near-clearing of psoriasis during an induction phase of cyclosporine treatment were randomly assigned to receive 1.5 or 3 mg/kg per day of cyclosporine or placebo for maintenance therapy. Sixty patients completed the 4-month study. Time to relapse was defined as the time from the beginning of maintenance treatment until a 2-point worsening of psoriasis on a 7-point scale.

Findings.—Patients receiving 3 mg/kg of cyclosporine had a significantly longer mean time to relapse than those given 1.5 mg/kg or placebo. Mean times to relapse were 12, 9, and 7 weeks, respectively. The groups given 1.5 mg/kg of cyclosporine or placebo did not differ significantly in relapse times. By the end of the study, 57% of the 3 mg/kg group had not relapsed, compared with 21% of the 1.5 mg/kg group and 5% of the placebo group. Longer remissions were associated with less psoriasis at the beginning of maintenance dosing, lower cyclosporine dose needed to obtain clearing or near-clearing during induction therapy, greater maintenance dosing, and smaller differences between the induction and maintenance doses. Laboratory values were improved compared with induction values. None of the patients had important clinical side effects during maintenance therapy.

Conclusions.—Maintenance therapy with 3 mg/kg of cyclosporine per day is effective after clearing or near-clearing of psoriasis in patients with severe disease. Remissions tend to be longer in patients who have greater clearing of psoriasis at lower induction doses.

▶ Cyclosporine seems to have a dramatic impact for the good in most patients with severe psoriasis, but it is not without risk. These authors have tried to determine what is a reasonable dose of this drug to maintain a cyclosporine-induced remission. They suggest 3 mg/kg per day.

L. Lasagna, M.D.

The Treatment of Scabies With Ivermectin

Meinking TL, Taplin D, Hermida JL, et al (Univ of Miami, Fla)
N Engl J Med 333:26–30, 1995   20–3

Background.—Anecdotal reports and a few clinical studies suggest that scabies can be treated effectively with ivermectin, an oral anthelmintic agent used successfully for treating onchocerciasis and other filarial infestations. The effectiveness of ivermectin was examined in treating scabies in both patients who were otherwise healthy and in patients with HIV.

Methods.—In this open-label study, ivermectin was given in a single oral dose of 200 µg/kg to 11 otherwise healthy patients and 11 who were HIV-positive, including 7 who had AIDS. Scabies severity ranged from

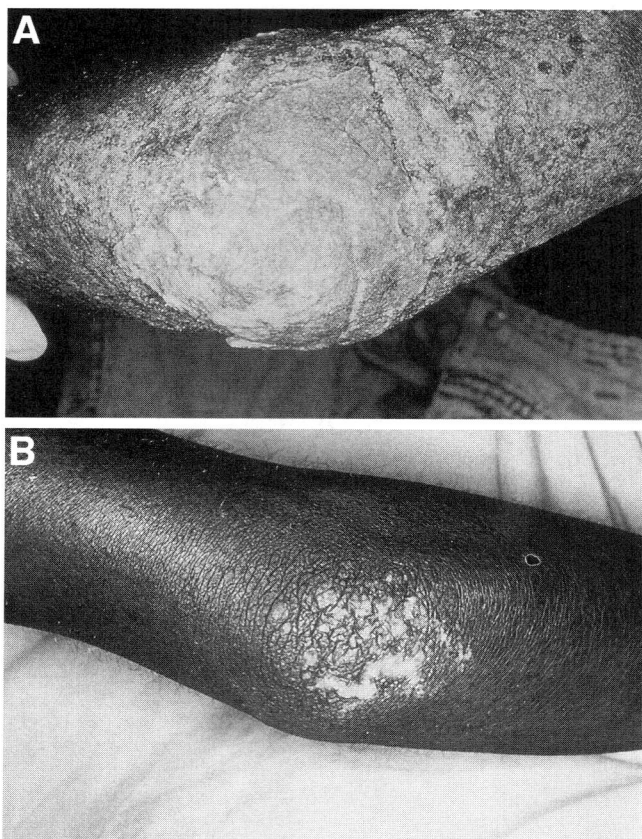

FIGURE 2.—The left elbow of a patient with AIDS before and after treatment for scabies. The patient had heavily crusted elbows before treatment (**A**), but was cured of scabies 6 weeks after the initial visit (**B**). She required 3 doses of oral ivermectin and topical treatment with 5% permethrin cream. (Courtesy of Meinking TL, Taplin D, Hermida JL, et al: The treatment of scabies with ivermectin. N Engl J Med 333:26–30, 1995. Reprinted by permission of The New England Journal of Medicine.)

mild to crusted lesions. Skin scrapings were examined for the mite at initiation and at 2 and 4 weeks after treatment. No other scabicides were used for 1 month before treatment or during the study. Individuals in close contact with the patients were treated with topical 5% permethrin cream to reduce chance of reinfestation.

Results.—At 4 weeks after treatment, all otherwise healthy patients were cured, as were 8 of the 11 patients with HIV. Of the remaining 3, 2 were given a second dose 2 weeks after the first treatment and were cured by week 4. The remaining patient, who had AIDS, tuberculosis, and heavily crusted lesions, improved dramatically after a second dose at week 2 but still had crusts on her elbows at week 4. Live mites were recovered and she was given a third ivermectin dose along with total body 5% permethrin cream; 2 weeks later she was cured (Fig 2).

Discussion.—There were no adverse effects, and pruritus diminished soon after initial treatment. One patient became reinfested 2 months after treatment, indicating that ivermectin has no residual activity against scabies 2 months after the initial dose. A single dose of 200 µg/kg seems to cure most cases of scabies, but crusted or other stubborn cases may require additional ivermectin and topical treatments.

▶ Ivermectin, an extremely useful antihelmintic, was discovered 20 years ago when Merck in the United States and the Kitasato Institute in Japan collaborated in a massive screening of more than 40,000 cultures of actinomycetes. Only 1 organism, *Streptomyces avermitilis*, produced the class of compounds known as avermectins.

Ivermectin is effective against a variety of parasites, notably canine heartworm, onchocerciasis, and filariasis. To those we can now add scabies—and with a single dose!

L. Lasagna, M.D.

Flutamide in the Treatment of Hirsutism: Long-term Clinical Effects, Endocrine Changes, and Androgen Receptor Behavior
Moghetti P, Magnani CM, Castello R, et al (Univ of Verona, Italy; Ospedale Maggiore, Verona, Italy; Univ of Padua, Italy)
Fertil Steril 64:511–517, 1995   20–4

Objective.—Antiandrogen drugs commonly used to treat hirsutism interfere with female hormone cycles and cause menstrual irregularities and breast tenderness. The nonsteroidal drug flutamide, an antiandrogen used to treat prostate cancer, has been used successfully to treat hirsutism but has yielded equivocal endocrine profile results. The long-term clinical and hormonal effects of low doses of flutamide and the effect of antiandrogen treatment on androgen receptor status in 18 hirsute women with regular ovulatory cycles were presented.

Methods.—Eighteen hirsute women (average age, 24 years) were given 125 mg flutamide 3 times daily for 12 months. Four of the women had acne. Clinical evaluations and hormone profiles were determined at baseline and at 4-month intervals. Serum sex hormone-binding globulins, 3α androstanediol glucuronide, and gonodotropin response to gonadotropin-releasing hormone (GnRH) stimulation were assessed at baseline and 3 months into treatment. Hirsutism was scored in 9 areas according to the Ferriman and Gallwey system. The androgen receptor content in mononuclear leukocytes was determined during both follicular and luteal phases of the menstrual cycle at baseline and 4 months into treatment.

Results.—An increase in serum transaminase caused 1 patient to drop out. All patients had normal menses and ovulation. Sixteen patients completed the study. Acne cleared up in all affected women 3 months into treatment. Ferriman-Gallwey scores decreased from 14.1 to 4.1 after 1 year of therapy. Patient-rated results were excellent for 10, satisfactory for 5, poor for 1, and absent for 1. Serum androgen levels were reduced. Basal and GnRH-stimulated gonadotropin levels, as well as cortisol and 17-hydroxyprogesterone responses to adrenocorticotropic hormone, remained unchanged. Although androgen receptor concentration before therapy was higher in the luteal than in the follicular phase, after treatment there was no significant difference in concentration between the 2 phases.

Conclusions.—Flutamide is effective in treating hirsutism and probably works by reducing serum androgen levels. Liver function must be monitored in these patients. Why the drug also affects androgen receptor concentration during the menstrual cycle is unclear.

▶ Lately, physicians have been asked to treat patients for a variety of symptomatic problems or for almost cosmetic-type indications. In each case, we have to ask ourselves whether the patient's problems and condition warrant treatment with a medication that might have serious side effects. We hope that the treatment-induced side effects are not as serious as the side effects of the disease itself. Hirsutism is one of those illnesses, particularly in these women, all of whom were fertile and who required contraception with barrier mechanisms or intrauterine devices. This took a lot of courage on the part of the physicians and did, I hope, indicate that the hirsutism was more serious than the side effects of flutamide.

M. Weintraub, M.D.

The Effect of Topical 0.75% Metronidazole Gel on Malodorous Cutaneous Ulcers
Finlay IG, Bowszyc J, Ramlau C, et al (Holme Tower Marie Curie Centre, Penarth, Wales; Univ School of Medicine, Poznan, Poland; Klinika Dermatologiczina AM, Bydgoszcz, Poland)
J Pain Symptom Manage 11:158–162, 1996   20–5

Background.—The unpleasant smell of infected fungating tumors and benign cutaneous ulcers is distressing. Anaerobic infection can also occur.

Studies have shown that topical metronizadole 0.8% gel reduces odor from fungating malodorous tumors.

Methods and Findings.—Forty-seven patients were enrolled in a prospective study to assess the subjective and bacteriologic response to 0.75% metronidazole gel and to determine whether tubes of gel become contaminated bacterially during use. All patients had foul-smelling benign or malignant cutaneous lesions. Smell, pain, appearance, and bacteriologic profile were assessed before entry and at 7 and 14 days after application. Ninety-five percent of the 43 patients evaluated at 14 days reported an improvement in odor. Anaerobic infection, initially found in 53% of the patients, was eliminated in 84%. After 7 days, patients reported a reduction in pain. Discharge and related cellulitis also decreased significantly.

Conclusion.—The deodorizing effect of topical metronidazole gel is accompanied by a reduction in lesion pain, discharge surrounding cellulitis, and wound colonization by anaerobic bacteria. Tubes of 0.75% metronidazole gel in use for several days show no evidence of bacterial contamination.

▶ In certain cases, all that you want to do with the treatment of skin ulcers or wounds is take care of the unpleasant odor. The decrease in odor may give people more self-confidence, as well as the ability to interact with their friends and caregivers. Controlling the odor may increase their appetite and sleep. We have to remember that these patients very rarely lose their ability to smell their skin lesions. In some senses, the other effects of medication are important: decreased pain, decreased discharge, and decreases in other bacteria colonizing the lesion. Not everything is concerned with curing cancer. Sometimes, reducing the smell of a lesion is just as valuable.

M. Weintraub, M.D.

Dramatic Response to Levamisole and Low-dose Prednisolone in 23 Patients With Oral Lichen Planus: A 6-Year Prospective Follow-up Study

Lu S-Y, Chen W-J, Eng H-L (Chang Gung Mem Hosp, Taiwan, Republic of China; Kaohsiung Med Ctr, Taiwan, Republic of China)
Oral Surg Oral Med Oral Pathol Oral Radiol Endod 80:705–709, 1995 20–6

Background.—Levamisole has been shown to potentiate numerous biological immune functions and alter the natural course of some chronic, recurrent, inflammatory diseases. Oral lichen planus (OLP) is a chronic, recurrent, inflammatory mucocutaneous disease that is often resistant to treatment. A patient with OLP had a dramatic response to combination therapy with levamisole and prednisolone, allowing reduction of the prednisolone dose. This prompted an investigation of the efficacy of combination treatment of OLP with prednisolone and levamisole.

Methods.—Twenty-three patients with OLP were treated with 50 mg of levamisole 3 times daily and 5 mg of prednisolone 3 times daily for 3 consecutive days per week until their symptoms were resolved. The disease-free duration after discontinuation of treatment was recorded.

Results.—Twelve of the 23 patients had a dramatic treatment response, and the other 11 had a partial response within 2 weeks of treatment initiation. Most patients had a dramatic response after 4–6 weeks of treatment and remained disease-free for 6–9 months without treatment. Patients also responded to the combination therapy during disease recurrences. Three patients had side effects: mild facial skin rash, headache, and insomnia.

Conclusions.—Levamisole, in combination with low-dose systemic prednisolone, appears to be effective in the treatment of OLP. Because the corticosteroid dose can be minimized, the side effects associated with long-term, high-dose prednisolone therapy can be avoided. Evaluation of the treatment regimen in a double-blind, placebo-controlled study is warranted.

▶ Levamisole started off its therapeutic career in animals as an antihelminthic medication. It was later tried in rheumatoid arthritis. More recently, it has been prescribed in bowel cancer, where it has become quite useful. I have often suspected that we do not know how to dose the drug for its immunomodulatory processes. We do not know whether to give it once a day, three times a week, or by some other schedule. However, it seems that, in conjunction with prednisolone, levamisole was very effective in lichen planus in a dose of 50 mg 3 times per day.

M. Weintraub, M.D.

Medication Use and the Risk of Stevens–Johnson Syndrome or Toxic Epidermal Necrolysis
Roujeau J-C, Kelly JP, Naldi L, et al (Université Paris XII; Boston Univ; Università degli Studi di Milano, Bergamo, Italy; et al)
N Engl J Med 333:1600–1607, 1995   20–7

Background.—Toxic epidermal necrolysis and Stevens-Johnson syndrome are rare, drug-induced cutaneous reactions that can be life-threatening. The association between specific drugs and these complications was quantified in a large, international, case-control study.

Methods.—Data on 245 patients hospitalized for toxic epidermal necrosis or Stevens-Johnson syndrome were obtained through surveillance networks in France, Germany, Italy, and Portugal. The control group consisted of 1,147 patients hospitalized for other reasons.

Findings.—The risks for toxic epidermal necrolysis and Stevens-Johnson syndrome were increased for several drugs used in the short term. These included trimethoprim-sulfamethoxazole and other sulfonamide antibiotics, with a crude relative risk of 172; chlormezanone, with a crude relative risk of 62; aminopenicillins, with a multivariate relative risk of 6.7; quinolones, with a multivariate relative risk of 10; and cephalosporins, with a multivariate relative risk of 14. The multivariate relative risk for acetaminophen was 0.6 in France but 9.3 in the other countries. Risk increases associated with drugs usually taken for months or years were confined mainly to the first 2 months of treatment. The crude relative risks were 90 for carbamazepine; 45 for phenobarbital; 53 for phenytoin; 25 for valproic acid; 72 for oxicam nonsteroidal anti-inflammatory drugs; 52 for allopurinol; and 54 for corticosteroids. The risks for toxic epidermal necrolysis and Stevens-Johnson syndrome were not increased significantly for other drugs used in the long term, including thiazide diuretics and oral hypoglycemic agents.

Conclusions.—The risk of Stevens-Johnson syndrome or toxic epidermal necrolysis is substantially increased with antibacterial sulfonamides, anticonvulsant agents, oxicam nonsteroidal anti-inflammatory drugs, allopurinol, chlormezanone, and corticosteroids. However, the increased risk did not exceed 5 cases per million users per week for any of these drugs.

▶ It's tricky linking cause and effect in cases of Stevens-Johnson syndrome, because it probably has infectious causes as well as drug causes, and antibiotics or other drugs are often given for the non skin manifestations as the disease is evolving.

L. Lasagna, M.D.

Photosensitivity Reactions: A Case Report Involving NSAIDs
Mammen L, Schmidt CP (Naval Med Clinic, Pearl Harbor, Hawaii)
Am Fam Physician 52:575–579, 1995   20–8

Introduction.—Nonsteroidal anti-inflammatory drugs are widely prescribed for the treatment of numerous conditions. Photosensitivity reactions associated with these drugs have been frequently reported. These reactions may be either phototoxic (a nonimmunologic reaction) or photoallergic (involving an immunologic mechanism). A case of photoallergy induced by nonsteroidal anti-inflammatory drug therapy was reviewed.

Case Report.—Woman, 42, was prescribed piroxicam, 20 mg daily, to relieve foot pain. A pruritic rash appeared on her face, arms, and neck in areas exposed to the sun within 3 days of the initiation of therapy. She also had multiple vesicles on the dorsum of her hands. Piroxicam therapy was discontinued. She was treated unsuccessfully with Benadryl, a topical corticosteroid cream, and avoided the sun. With 3 weeks of tapered treatment with prednisone, her symptoms resolved. Results from a skin biopsy showed epidermal spongiosis and a perivascular lymphocytic infiltrate in the superficial derma, suggesting a diagnosis of photoallergy.

Discussion.—Photosensitivity in this case could have been induced by either piroxicam itself or metabolites produced photochemically. Photosensitivity should be suspected when a rash location corresponds to sun-exposed areas of the skin. Treatment of a rash is determined by the type of reaction. Phototoxic reactions are treated with routine burn care and avoidance of inducing agents. Photoallergic reactions may be adequately treated with avoidance of both the sun and the photosensitizing agent. Other patients may need topical corticosteroids and antihistamines to relieve itching. Patients with severe symptoms can be treated with prednisone.

▶ Over-the-counter analgesics are deservedly popular and, for the most part, benign. This case report documents an exception to this generality, and shows the need to consider a photosensitivity reaction when a patient is seen with a rash affecting sun-exposed skin areas.

L. Lasagna, M.D.

Contact Allergy to Topical Corticosteroids and Systemic Contact Dermatitis From Prednisolone With Tolerance of Triamcinolone
Bircher AJ, Levy F, Langauer S, et al (Univ Hosp, Basel, Switzerland; Clinique Dermatologique, Strasbourg, France)
Acta Derm Venereol 75:490–493, 1995   20–9

Background.—Contact hypersensitivity to corticosteroids is an important clinical problem. A patient who initially had allergic contact dermatitis to topical corticosteroids, then a generalized exanthem to oral prednisolone, was described.

Case Report.—Woman, 27, had an allergic contact dermatitis to topical agents in corticosteroid groups A and D. A disseminated exanthem began within 24 hours of the start of oral therapy with prednisolone. Patch testing showed sensitization to group A, C, and D corticosteroids, including prednisolone-21-acetate and betamethasone valerate. The patient was not sensitive to group B agents, such as triamcinolone. The exanthem flared again after intradermal corticosteroid testing. Oral triamcinolone treatment was initiated, and her symptoms improved rapidly.

Conclusions.—Exanthematous reactions after systemic treatment with corticosteroids have rarely been reported in the literature. A safe corticosteroid should be identified for such patients by patch and intradermal testing because corticosteroids are essential emergency drugs.

▶ Although exanthemata systemic corticosteroids are rare, positive patch tests have been reported in 0.2% to 5% of patients, and allergic contact dermatitis occurs after topical use. This paper suggests that skin tests (patch or intradermal or both) can be helpful, albeit imperfect, in choosing a safe corticosteroid.

L. Lasagna, M.D.

21 Surgery

Randomised Controlled Trial of Single-dose Antibiotic Prophylaxis in Surgical Treatment of Closed Fractures: The Dutch Trauma Trial
Boxma H, Broekhuizen T, Patka P, et al (Zuiderziekenhuis, Rotterdam, The Netherlands; Univ of Amsterdam; Free Univ, Amsterdam)
Lancet 347:1133–1137, 1996   21–1

Background.—Because of the dearth of published prospective studies, the role of antibiotic prophylaxis in fracture surgery is controversial. The efficacy of single-dose prophylactic cephalosporin in primary surgical treatment of closed fractures of the limbs was evaluated in a randomized, double-blind, placebo-controlled, prospective study.

Methods.—Adult patients undergoing primary osteosynthesis or the placement of a prosthetic device to treat closed limb fractures were randomly assigned to receive a single 2-g dose of ceftriaxone or placebo at the induction of anesthesia. The development of wound infection was evaluated clinically at 10, 30, and 120 days postoperatively. Nosocomial infection within the first postoperative month was also monitored.

Results.—Of the 2,195 patients with 2,299 closed fractures, 1,090 received placebo and 1,105 received ceftriaxone. The 2 groups had comparable demographic and clinical characteristics. At day 10, the wound infection rates were 4% in the placebo group and 0.5% in the ceftriaxone group. Thereafter, new infections developed in similar numbers in the 2 groups. However, the overall infection rates at 4 months were 8.3% in the placebo group and 3.6% in the ceftriaxone group, a significant difference. Risk factors for infection included age older than 65 years, prosthetic hip surgery, and surgery lasting more than 2 hours. Stepwise logistic regression analysis revealed a significant benefit associated with ceftriaxone prophylaxis. Ceftriaxone prophylaxis was also associated with a significantly lower incidence of nosocomial infection during the first postoperative month.

Conclusions.—All patients undergoing surgical treatment of closed fractures should be given adequate antibiotic prophylaxis with a long-acting, broad-spectrum antibiotic.

▶ The literature on the value of antibiotic prophylaxis in bone and joint surgery is variably supportive of the value of such an approach. Some of the disagreement can be explained by differences in the experimental populations studied. (Elective surgery poses different threats from those seen in acutely traumatized patients.) Some of the negative trials may have been "underpowered" because of inadequate sample size, especially because the incidence of infection is low in clean operations.

The authors of this article argue persuasively that routine prophylaxis is justified and cost-effective.

L. Lasagna, M.D.

Subject Index*

A

Abdominal
  hysterectomy (see Hysterectomy,
    abdominal)
  infection, surgically treated,
    piperacillin/tazobactam therapy of,
    95: 342
  operations, upper, ceftriaxone vs.
    cefoxitin prophylaxis for chest and
    wound infections after, 95: 341
  pain
    after mesalamine, oral, in ulcerative
      colitis, 97: 175
    after triple therapy for Helicobacter
      pylori, 95: 161
  surgery, lower, effect of pre-emptive
    lumbar epidural anesthesia on
    postoperative pain and
    patient-controlled morphine
    consumption after, 96: 305
Abortion
  early, methotrexate/misoprostol for
    acceptability of, 97: 268
    safety and efficacy of, 97: 269
    vs. misoprostol alone, 96: 292
  legal, contraceptive methods among
    women seeking, 96: 288
  misoprostol for, 95: 253
Abscess
  lymphoglandular swelling with, after
    • BCG vaccination, in children,
    95: 194
Abuse
  alcohol, and lack of cognitive recovery
    after withdrawal from long-term
    benzodiazepines, 95: 47
  clonidine as drug of, 96: 91
  cocaine
    behavioral treatment of, outpatient,
      incentives improve outcome,
      96: 90
    buprenorphine dosage and, 95: 18
  drug, 97: 33–65; 96: 47–93
    propofol potential for, 95: 17
  opioid, and buprenorphine dosage,
    95: 18
  reabuse of heroin after detoxification,
    naltrexone in prevention of, 96: 89
Acanthosis nigricans
  niacin causing, sustained-release,
    95: 147

Acarbose
  in diabetes, insulin-requiring type II,
    97: 148
  effect on serum acetate in diabetics,
    96: 182
Acenocoumarol
  bleeding complications of, risk factor
    analysis, 95: 87
  long-term, after myocardial infarction,
    effect on mortality and
    cardiovascular morbidity, 95: 111
Acetaminophen
  antipyretic effect in endotoxin-induced
    fever, 96: 35
  cancer and
    colorectal, 96: 255
    renal pelvis and ureter, 97: 310
  in headache, episodic tension-type,
    97: 302
  for pain, postoperative, 95: 275
    with oxycodone, 95: 275
  pretreatment regimens for adverse
    events related to infusion of
    amphotericin B, 96: 61
  risk of Stevens-Johnson syndrome or
    toxic epidermal necrolysis with,
    97: 349
  for self-poisoning, 96: 75
  use, long-term, and risk of colorectal
    neoplasia, 97: 242
  vs. aspirin, 97: 300
  vs. NSAID in osteoarthritis, 96: 354
Acetate
  serum, in diabetics, effect of acarbose
    on, 96: 182
Acetazolamide
  in COPD, effects on gas exchange,
    95: 320
  in sleep apnea, obstructive, 96: 341
Acetylator
  slow, phenotype, as risk factor for
    hepatotoxicity from
    antituberculosis drugs, 97: 201
Acetylcholinesterase
  inhibitors in dementia, 97: 322
Acetylsalicylic acid (see Aspirin)
N-Acetyltransferase
  2 polymorphism in HIV-infected
    patients, 97: 73
Achalasia
  botulinum toxin in, 96: 198

---

* All entries refer to the year and page number(s) for data appearing in this and previous
editions of the YEAR BOOK.

Flu
-like symptoms after cisplatin and
  interferon-α2b in penile carcinoma,
  96: 277
syndrome after oral mesalamine in
  ulcerative colitis, *97:* 175
Fluconazole
activity against *Candida* species, in vitro
  and in vivo (in mice), *96:* 222
/flucytosine for cryptococcal meningitis
  in AIDS, *96:* 105
prophylactic
  for fungal infections after marrow
    transplantation, *96:* 247
  in neutropenic cancer patients,
    96: 246
-resistant mucosal candidiasis, in AIDS,
  96: 106
salivary concentrations of, *96:* 248
vs. amphotericin B in candidemia in
  patients without neutropenia,
  96: 245
Flucytosine
activity against *Candida* species, in vitro
  and in vivo (in mice), *96:* 222
/fluconazole for cryptococcal meningitis
  in AIDS, *96:* 105
Fludarabine
in lymphoma, follicular, *97:* 247
potential as immunosuppressive agent,
  97: 231
in Waldenström's macroglobulinemia,
  resistant, *96:* 275
Flumazenil
in benzodiazepine overdose, *97:* 38;
  95: 50
Fluorescence
in high-performance liquid
  chromatography for urinary
  dextromethorphan and
  dextrorphan, *95:* 20
Fluoroquinolone
combined with penicillin V for
  reduction of fever and streptococcal
  bacteremia in granulocytopenic
  patients with cancer, *96:* 238
resistance, development during
  treatment, *96:* 28
5-Fluorouracil
in breast cancer
  advanced or recurrent, with
    medroxyprogesterone, *96:* 260
  carboplatin and cyclophosphamide
    combined with, *95:* 214
  node-positive, combined with
    cyclophosphamide and
    methotrexate, *96:* 258
  obesity and, *95:* 213

/cisplatin in advanced head and neck
  cancer, radiation after, *95:* 225
/folinic acid in colon cancer, *95:* 221
infusion
  in colorectal cancer, *97:* 244
  continuous, causing gastric mucosal
    lesions, *95:* 60
  protracted, combined with
    postoperative radiation for rectal
    cancer, *96:* 256
in keratoses, actinic, *96:* 363
/levamisole after resection of stage III
  colon carcinoma, *96:* 257
/methotrexate in metastatic colorectal
  cancer, *95:* 222
toxicity, age and sex as predictors of,
  96: 67
Fluoxetine
in dysphoria, premenstrual, *96:* 328
effect on resting energy expenditure and
  basal body temperature, *96:* 173
inadequate, outcomes of, *97:* 317
in obesity, *95:* 137
in obsessive-compulsive disorder,
  95: 313
in trichotillomania, *97:* 325
Flurbiprofen
oro-genital ulcerations after, recurrent,
  96: 54
Flutamide
/finasteride in advanced prostate
  carcinoma, *97:* 233
in hirsutism, *95:* 336
  long-term clinical effects, endocrine
    changes, and androgen receptor
    behavior after, *97:* 345
in Tourette's syndrome, *95:* 244
withdrawal in advanced prostate cancer,
  97: 192
Fluvastatin
/cholestyramine, low-dose, in
  hyperlipidemia, *95:* 150
Fluvoxamine
in obsessive-compulsive disorder,
  95: 313
Folate
supplementation
  in prevention of fetal neural tube
    defects, minimal compliance with
    Department of Health
    recommendation for, *96:* 41
  in vivo, effect on in vitro
    methotrexate toxicity in Down
    syndrome, *96:* 38
synthesized by bacteria in upper small
  intestine assimilated by host,
  97: 23

Medicaid
  population, costs of interrupting
    antihypertensive drug therapy in,
    95: 91
Medical
  center, university, vancomycin use in,
    97: 197
  effects of anabolic-androgenic steroids,
    95: 28
  history, comparison of self-reported and
    physician reported, 95: 6
Medically ill
  elderly, depressed, methylphenidate for,
    96: 324
Medication(s)
  (*See also* Drugs)
  administration, causing death, 95: 35
  asthma, inhaled, compliance in
    preschool children, 97: 78
  compliance after renal transplantation,
    97: 14
  delivery to children in summer camps,
    safe, 96: 16
  errors
    adverse drug events and, 96: 49
    pediatric, predicting and preventing,
      96: 14
  headache, symptomatic, chronic use of,
    97: 301
  herbal (*see* Herbal, medication)
  over-the-counter (*see* Over-the-counter,
    drugs)
  patient's, brought to hospital, an
    overlooked resource? 95: 5
  regimens, compliance with
    effects of self-medication program on,
      in elderly, 96: 13
    in older patients, capacity to comply,
      96: 12
  self-medication
    future for, 97: 12
    program, effects on knowledge of
      drugs and compliance with
      treatment, in elderly, 96: 13
  taking behaviors in high- and
    low-functioning elderly, 96: 11
  use
    falls and, in elderly, 97: 319
    impact of migraine and tension-type
      headache on, 95: 236
    risk of Stevens-Johnson syndrome or
      toxic epidermal necrolysis and,
      97: 348
Medicine
  emergency medicine residents and
    pharmaceutical representatives,
    95: 9

  homeopathic, in acute childhood
    diarrhea, 96: 18
Medrogestone
  replacement therapy for menopause,
    effects on mechanical properties of
    skin, 96: 364
Medroxyprogesterone
  /chemotherapy for advanced or
    recurrent breast cancer, 96: 260
  cyclic, effect on bone density, 96: 301
  depot
    effects on bone density, in
      premenopausal women, 97: 273
    metabolic parameters, bleeding, and
      weight changes in women using,
      96: 290
    in prostate hyperplasia, benign,
      97: 184
  /estrogen, continuous combined, effects
    on lipid levels in
    hypercholesterolemic
    postmenopausal women, 97: 278
  less than monthly, in postmenopausal
    women given estrogen replacement,
    96: 300
  replacement therapy, development of
    endometrial cancer during, 96: 296
  in sleep apnea, obstructive, 96: 341
Mefenamic acid
  undeclared, in Chinese herbal
    medications, complications from,
    96: 24
Megestrol acetate
  in anorexia, HIV-associated, in children,
    96: 112
  /cisplatin/etoposide in extensive-stage
    small cell lung cancer, 97: 239
Melanoma
  antibody response polyvalent melanoma
    vaccine in, and improved survival,
    96: 265
Melatonin
  secretion, nocturnal, and winter
    depression, 96: 324
Melphalan
  in multiple myeloma
    in high-dose sequential
      chemoradiotherapy, 95: 231
    late, 95: 230
Membranes
  intact, antibiotic treatment of preterm
    labor with, 95: 259
Memory
  improvement during chronic, low dose
    IV arecoline in Alzheimer's disease,
    95: 298

Monosialoganglioside
in Alzheimer's disease, 95: 299
Mood
disorders
state regulation of benzodiazepine
prescriptions and, 95: 288
steroids causing, anabolic, 95: 28
MOPP therapy
for Hodgkin's disease, male
reproductive potential after,
96: 186
Moraxella catarrhalis
ampicillin-resistant, causing acute otitis
media, 97: 135
Morbidity
cardiac, after tamoxifen in breast
cancer, 97: 236
cardiovascular, after myocardial
infarction, effect of long-term oral
anticoagulants on, 95: 111
febrile, after prophylactic ceftizoxime in
hysterectomy, 95: 258
of myocardial infarction patients with
clinical evidence of heart failure,
effect of ramipril on, 95: 117
vascular, after tamoxifen in breast
cancer, 97: 236
Morning
stiffness in rheumatoid arthritis patients,
effects of triazolam on, 97: 312
Morphine
acute effects in opioid-dependent
patients, 95: 266
analgesic effect, ephedrine enhancement
of, 95: 269
concentrations, plasma and CSF, after
oral morphine, 96: 37
dose
serial IV, in postoperative pain in
outpatients, 95: 270
single, effect on vomiting after
outpatient inguinal surgery, in
children, 96: 307
epidural
patient satisfaction with, 95: 281
pretreatment for postepisiotomy pain,
96: 306
glucuronides, plasma and CSF
concentrations, after oral
morphine, 96: 37
intraarticular
effects on analgesic requirements after
anterior cruciate ligament repair,
95: 277
in knee arthroscopy, 95: 276
intramuscular, *vs.* oral ketorolac for
pain after orthopedic surgery,
95: 273

oral
for cancer pain, 95: 275
plasma and CSF concentrations of
morphine and morphine
glucuronides after, 96: 37
overdose
massive intrathecal, successful
treatment of, 96: 79
from patient-controlled analgesia
pumps, 97: 292
patient-controlled, consumption after
lower abdominal surgery, effect of
pre-emptive lumbar epidural
anesthesia on, 96: 305
requirements, postoperative, age as
predictor of, 97: 283
respiratory depressant effect of, 95: 24
response to, ethnic differences in,
95: 18
in ureteric colic (in dog), 95: 177
vs. ketorolac after tonsillectomy, in
children, 97: 289
Mortality
(*See also* Death)
alcohol intake and, 95: 13
among women, 96: 22
asthma, and sales of inhaled
bronchodilators and anti-asthmatic
drugs, 96: 116
in asthmatics on inhaled beta-agonists,
95: 74
after cholesterol reduction, serum,
95: 108
after gemfibrozil, in Helsinki Heart
Study follow-up, 95: 107
meningitis, *Haemophilus influenzae*,
among children, 95: 196
of myocardial infarction
effect of anticoagulants on, long-term
oral, 95: 111
effect of aspirin use and smoking
status on, 96: 31
in patients with clinical evidence of
heart failure, effect of ramipril on,
95: 117
treated with thrombolytic therapy,
gender differences in, 97: 108
risk, predicted, use to evaluate efficacy
of anticytokine therapy in sepsis,
97: 202
in surgical patients, high-risk, effect of
deliberate perioperative increase of
oxygen delivery on, 95: 340
Mothers
adolescent, Norplant in, 96: 287
Mountain sickness
acute, no effect of nifedipine on,
96: 339

outcome, and antiepileptic drugs,
95: 234
rate after captopril in male infertility,
95: 184
vaginitis and, candidal, 95: 255
Premature infant
patent ductus arteriosus and respiratory
distress syndrome in, aspirin *vs.*
indomethacin for, 97: 333
poliovirus vaccine in, inactivated, early
immunization with, 97: 214
Premenopausal women
differential effects on bone density of
progestogen-only oral
contraceptives in, 97: 273
levodopa/carbidopa in winter seasonal
affective disorder in, 95: 296
Premenstrual
dysphoria, fluoxetine in, 96: 328
syndrome treatments, clinical trials of,
96: 327
Prenatal
maternal indomethacin use causing
prolonged neonatal renal
insufficiency, 95: 42
Prepyloric
gastric ulcer, effect of omeprazole and
sucralfate on, 96: 194
Preschoolers
compliance with inhaled asthma
medication in, 97: 78
over-the-counter medication use in,
96: 30
vaccination levels in
in Los Angeles public health centers,
97: 207
low, in U.S., 95: 191
Prescribing
among elderly, potentially undesirable,
95: 7
analgesic, improvement in general
teaching hospital, 97: 286
antimicrobial drug, trends among
office-based physicians, 96: 220
of cholesterol-lowering drugs, influence
of method of reporting study
results on decision of physicians to
prescribe, 96: 7
errors, death due to, 95: 35
inappropriate, for community-dwelling
elderly, 96: 10
of NSAIDs in general practice, 96: 8
patterns, prophylactic antibiotic, in
orthopedic surgery, 95: 337
Prescription(s)
(*See also* Drugs, prescription)
asthma, compliance with, 95: 71

benzodiazepine, state regulation of,
clinical profile of patients affected
by, 95: 288
of estrogen replacement therapy, effect
of physician gender on, 97: 275
of lipid lowering agents, general
practitioners' policies in, 96: 6
for nitrates, implication of, 95: 102
patterns of NSAIDs and
gastroprotective agents, 96: 344
recommendations for
cholesterol-lowering drugs,
cost-effectiveness of, 97: 113
Pressure
urticaria/angioedema, delayed,
sulfasalazine in, 97: 337
Preterm labor
with intact membranes, antibiotic
treatment of, 95: 259
threatened, indomethacin and sulindac
therapy for, fetal cardiac function
and ductus arteriosus during,
97: 271
Pretreatment
regimens for adverse events related to
infusion of amphotericin B, 96: 61
Preventive care
underimmunization as marker for
insufficient utilization of, 97: 207
Price
(*See also* Cost)
stickers do not alter drug usage, 96: 2
Primary care
underimmunization as marker for
insufficient utilization of, 97: 207
Prisolec (*see* Omeprazole)
Probucol
therapy, QT prolongation during,
95: 99
Procainamide
in cardiac arrest survivors, 95: 99
Procarbazine
in Hodgkin's disease
male reproductive potential after,
96: 186
stage IIIA, with radiotherapy, 96: 271
in lymphoma, primary CNS, in AIDS,
96: 111
Procyclidine
dysphagia due to, severe, 96: 80
Product
risk, examining in context, 95: 1
Progenitor cells
blood, transplantation in multiple
myeloma, 95: 231

patients, elderly, inadequate emergency department analgesia in, 97: 282
spinal detrusor hyperreflexia due to, chronic, intravesical capsaicin in, 97: 307
stress disorder after, amitriptyline in, 95: 314
subarachnoid hemorrhage after, nimodipine in, 95: 247
Travelers' diarrhea
ciprofloxacin in, single-dose, 96: 244
norfloxacin in, 95: 157
Trazodone
in anxiety disorder, generalized, 95: 309
-yohimbine in psychogenic impotence, 96: 209
Tremor
in Parkinson's disease, clozapine for, 96: 284
Tretinoin
topical, neurotoxicity of, 97: 43
Trial(s)
clinical
obstetric, pill counts as measures of compliance in, 95: 251
randomized, in single patients during 2-year period, 95: 11
translation into practice, for thrombolysis in myocardial infarction, 97: 105
corticosteroid, comparative inhaled, sample sizes with emphasis on showing therapeutic equivalence, 97: 9
crossover, with binary response, 97: 10
discordance between meta-analyses and large-scale randomized, controlled trials in management of myocardial infarction, 97: 104
multiple sclerosis, placebo-controlled randomized, impact of blinding on results of, 95: 3
randomized, current and ongoing, in heart failure and left ventricular dysfunction, 95: 116
Triamterene
/hydrochlorothiazide, plasma sodium levels after, in elderly, 95: 31
Triazolam
in rheumatoid arthritis, effects on sleep, daytime sleepiness and morning stiffness, 97: 312
in sleep apnea, obstructive, 96: 77
Trichotillomania
fluoxetine in, 97: 325

Tricyclic
antidepressants, discontinuation, *vs.* discontinuation of serotonin reuptake inhibitors, 97: 318
Trifluride
topical, in acyclovir-resistant herpes simplex and varicella-zoster virus infections, 95: 68
Triglycerides
effects of fish oil concentrate on, low-dose, 96: 154
effects of pravastatin on, in elderly, 96: 154
Triiodothyronine
therapy, effect on atrial fibrillation after cardiac operations, 97: 124
Trimethoprim
reactions to, cutaneous, 96: 48
-sulfamethoxazole
in *Cyclospora* infection in HIV infection, 96: 107
hyperkalemia due to, 97: 54; 95: 53
for *Pneumocystis carinii* pneumonia in AIDS, adjunctive folinic acid with, 96: 103
for *Pneumocystis carinii* pneumonia prophylaxis in HIV-infected children, 96: 104
prophylaxis against relapses of Wegener's granulomatosis, 97: 226
resistance, development during treatment, 96: 28
Streptococcus pneumoniae susceptibility to, 96: 237
suspension, oral, variation in acceptance of, 96: 27
thrombocytopenic purpura due to, 95: 57
use and risk of Stevens-Johnson syndrome or toxic epidermal necrolysis, 97: 348
in Whipple's disease, *vs.* tetracycline, 96: 202
Trimipramine
in suicide, 96: 322
Troglitazone
pharmacokinetics, prediction of, 97: 154
L-Tryptophan
eosinophilia-myalgia syndrome due to, status and treatment results 2 years after onset, 96: 357
Tuberculin
positivity and conversion in long-term care facility, choosing appropriate criteria for, 95: 195

Author Index